MOUNTAIN STATES

MEDICINAL PLANTS

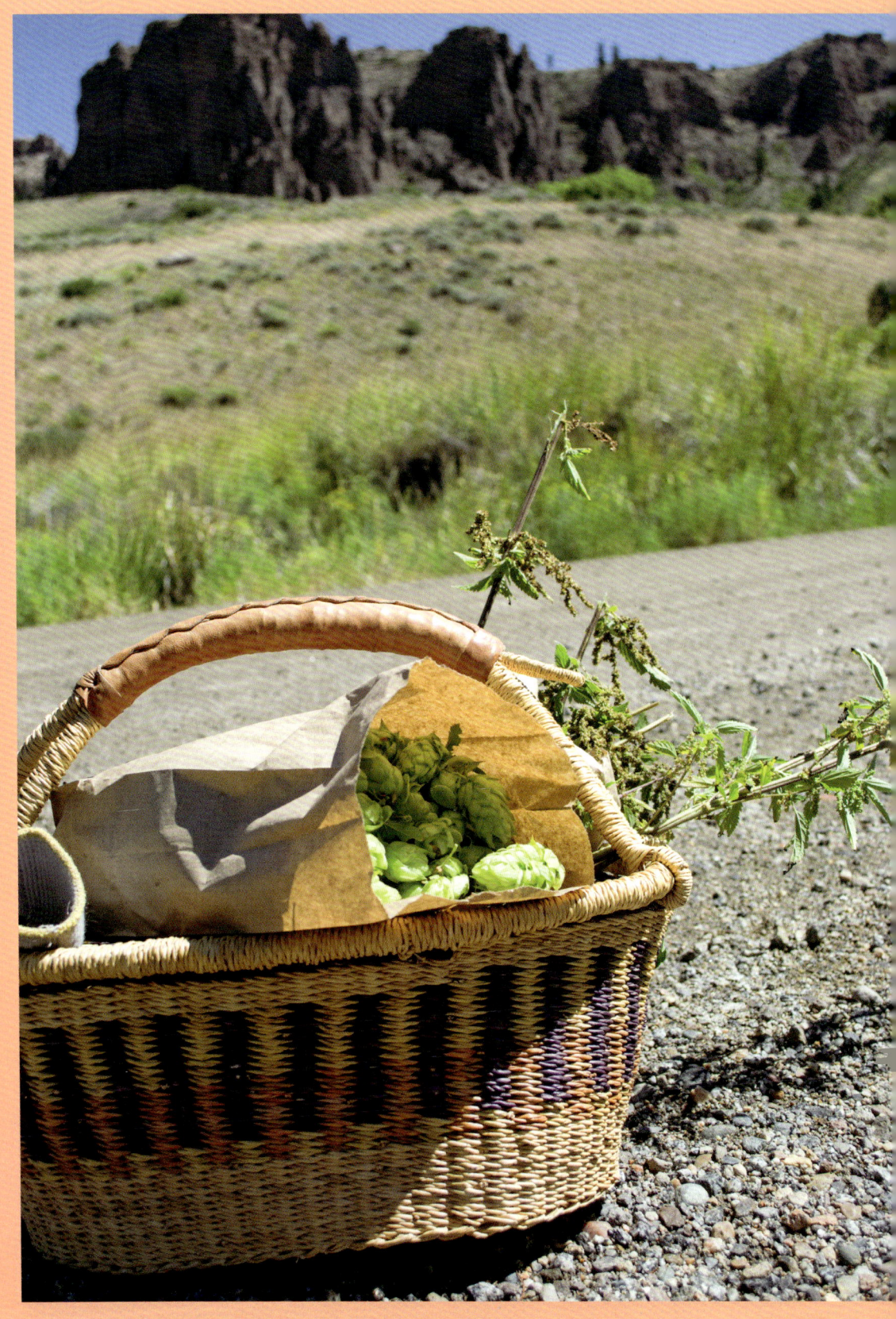

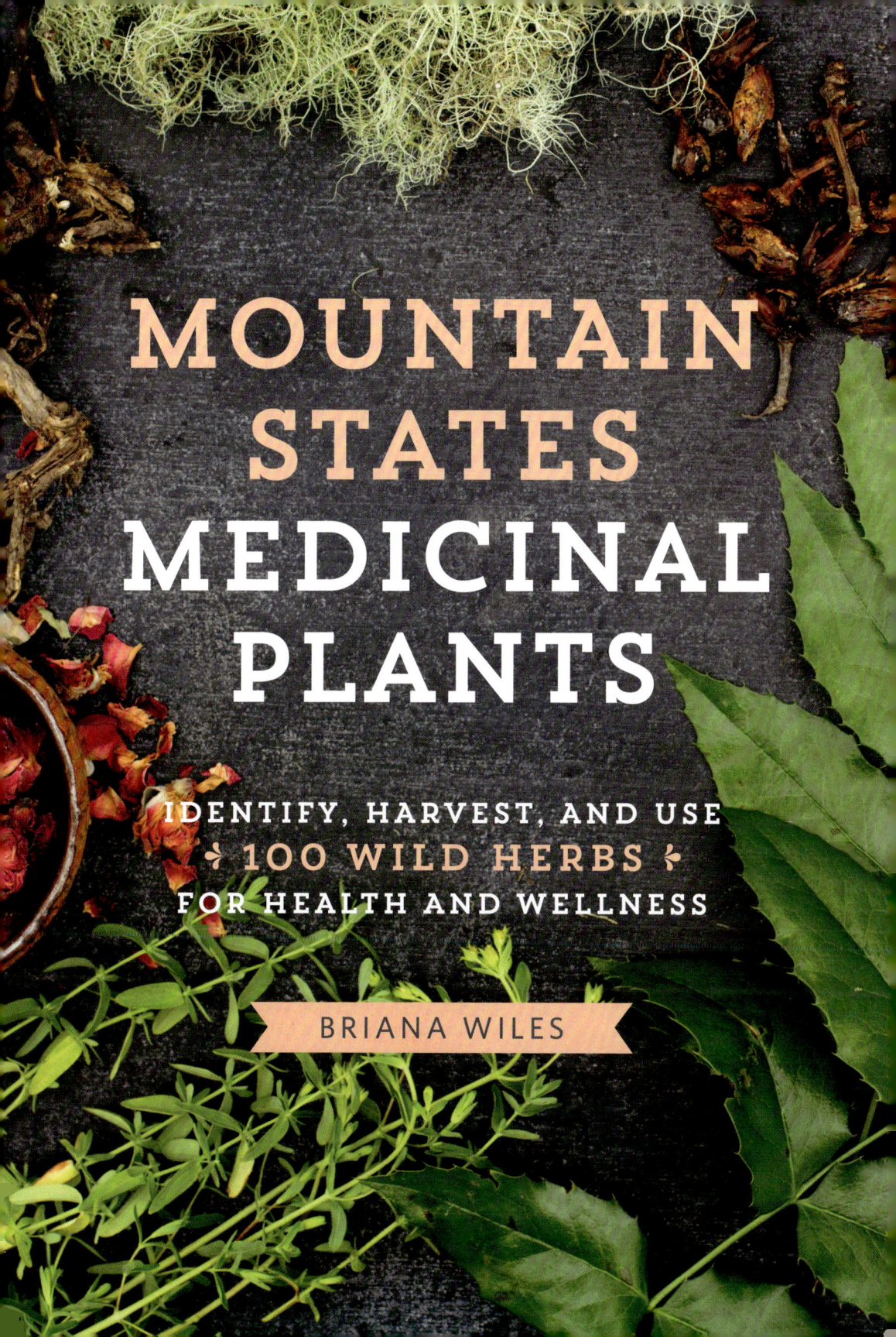

MOUNTAIN STATES MEDICINAL PLANTS

IDENTIFY, HARVEST, AND USE ❧ 100 WILD HERBS ❧ FOR HEALTH AND WELLNESS

BRIANA WILES

Timber Press
Workman Publishing
Hachette Book Group, Inc.
1290 Avenue of the Americas
New York, New York 10104
timberpress.com

Timber Press is an imprint of Workman Publishing,
a division of Hachette Book Group, Inc. The Timber Press name and logo
are registered trademarks of Hachette Book Group, Inc.

Printed in China on paper from responsible sources
Fifth printing 2024
Text and cover design by Adrianna Sutton

The publisher is not responsible for websites (or their content) that are not
owned by the publisher. The Hachette Speakers Bureau provides a wide range of
authors for speaking events. To find out more, go to hachettespeakersbureau.com
or email hachettespeakers@hbgusa.com.

A catalog record for this book is available from the Library of Congress.

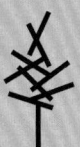

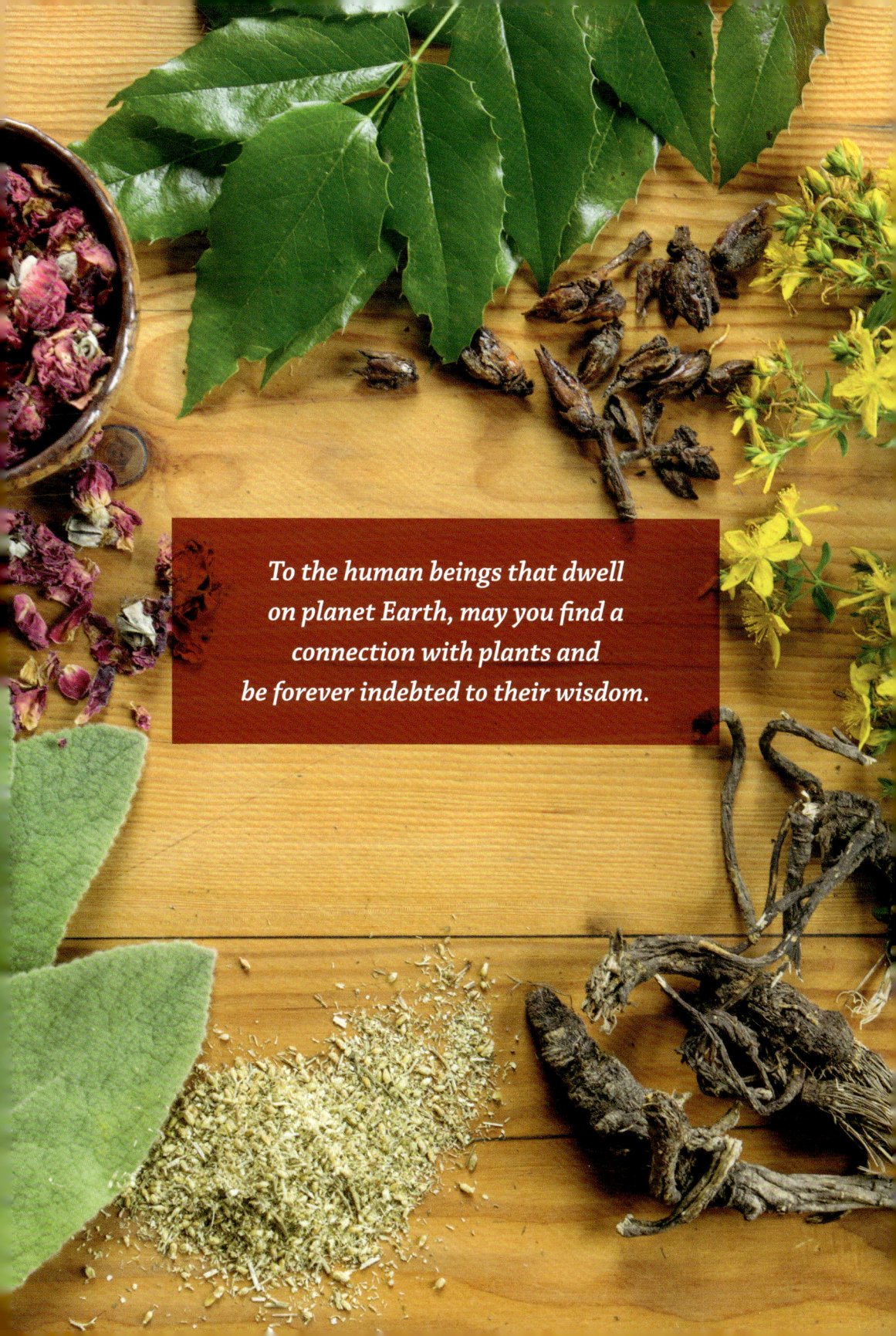

To the human beings that dwell on planet Earth, may you find a connection with plants and be forever indebted to their wisdom.

CONTENTS

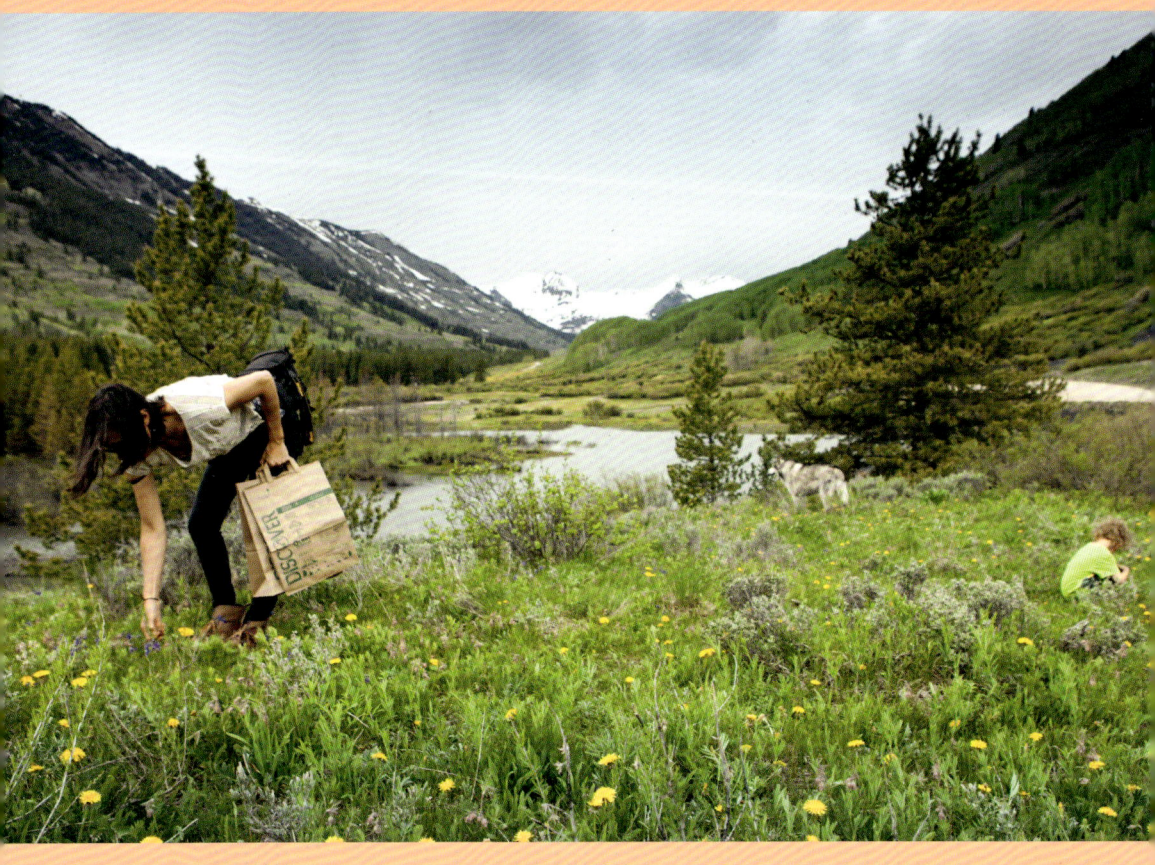

Gathering dandelion heads, high in the mountains with my usual posse: Salix, my son, and Bella, our Alaskan malamute.

❧ PREFACE ❧

I have been trying to teach my son something (everything!), and it is this: each and every time you go out into nature, an exchange takes place. You are joining an age-old dance we do together with plants to unite the powers we both hold within our cells. Your feet are in step with the rhythm of life—with each impression of the soil you could be setting a seed to the right depth for germination. Every time you touch a plant it has a response, and so do you, if you take the time to notice it.

This exchange becomes deeper when you begin to harvest on your own, the interaction becomes more physical, and the connection can last a lifetime. Some of your harvests you dry for future use in tea blending or oil infusions. Others you quickly place in alcohol or vinegar to preserve their highest offerings, possibly for decades to come. An impression has formed between you and this plant. You have learned to recognize it, to trust your instincts and your knowledge. You trust yourself with the primal wisdom that has been passed down for as long as we humans have existed—this is medicine.

This exchange can be mutual if we take the time to honor each plant and its lineage, to thank it for allowing us to participate in its life cycle. Check in mentally or verbally with every plant you are considering gathering. Many will tell you "no," and you need to respect that. The plants that do give you permission to harvest need to be thanked. When out wildcrafting, offer the plants a gift—of song, water, attention, intention—before or after you begin to clip or dig.

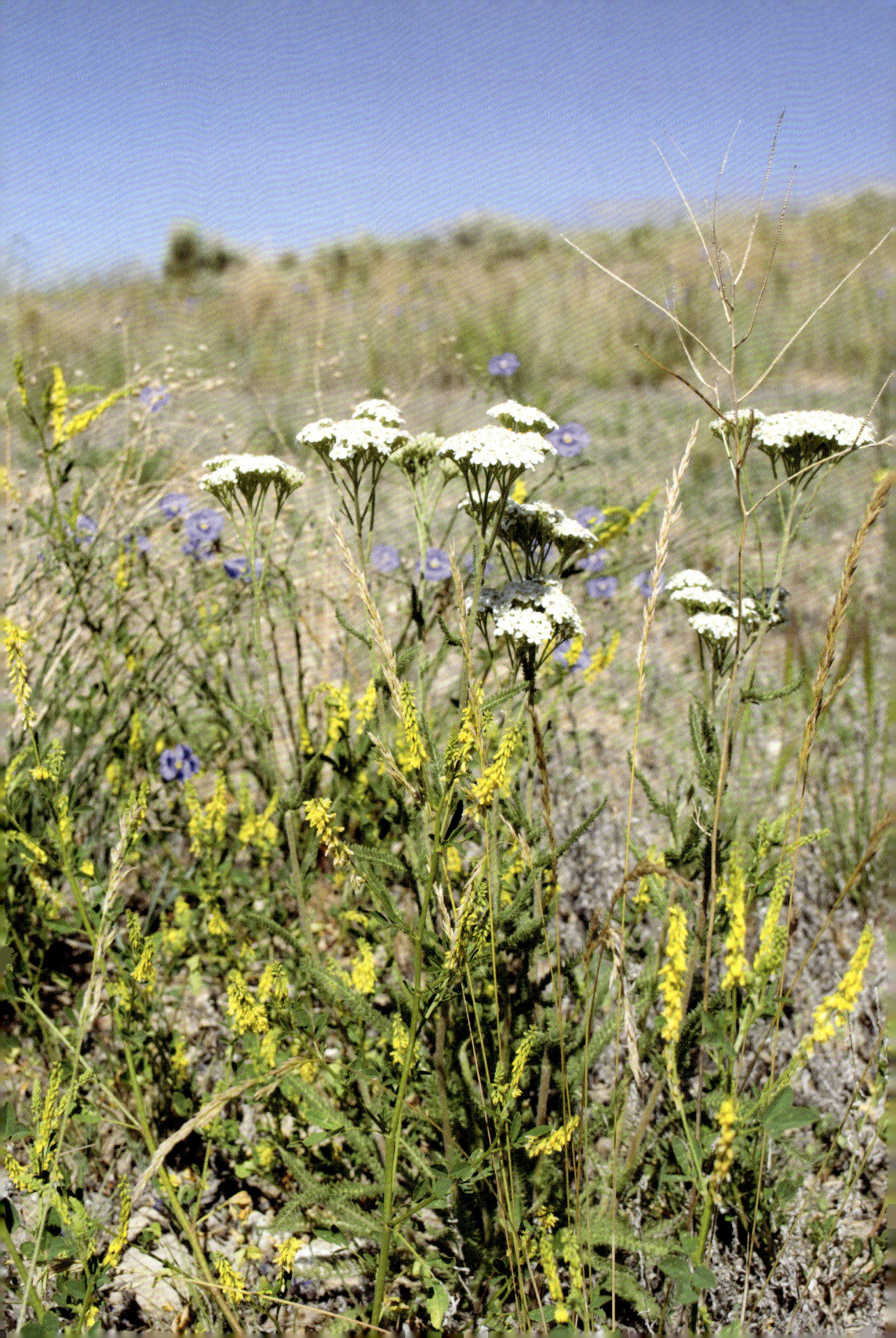

INTRODUCTION

WILDCRAFTING YOUR MEDICINE

Something brought this book into your hands, that innate need for learning, a passion for plants, or a desire to understand how to make simple, pure medicines. With this book, you will be able to identify and recognize plants you may have walked past before or even thought of as weeds. Just getting outside into nature to meet any of these plants is therapeutic and mind-altering. You will start to hear and participate in the communication that takes place between humans and plants. Gathering information and inspiration on which plants grow near you, or which ones you want to search for, will connect you to the earth in a powerful way. Likewise, there is much empowerment in taking charge of your health and what enters your body.

MOUNTAIN WEST

Mountain ranges of the Rockies span through each of the states and provinces covered in this book. The mountain west starts to the south in Colorado, Utah, and Nevada; moves north through Wyoming, Montana, and Idaho; slides west into the eastern sides of Oregon and Washington; and reaches further north into southern Alberta and Saskatchewan. In this territory all the plants in this book can be discovered; however, each herb does not grow in every part of this territory. The mountain west holds a great variety of elevations and ecosystems. Some plants grow only in the southern states, others only in the north; many plants are found either below a certain elevation or above it. An hour's drive can bring you thousands of feet lower or higher and to a whole new land of plants. This is an added benefit to living at altitude—you can chase the seasons. Spring starts low and ends high, meaning just as one season ends at 5000 feet, it is just beginning again at 7000 feet.

GUIDANCE FOR THE WILD HARVEST

Let this book give you guidance, not only on where to find medicinal plants but also on how to approach your search. Let it also provide you with inspiration to prepare herbs for medicine-making, eventually leading you to concoct your own unique remedies. This book is full of rules and recipes to follow, but they were made to be tweaked. When you don't find the plants you're looking for, research the ones you do have near you. Be aware of variations in climate and in the plants themselves. Always harvest with these variations in mind—if it's a meager-looking plant, let it be and find one that has more vitality, which also means more medicine. I always say, the altering of recipes often begins with the plants themselves.

Wildcraft safely

Be careful. Always use multiple references when learning to identify a new plant. Bring your books and notes with you into the field. Learn which plants not to harvest, because they are poisonous, or threatened, or because taking them away would damage the surrounding ecosystem. When reading about a plant, always check the potential cautions for harvesting and ingestion.

Harvest wisely. Make sure the plant you are gathering is the one you are after. Be mindful of any other plants that make it into your basket. Some may be unintended or downright undesirable. Take the time to garble your plants, separating out the parts you are going to use, and process them with care.

Be leery of contaminated grounds

Even in the wide open spaces of the mountain west, we need to be mindful of where we harvest. Stay well away from polluted lands and waterways. Ranches and farms can send fertilizers, manure, and other contaminants leaching into waterways downstream. Mining and factories have caused water and land to carry heavy metals and other pollutants. Look for signs of mining in the landscape and steer clear of harvesting here. Know which plants are targeted for eradication so as to avoid harvesting plants in an area that has been or is being sprayed. Always harvest away from roads, railways, municipal facilities, golf courses, and landscaped buildings, as these are usually kept green and pristine with chemicals.

Tend nature's garden

Nature surrounds us, whether in the cracks of our concrete world or the extensive (and too often unseen) wilderness that cushions and supports our lives. Wherever it occurs, tend to it with love, respect, and care. Walk through it without leaving a trace, and harvest your plants in the same manner. It should not be possible for anyone to know you were even there.

If you are digging a root for your harvest, fill that hole with dirt and replace any roots of neighboring plants that were displaced.

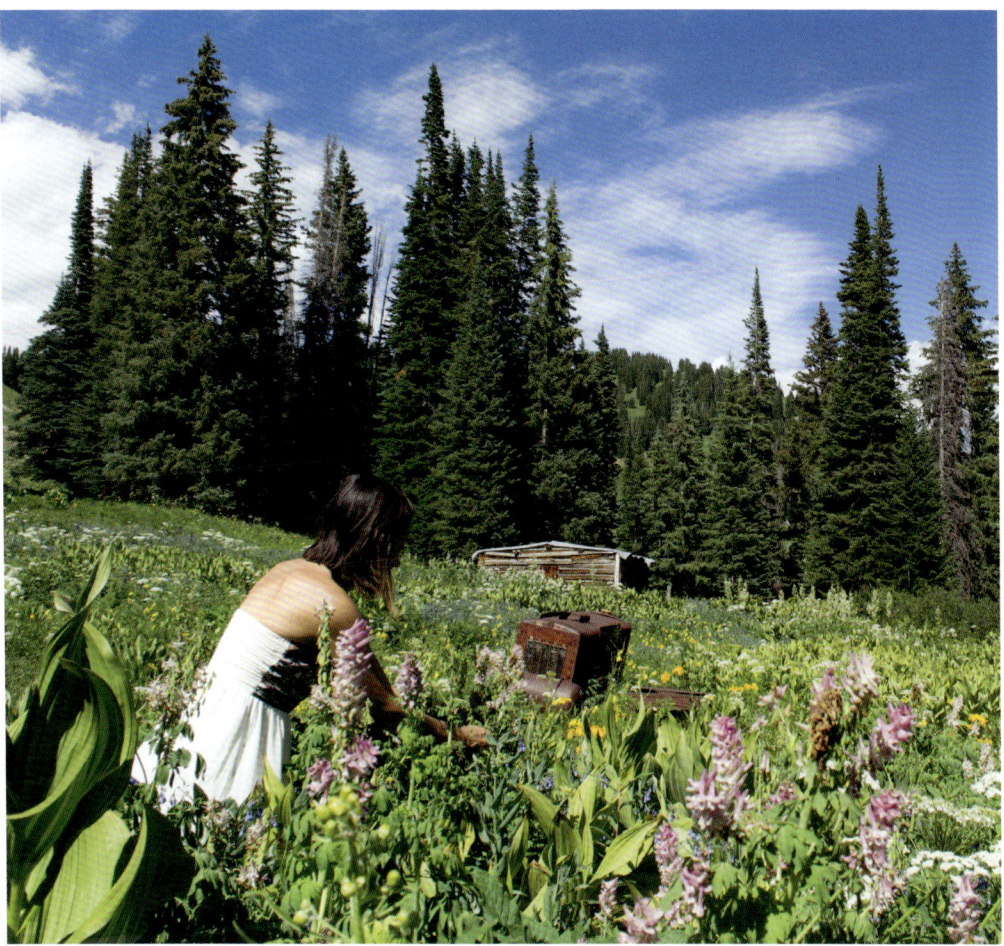

Moving through a meadow of alpine wildflowers, gathering the flowers from bluebells and leaves from many plants.

Make sure to cut the root clean with a knife or clippers if you cannot dig up the entire root; this will minimize injury and keep the root healthier. When trimming tree branches or twigs, prune to bring more light to the plants below. Harvest flowers with the knowledge that you are taking from the bees and potentially an animal; space out your gathering so many flowers still fill the area. Take in the sounds surrounding you, and take time to thank any pollinators that are about for trying to keep the balance in nature. If the season is right, sprinkle some seeds from a nearby seedhead of the plant you took. When gathering fruits, drop some to the ground as you move through for the hope of future germinating. Never just rip plants from the ground, but if you do so accidentally, replant them. Be a steward to the land. Take only what you can process; more than you need is a waste.

Keep it legal
Public lands dominate much of the rural west, which is great for the wildcrafter, but be aware: restrictions often apply. Each

DON'T PICK POISONS

*Always know your poisonous plants first. You need to learn which plants to keep **out** of your basket before you can know which ones to put in. These are some poisonous plants commonly found throughout the states and provinces of the mountain west.*

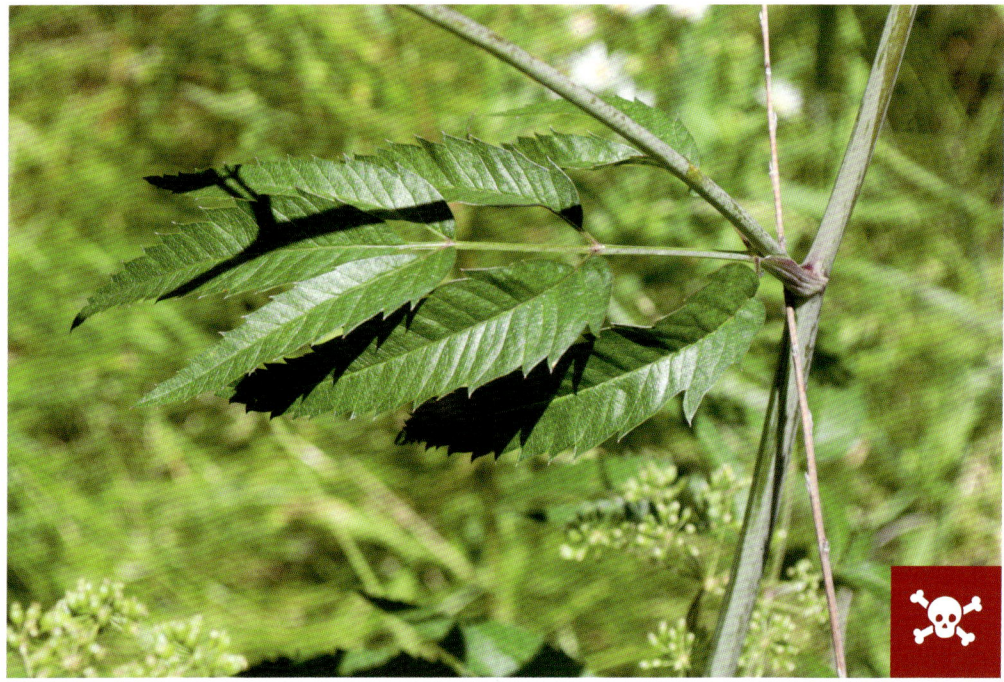

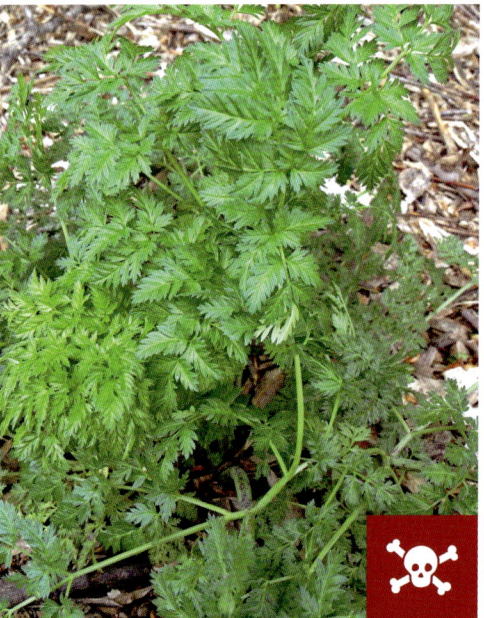

(ABOVE) Take a good look at the shape of water hemlock (*Cicuta* species) leaves; they are the first thing you want to be able to recognize on these toxic plants. Also, become familiar with identifying the ribbed and plumply crescent-shaped seeds. Water hemlock can be confused with *Angelica* species.

(LEFT) Poison hemlock (*Conium maculatum*) can grow very tall and take over entire fields. Learn to identify it for certain, as it looks very similar to osha's leaves and flowers.

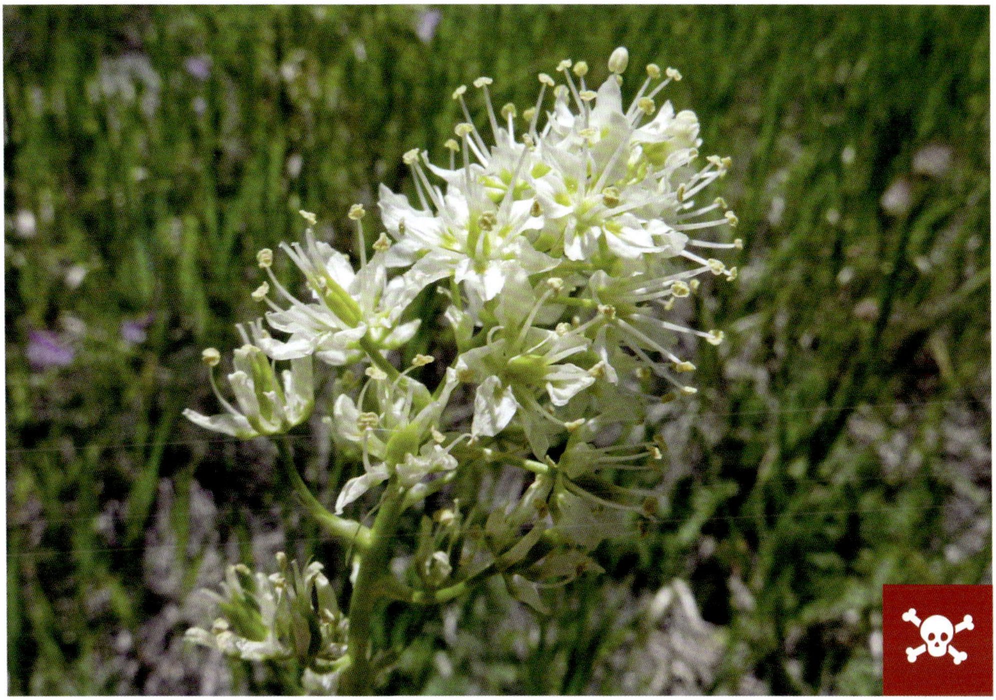

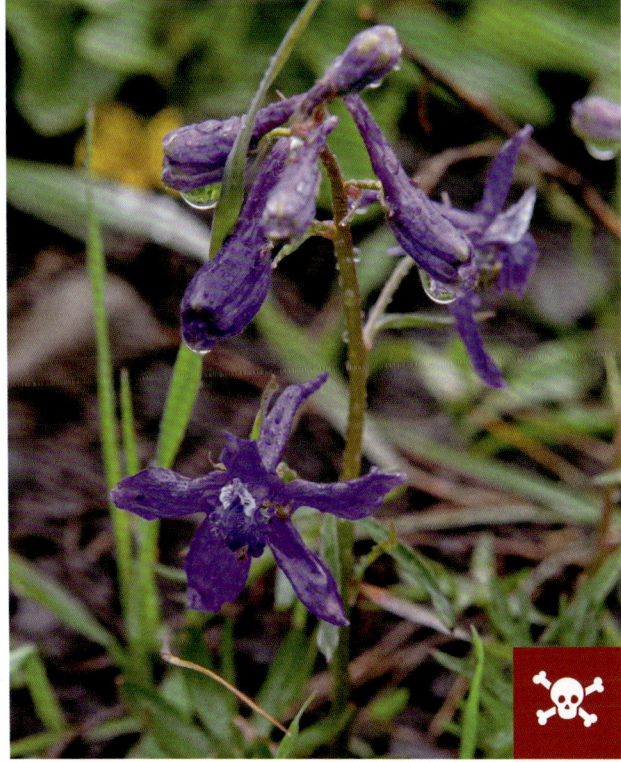

(ABOVE) Meadow death camas (*Toxicoscordion venenosum*), pictured, and mountain death camas (*Anticlea elegans*) should never be mixed with the medicinal herbs you are gathering. They resemble wild onion more than anything else and can grow among common medicinal species, such as those of *Arnica* and *Mertensia*.

(LEFT) Larkspurs (*Delphinium* species) are beautiful but not used for medicine.

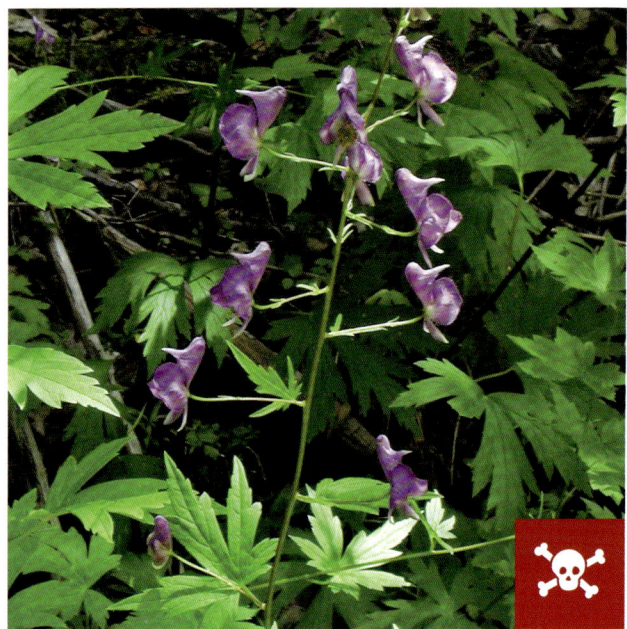

All parts of monkshood (*Aconitum columbianum*) are poisonous; avoid them while harvesting plants for medicine-making.

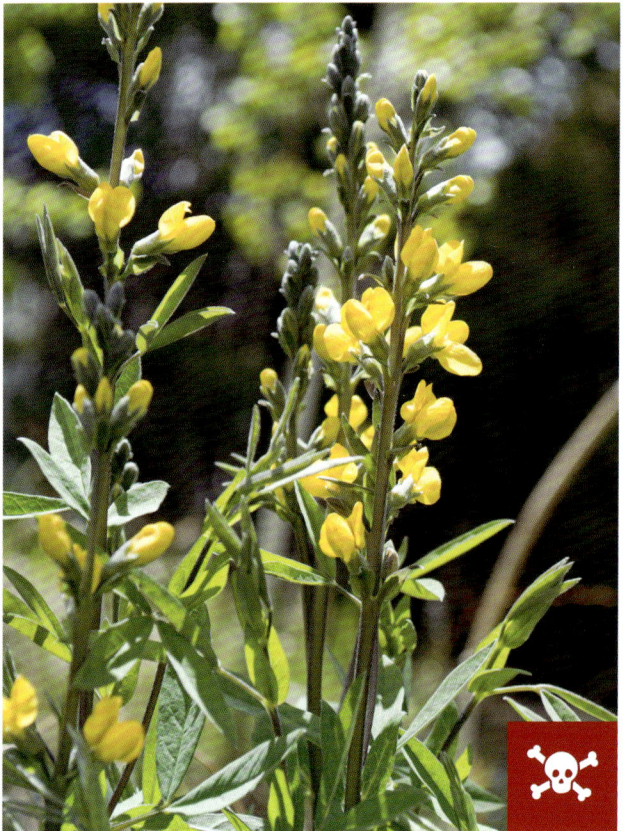

Young leaves of golden banner (*Thermopsis* species) can resemble alfalfa, sweet clover, and other clovers.

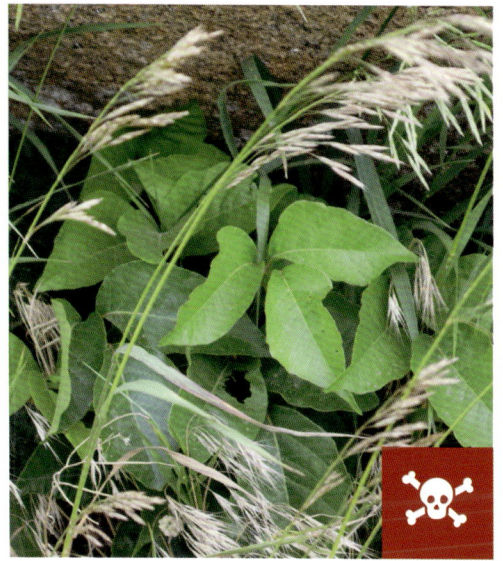

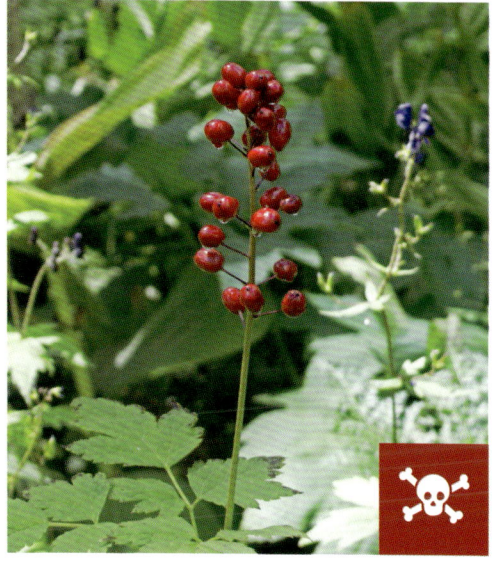

(ABOVE, LEFT) See those "leaves of three"? Poison ivy (*Toxicodendron* species) is a plant you do not want to grab hold of.

(ABOVE, RIGHT) Baneberries (*Actaea* species) can be red or white. Either way, avoid them.

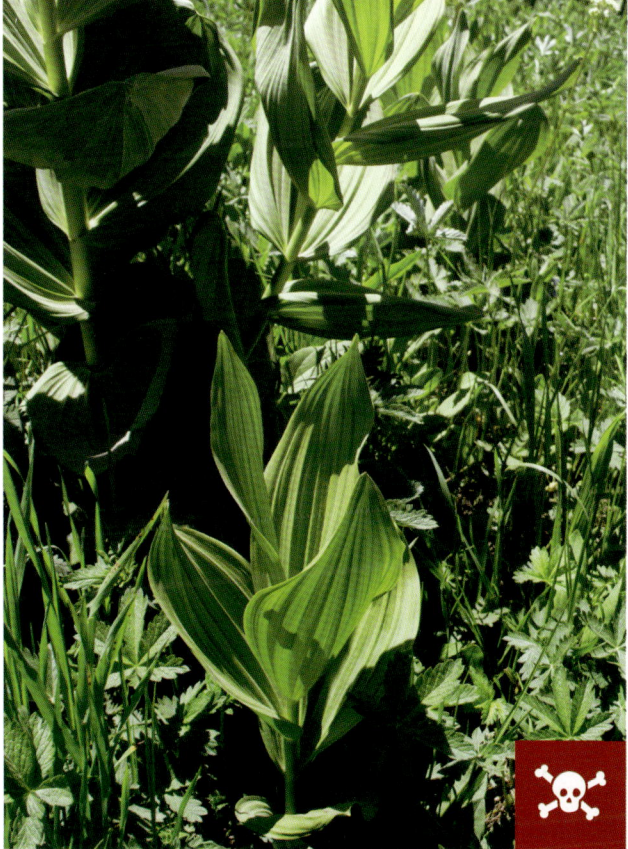

(LEFT) The light green shoots of false hellebore (*Veratrum* species) should not be confused with *Maianthemum* species.

public land agency—such as the Bureau of Land Management (BLM), the United States Fish and Wildlife Service, and national, state, and provincial park services—has different rules and regulations about harvesting on its lands. In addition to federal or Crown lands, states and provinces also manage open spaces and have their own sets of rules. Always check with your local office to learn what the regulations are and to acquire permits if needed.

Be aware of private properties, such as ranches and mining claims. It is your duty to know if you are trespassing. Even within neighborhoods or down alleyways, always ask permission to harvest from someone else's property.

Wildcraft the weeds

Become familiar with the weedy plants that can withstand being harvested in bounty. Burdock, dandelion, and chicory have roots so vigorous that they will probably be back next year, even when you think you got the whole root out. Stick to the weeds for most of your needs, and save the sacred medicinals for special remedies.

ESSENTIAL TOOLS AND GARB FOR GATHERING

The mountain west has weather that can shift suddenly as daylight fades away. Always be prepared by dressing in layers, bringing something warm or dry for later. You never know when you'll need to cross a river fully clothed or warm yourself from a sudden cold wind.

Be sure to have proper shoes if barefoot is not your style. Rubber boots are amazing for tromping through the wet, riparian zones. While sandals can get you most places, a closed-toe shoe helps to keep out poky debris and stones.

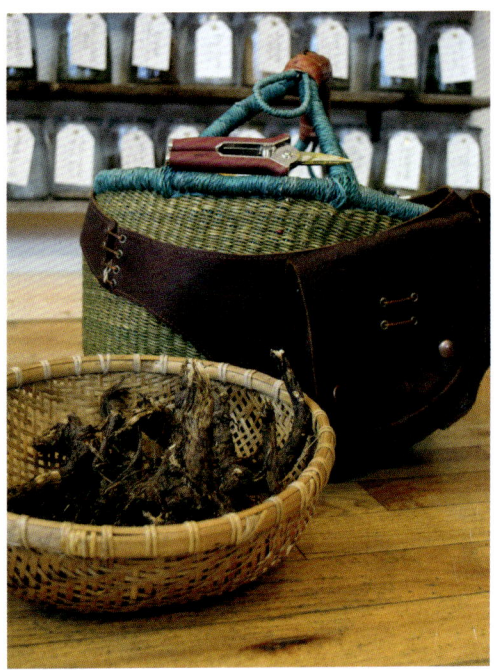

When heading out into the hills, I bring baskets, pruners, usually a shovel, and always my hip pouch for stashing away my tools.

Protect yourself with a hat, sunglasses, sunblock, and a raincoat for the summer monsoons. Always be well prepared with drinking water, as altitude makes the sun fiercer and our bodies work harder.

My favorite things to lug around are tools and baskets. I always set out to gather prepped with a hip pouch for holding my pruners, knife, and hori-hori, or soil knife, and a basket for holding paper bags and a small digging shovel. Paper grocery bags, baskets, or pillowcases make excellent vessels for keeping harvested plants separate and allowing them to breath. Avoid using plastic altogether for your harvest storage.

HANDLING THE HARVEST

Now that you have your freshly gathered plants, it's time to take care of the preservation and concocting of the herbs.

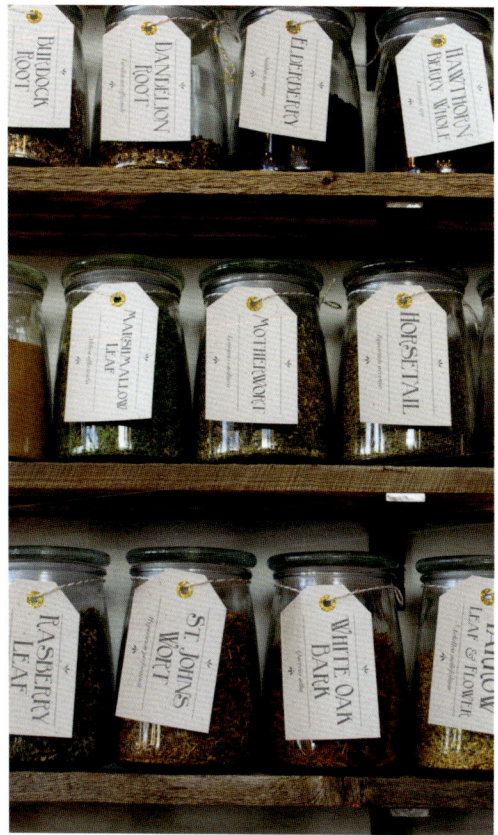

A wall of delicately dried and well-marked herbs at the apothecary.

Winnowing

Winnowing is the process of removing seeds from the bracts or casings that enclose them. Try this with small seeds like alfalfa, amaranth, burdock, and stinging nettle. Garble your seedheads off the plants and set them aside in a bowl or basket. Begin winnowing outside, where you can let the chaff float away in the wind. With your harvesting basket or bowl at your side, stand over a bucket. Take a scoop of seedheads in one hand, then take both hands and rub them together slowly. This lets the desired seeds fall into the bucket, a foot or so below, while simultaneously allowing the chaff and other plant debris to blow away in the wind.

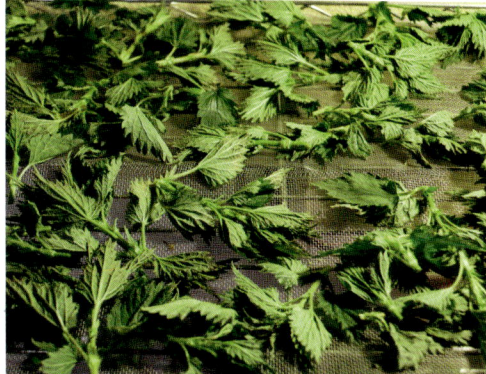

Stinging nettle leaves laid out to dry on a wire mesh screen.

Dehydrating and drying

Storing up your collection of herbs starts with good drying practices. Don't worry if you are not equipped with a fancy dehydrator. Your kitchen table, oven, shed, or broken-down car will work just fine.

If you have a dehydrator, use your lowest setting for bark, leaves, and flowers. Roots, berries, and small fruits may be able to withstand a warmer temperature. Always use the lowest temperature setting if using an oven, which is generally around 170°F.

My favorite way to dry plant matter is to spread it all out on mesh screens, hanging baskets, or stretched-out linen sheets; the herb can then be jostled every so often to keep the drying evenly distributed. Try to find a place outside that is in the shade, so the plants do not scorch in the sun. Doing the drying inside is absolutely fine but can sometimes result in a home bug infestation.

Always harvest your herbs at their most vibrant color and smell for the best dried medicinals. Roots will usually need to be chopped up while still fresh to the desired size for storing. Leaves, stems, or twigs can also be clipped into smaller pieces before storage, or whole leaves and flowers can be dried then crumbled by hand to store.

PLANT TALK

Plants have characteristics all their own, and learning some easy terminology will help you to identify which to gather. Because plants bear leaves most of the harvesting season, even without flowers or fruit, leaves are key to identifying and distinguishing plants. Take a look at the shape of the leaves, and the pattern in which the leaves are arranged. For a better botanical understanding, here are some examples of common leaf arrangements, shapes, and margins.

OPPOSITE

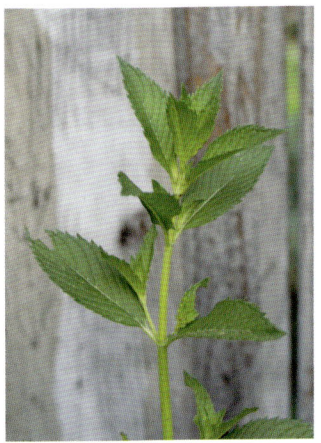

Mint leaves grow in pairs, joining at the same node on the stem.

ALTERNATE

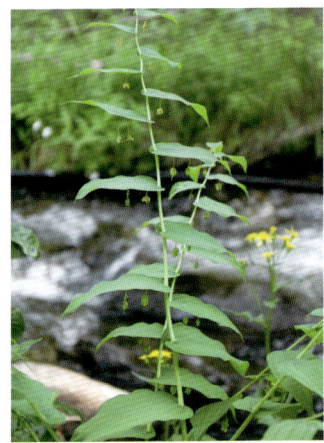

The leaves of twisted stalk grow along the stem, one at each node.

WHORLED

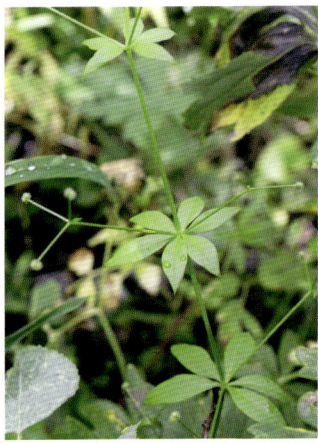

Cleavers has three or more leaves arranged around one node on a stem.

ROSETTE

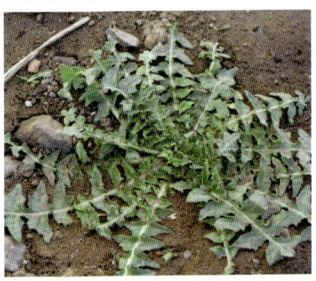

Tumble mustard leaves are arranged around the base of the plant, forming a dense mat of leaves on the ground.

COMPOUND

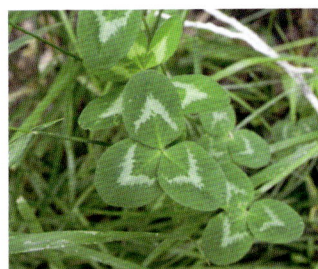

Red clover leaves are separated into three leaflets.

PINNATE

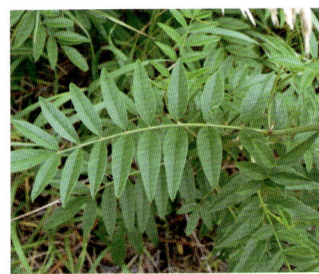

Wild licorice has a compound leaf with opposite leaflets along the axis.

OBLONG

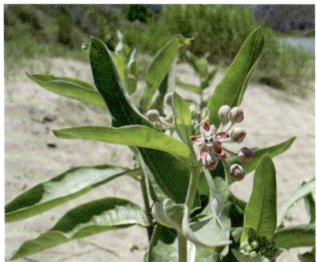

Showy milkweed leaves are longer than they are wide.

LANCEOLATE

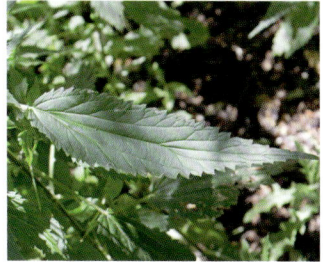

Stinging nettle leaves are longer than they are wide, with a speared tip.

OVATE

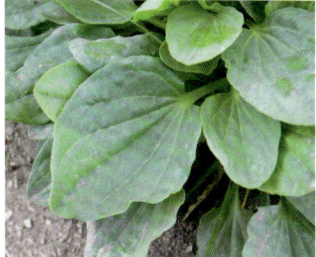

Broadleaf plantain has oval or egg-shaped leaves.

PALMATE

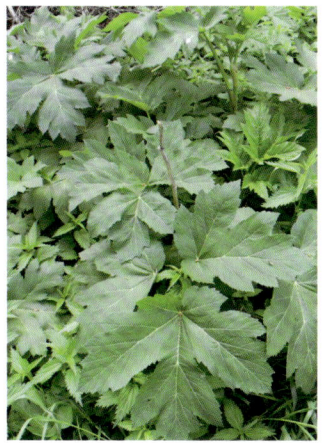

Cow parsnip veins radiate from a central point into lobes.

ENTIRE

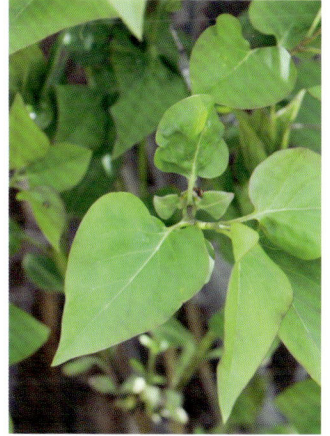

Lilac leaves are smooth around the margin.

SERRATED

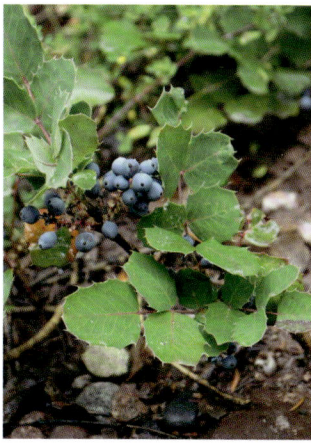

The margins of Oregon grape leaves are jagged or toothed.

LOBED

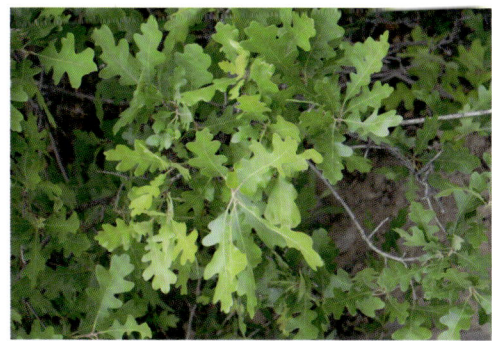

Scrub oak leaves have deep rounded margins.

Garbling Plants

To garble a plant is to separate the directly medicinal parts of the plant from the less usable or nonmedicinal portions. For example, garbling elderflowers or elderberries would mean that you pick off only the flowers or fruit, keeping all the big stems out of your harvest pile—the stems of elderberry are slightly toxic and can upset your stomach.

It also means going through your harvest basket and making sure that you gathered only the plants you meant to harvest, removing any plants that are not identified or debris that is undesirable.

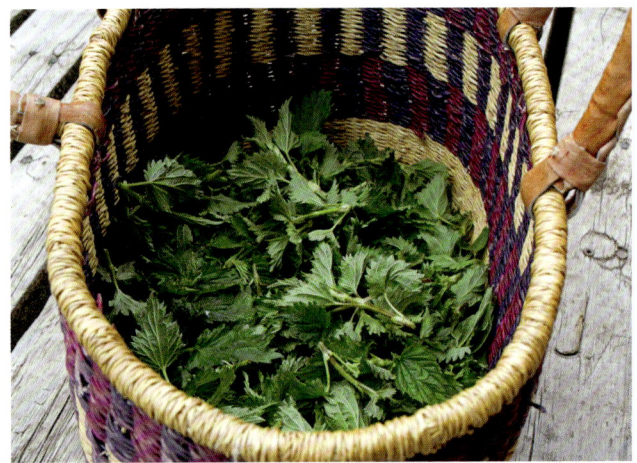

A load of stinging nettles, ready to be picked through to make sure no grass shards or unwanted plants made it into the gathering basket.

HERBAL PREPARATIONS

The different herbal preparations have a great deal of influence on the expression of a medicine. Factors such as condition of the plant, time of year, and a person's constitution are all influences in choosing which preparation to use. Also consider the best way to administer the medicine, and that different extraction methods vary in how potently they carry the medicinal constituents of an herb.

Decoctions and infusions in hot or cold water are forms of noncaffeinated tea, otherwise know as herbal tisanes. These are taken internally, warmed, cooled, or sweetened, and are the premier carrier of water-soluble herbal extractions. A sitz bath soak or wash is a tea meant to be used externally.

Tinctures and liniments are extractions of herbs made in alcohol of any sort. Vinegar is an alternative to alcohol and is preferable for extracting herbs with high vitamin and mineral content. Infusing herbs in honey is a delicious way to administer their medicine orally; oil infusions and liniments offer more ways to address topical issues. Many herbs extract well in oil and can be made into rubs, salves, or skincare products.

Infusions

Sipping on herbs is one of my favorite ways to get to know the actions and energetics of a plant. Hot or cold infusions work best with leaves and flowers of plants, fresh or dried. Roots, barks, and berries can be brewed as infusions when fresh, but once dried they extract better when decocted. Resins tend to be much less water-soluble, so for things like pine resin or gumweed an alcohol extraction is best.

A hot infusion is almost as simple as brewing a cup of tea. For most herbs, use 1 tablespoon per cup of water and steep for 5–15 minutes.

Allowing your infusion to steep longer than 15 minutes, even overnight, extracts more medicinal properties from inside the plant matter. The simplest way to do this is to dedicate a French press for the purpose of making tea. Don't share this with the coffee-loving people in your life. Most French presses are about a quart in size. A quart-sized jar also works well; you will just have the extra step of finding a strainer or investing in some reusable cloth tea bags. Use ½–1 ounce, or 4 tablespoons, of herbs per quart of boiled water.

This cooled infusion can be strained and added to a pot to reheat, or it can be chilled in the refrigerator. Squeeze in a lemon for

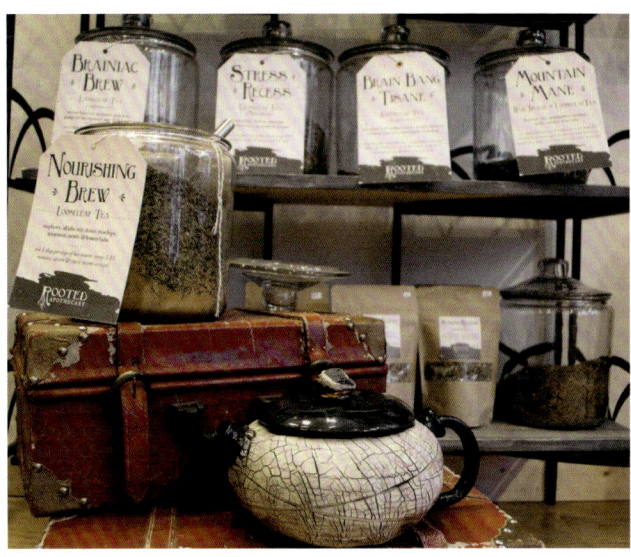

Brews, teas, and tisanes are all different names for infusions. A tisane is an herbal infusion that has no caffeine, while a tea generally refers to an infusion that has a caffeinated herb, such as *Camellia sinensis*.

your morning drink. Or, after straining, boil more water and give the herbs one final brew for a hot morning drink.

Hot infusions are the best preparation for herbs that are rich in vitamins, minerals, and nutrients, such as amaranth, chickweed, horsetail, and northern bedstraw. Become accustomed to making tea not just for a caffeinated sipping beverage or a warm comforting drink but as a nourishing tonic blended just for you.

A cold infusion is when you use unheated water to brew your tea. Place 1 tablespoon of herbs in a cup of water and stir well. Let the herbs steep for at least 15–25 minutes, or for a few hours to overnight. You could place your infusion in the warm rays of the sun for the day and dub it sun tea.

Herbs prepared in a cold infusion will not be as strongly aromatic or bitter. Artemisias and yarrow, for instance, are less potent when brewed cool. Conversely, for herbs that harbor demulcent properties, the cold water lets the mucilaginous properties extract more or less intact. Cold infusions are preferred for plants like mallow, Siberian elm, globemallow, violet, and plantain.

Decoctions

When using barks, twigs, roots, and most dried berries you need to use a little more force than just pouring hot water over the herbs. A decoction is the key to releasing the properties of these plant matters.

To make a decoction, get out a pot, pour 1–2 quarts of water in, and bring it to a boil. Add 1–4 ounces of herbs and place the lid on tight. Turn the burner down to low and gently let the herbs simmer for 25–40 minutes.

Strain out the herbs and add a creamer, or try an infused honey, if necessary, to balance flavor or to bring more medicine into your blend. Sip on the quart over the course of the day; leftover decoction can be stored in the fridge for a day or two.

Sitz bath

A sitz bath soak or wash is a tea of herbs—whether decoction, infusion, or a mix of the two processes—you can use for your external parts, by sitting in a tub of it, placing a limb in a pot of it, or using a soaked cloth to cover the affected area. A bathtub or bowl can be the vessel that holds the liquid. These herbs are used to bring pain relief, promote healing, or fight infections of the pelvic region. It can be very useful postpartum, for hemorrhoids, pelvic inflammations, or genital infections.

To create a sitz bath, fill a large pot with water, add your herbs that need decocting first, like cottonwood or aspen bark and Oregon grape, simmer for 25 minutes with the lid on, and turn the heat off to add the herbs that will need infusing, such as strawberry leaves, plantain, rose petals, or yarrow. Steep

Oxymel Creations

An oxymel is the union of honey and vinegar for an herbal extraction. Extract either a single plant or a combination of herbs in the honey and vinegar individually, then add the honey to the vinegar to taste. This can vary substantially from a few tablespoons to several ounces in a quart-sized jar.

An oxymel can be a blend using the same herb for both the honey and vinegar, or it can involve a combination of herbs. For example, try a decadently heart-opening oxymel of fresh rose petals extracted in vinegar early in the summer, adding a honey extraction of the fresh rosehips come fall. Or twist into formulating with herbs, offering honey infused with a blend like chokecherry and grindelia combined with vinegar of wild hops and peach fruit for soothing an incessant cough.

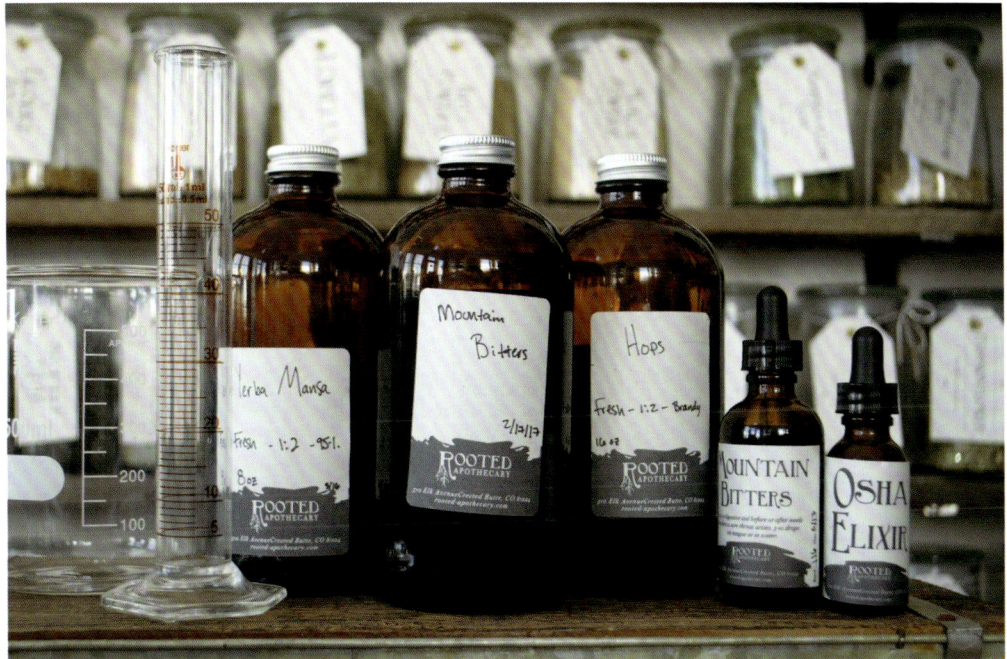

Tinctured herbs bottled for storage. Using amber jars helps to keep out light, more thoroughly preserving the medicinals extracted in alcohol.

with the lid on again for another 15 minutes. Use 3–4 ounces of herb per gallon of water.

Strain the herbs well, pour into whatever you can sit in, and soak for at least 20 minutes. Whatever vessel you use, the idea is to at least partially submerge your pelvic area—usually a few inches of depth is enough. Repeat as often as needed, but try to do it 3 times a day.

Extractions

Extractions of herbs in alcohol are a very concentrated form of herbal medicine. They are valued as a way to extract the constituents from the plants most potently. For those plants high in minerals and vitamins, however, vinegar is preferable to alcohol as the extracting medium. Extractions are made with fresh or dried herbs and a menstruum, or solvent, that contains a certain percentage of alcohol and water, or vinegar. Alcohol

extractions are used externally as a liniment or, if the herb is safe for consumption, internally as a tincture.

Tinctures are an alcoholic extraction of herbs. Dried herbs extract well in any flavor of alcohol from rum, to tequila, to vodka. Fresh herbs generally should be extracted in a higher proof of alcohol, such as Everclear, but they too can be utilized with a lower proof booze.

Fresh herb tinctures are generally made at a 1:2 ratio—1 part herb to 2 parts alcohol and water—using an alcohol higher than 75%. For this menstruum I use Everclear and dilute it with 25% water. If Everclear is not available to you, the highest proof alcohol you can find should also work. If using a lower proof alcohol, do a 1:3 or 1:4 ratio for fresh plant extractions.

Tinctures of dried herbs are made at a 1:4 or 1:5 ratio, meaning the formula is 1 part herb and 4 or 5 parts alcohol. Since there is no water being extracted out of the herbs, the lower proof of alcohol is completely suitable. Leave the herbs to macerate in the alcohol for 2–4 weeks.

A liniment is an external application of a tincture. Use the same extraction methods with liniments as with tinctures. Some people suggest using rubbing alcohol for extraction. Liniments are most popular with herbs that are not advised for internal use, such as arnica.

Vinegar offers another, alcohol-free method of extraction. This menstruum is most viable for herbs that are rich in vitamins, minerals, and other nutrients. Most herbs can be extracted in vinegar if alcohol is an issue for administration, though the medicinal potency will not be as strong for

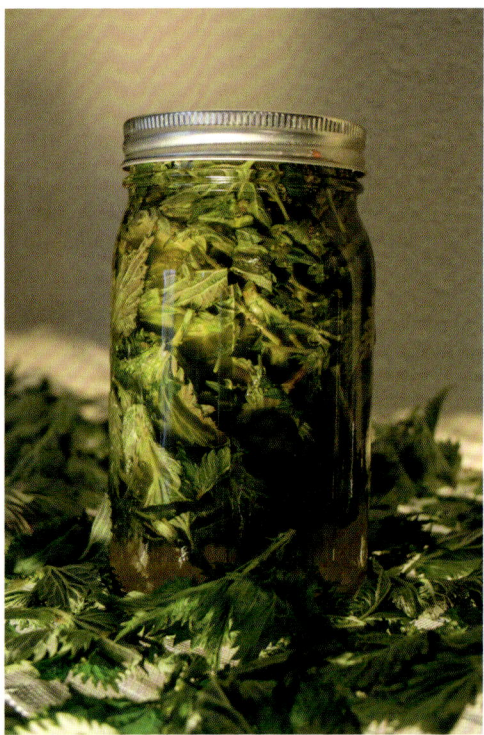

Fresh leaves of *Urtica dioica* extracting into raw, local apple cider vinegar.

some herbs as with a tincture. The ratio for vinegar extractions is usually 1:4 using fresh or dried herb. Let the mixture steep 1–2 weeks.

Oil infusions

Infusing herbs into oil brings their medicine to soothing topical applications, such as chest rubs, massage oils, salves, and skincare products. You may use any organic base oil, such as safflower, olive, almond, or even the semisolid coconut. Oils infused with dried plants work just fine, but I find oils infused with fresh plants to be a bit more potent. The one limitation with using fresh plant material is that you'll need to make your infused oils at different times of year, as each herb becomes available.

There are a number of methods for infusing oil, and each herbalist has their own preference. When using fresh plant material, a method involving heat is usually best. Some fresh herbs do better if they are fogged the night before. This means you dampen the herb with alcohol, to extract more of the resinous medicinals. This works well with plants like Saint John's wort and cottonwood buds. Make sure to keep your lid on your jar overnight while fogging, so the alcohol doesn't evaporate. In the morning, pour your oil over top and place the oil on a heated double boiler to cook off the alcohol.

When making fresh herb oil infusions you must follow through with some steps in order to prevent your oil from spoiling. Chop the plant up first and let it wilt overnight. Place plant matter in a jar and cover with plenty of oil at a ratio of 1:3. Place jar into a crock pot or pan of water, or if you have a double boiler, go ahead and use it. Never put a lid on the jar of a fresh plant oil infusion.

Keep the temperature of the oil below 100°F. Steep in warm oil for at least a day.

Making Salves

Salves can be made by using 1 cup of oil per 2 ounces of beeswax or shea or cocoa butter. This will make your salve a solid consistency. Adding castor oil or butters can give your salve a smoother consistency and a better glide. Many infused herbal oils can be combined to make a host of salves for many different ailments. Carrier oils, such as coconut and safflower, can be combined in various ratios to provide the exact oily feel you want. Always test your melted salve with a cold spoon—dipping it into the mixture will give you an idea of consistency. This is the opportunity to add more oil, beeswax, or butters.

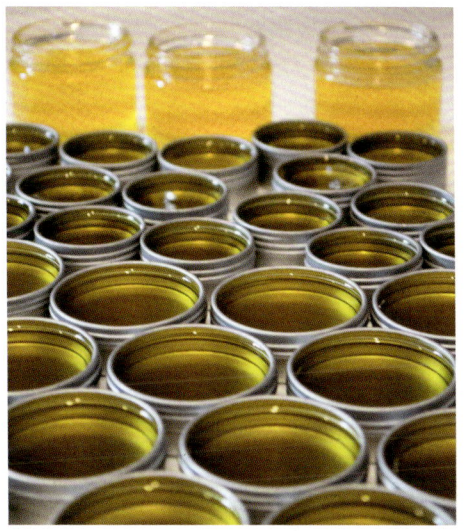

Cooling salves poured into metal tins and glass jars.

Turn off the heat and let it steep overnight. The next day, heat the oil again for a few more hours. Strain the herb from the oil and pour the oil into a clean jar. Heat up the oil without a lid for another hour to dispel and separate the water that extracted from the plant.

The last step is to pour out the oil into another clean jar, leaving behind the water or other residue that has sunk to the bottom. This step may require an extra strain through a fine coffee filter or tea bag. Add vitamin E oil, essential oils, or an oil or alcohol extraction of cottonwood buds to preserve your oil.

All steps are the same for dried herb oil infusions as for fresh plants, except you have no need to wilt the plant and no need to decant after straining, because there is no leftover water from dried plants. Dried herbs can be covered in oil at a 1:4 ratio. Instead of placing them in a heated double boiler, try placing them in a warm spot for a few weeks to infuse.

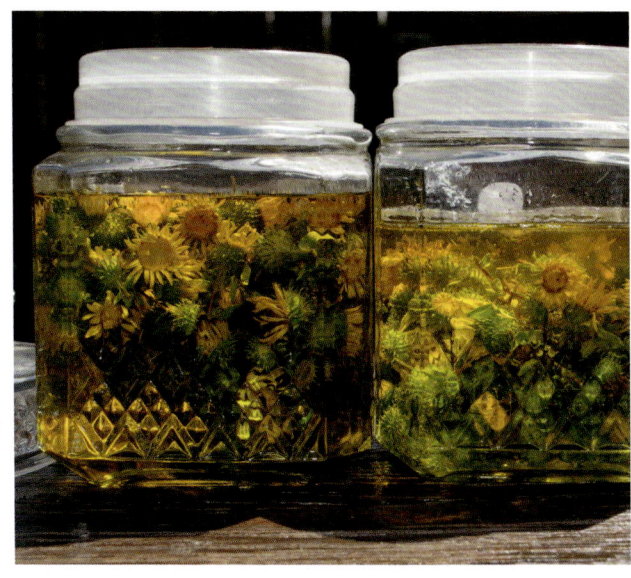

Fresh grindelia, sun-infusing in jojoba and safflower oils.

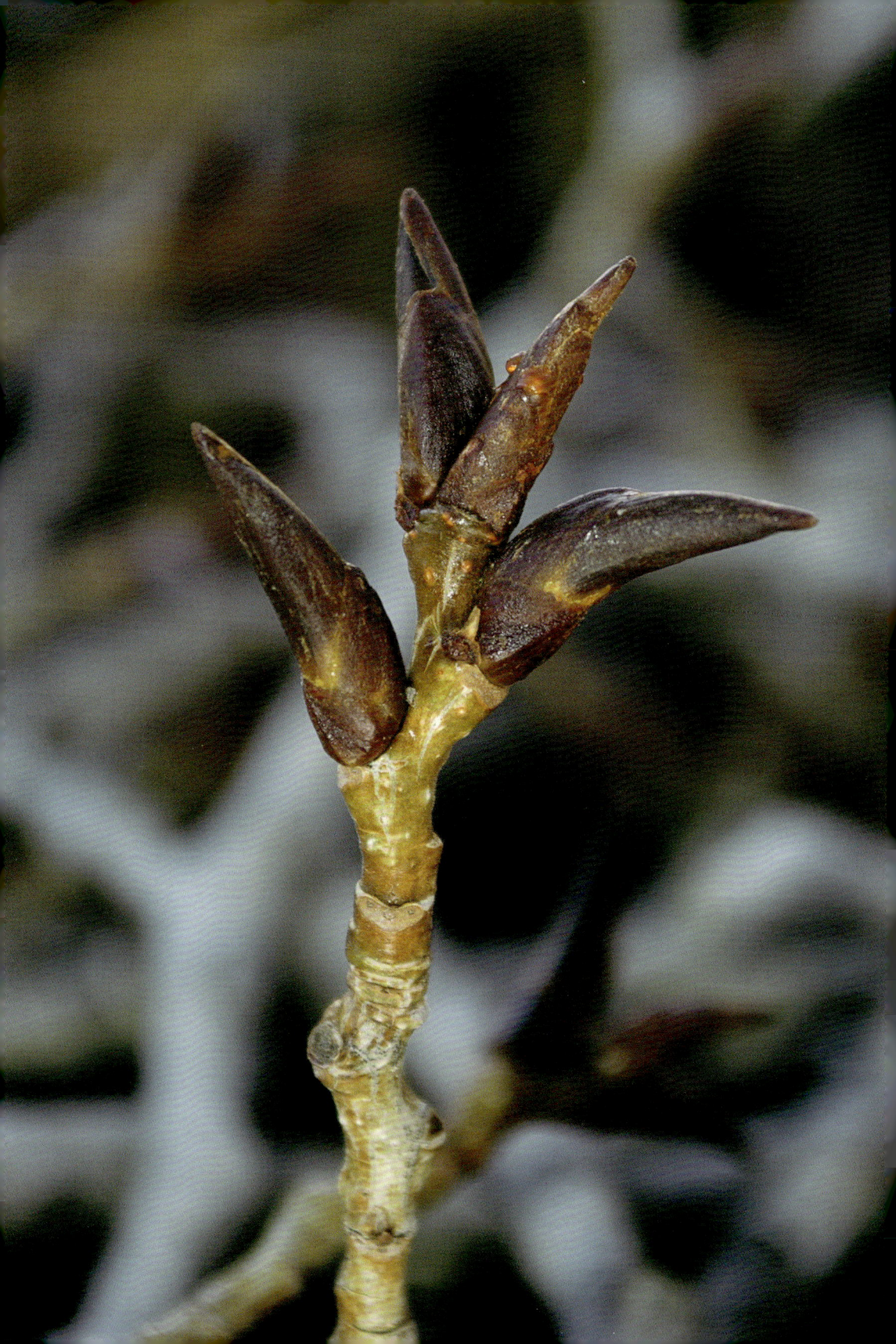

TIMING YOUR HARVEST

A GUIDE TO SEASONAL WILDCRAFTING

How easily a vast body of knowledge can slip away and be lost in a single lifetime. Don't let it happen! We can make the choice to pick up a forgotten tradition, rediscovering an old language of folk remedies, recipes, and ideas of how to treat common illness without the use of modern, over-the-counter medicines, many of which are in fact plant-based.

Attuning yourself to the change of seasons can prepare you for what is in store in Mother Nature's medicine chest. This is where your own personal journey of journaling can begin. Sit in the field and draw the plant that you are learning. Take a photograph of it and write a description with location and time of year for your reference.

The following pages are your guide for exploring what to gather in the wild, but know that plants are as various as the places they dwell, and in many genera, different species grow in different ecosystems. I have listed plants according to the ecosytems in which you are most likely to find them in a given season, limiting myself to listing each plant just once per season.

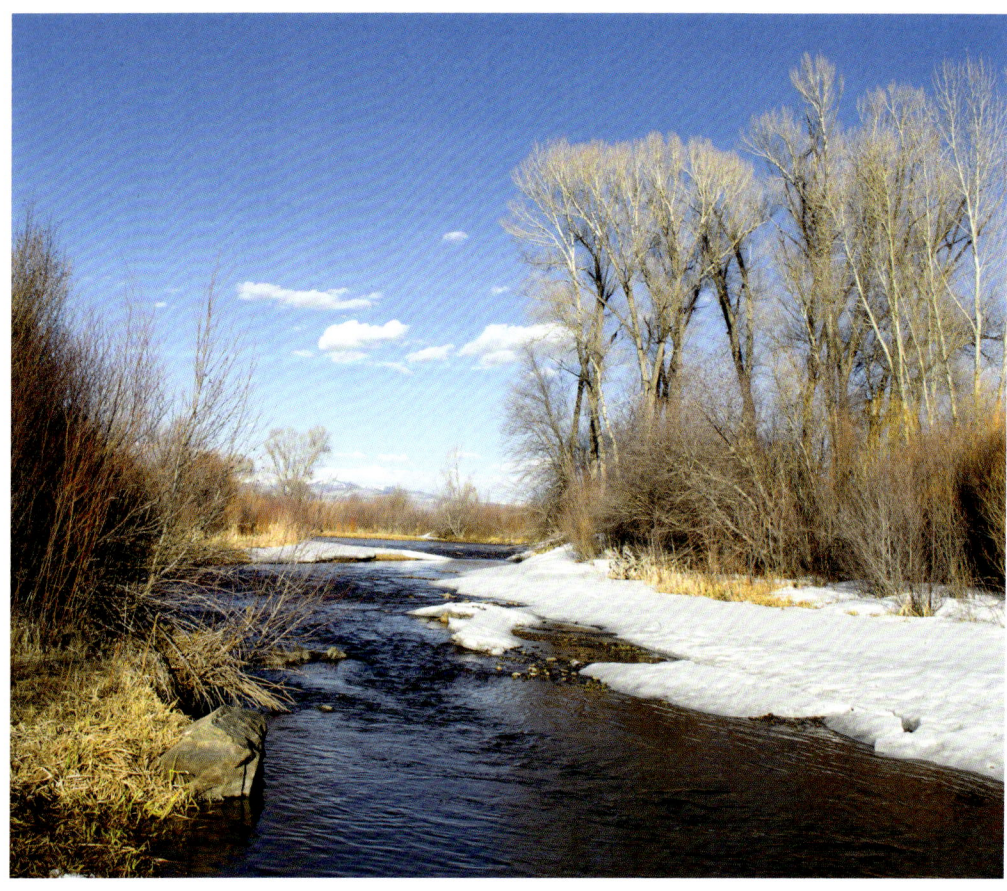

Snow thawing at the creek's edge while willow twigs and cottonwood buds are prime for gathering.

EARLY SPRING

Depending on where you live in our region, early spring doesn't arrive until the snow melts in May or June. Mid- to late spring sometimes hardly has an existence in the mountains, as winter turns quickly to summer. With such a large variance in elevation in the mountain west, you most likely will find these plants first on the lower slopes and flatlands between the Rocky Mountain ranges. It's a giddy feeling each spring identifying the first tips of plants such as shepherd's purse peaking through the soil, or resuming the annual binge of harvesting cottonwood buds before they begin to flower and sprout leaves.

Where to find early spring plants

Open Meadows, Disturbed Soils, or Forest Edges

apple: bark, twigs
beebalm: leaves
burdock: leaves, roots
catnip: leaves
chicory: roots
dandelion: leaves, roots
dock: leaves, roots
glacier lily: leaves
mallow: leaves, roots
motherwort: leaves
mullein: leaves, roots
peach: twigs

plantain: leaves

shepherd's purse: leaves, roots

teasel: roots

valerian: leaves, roots

wild lettuce: leaves

wild licorice: roots

wild strawberry: leaves

yarrow: leaves

Desert, Among Sagebrush, or Rocky Soil

chaparral: leaves

juniper: leaves, twigs, fruit

Mormon tea: stems

oak: bark, twigs

Oregon grape: leaves, roots

piñon: needles, resin, twigs

prickly pear: pads, flowerbuds

sagebrush: leaves, stems

yucca: leaves, roots

Near Wetlands, Riverbanks, Lakesides, or Bogs

alder: bark, twigs, catkins

angelica: roots

cottonwood: bark, twigs, buds

stinging nettle: leaves, roots

veronica: leaves

wild asparagus: roots

wild mint: leaves, stems

willow: bark, twigs

willowherb: leaves

yerba mansa: leaves, roots

Woodlands or Partially Shaded Places

alumroot: roots

aspen: bark, twigs, buds

chickweed: leaves, stems, flowers

cranesbill: leaves, roots

Douglas fir: needles, resin, twigs

fir: needles, resin, twigs

osha: leaves, roots

pine: needles, resin, twigs

redroot: roots, bark, twigs

Siberian elm: bark, leaves

Solomon's plume: roots

spruce: needles, resin, twigs

spikenard: roots

starry Solomon's seal: roots

sweet root: leaves, roots

usnea: all

uva-ursi: leaves

violet: leaves

wild cherry: bark, twigs

MID- TO LATE SPRING

That in-between season when it is almost summer in many places and still snowy high up in the mountain peaks, mid- to late spring is full of blooming flowers, budding plants, and fresh young leaves that can be gathered in bounty. Roots may still be dug in the high places before the plants flower, and the young tips of conifers can be clipped while they are still young and fresh. With the days getting long and the sun's rays strong and warm, there is plenty of time to spend in the wilderness.

Where to find mid- to late spring plants

Open Meadows, Disturbed Soils, or Forest Edges

alfalfa: leaves

amaranth: leaves

apple: leaves, flowers, bark, twigs

beebalm: leaves

bluebells: leaves, flowers

burdock: leaves, roots

catnip: leaves

chicory: roots

crabapple: leaves, flowers, bark, twigs

dandelion: leaves, flowers, roots

dock: leaves, roots

estafiate: leaves, stems

fireweed: leaves

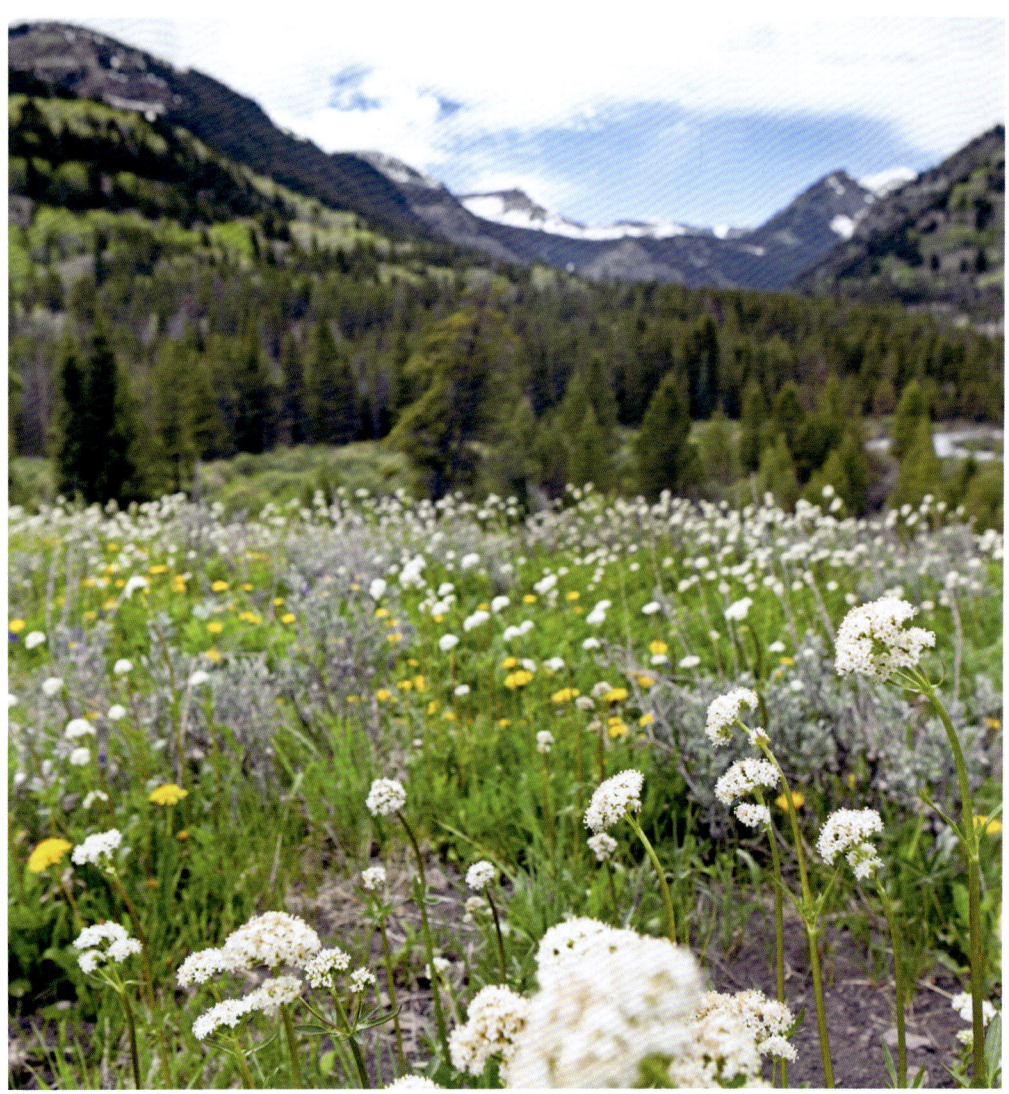

An abundance of valerian flowers in late spring.

glacier lily: leaves

horehound: leaves, flowers, stems

hyssop: leaves

mallow: leaves, flowers, roots

motherwort: leaves

mullein: leaves, roots

northern bedstraw: leaves, stems

peach: leaves, flowers, twigs

plantain: leaves, flowers, seeds

raspberry: leaves, stems, roots

red clover: leaves, flowers

Saint John's wort: leaves, flowers, flowerbuds

shepherd's purse: leaves, flowers, stems, seedpods

sweet clover: leaves

teasel: roots

valerian: leaves, flowers, roots, stems

wild caraway: leaves

wild lettuce: leaves, stems

wild licorice: roots

wild strawberry: leaves, flowers

wormwood: leaves, stems

yarrow: leaves

Desert, Among Sagebrush, or Rocky Soil

balsamroot: leaves, flowers, roots

chaparral: leaves

globemallow: leaves, flowers, seedpods, roots

juniper: leaves, twigs

Mormon tea: stems

oak: bark, twigs

Oregon grape: leaves, roots

piñon: needles, resin, twigs

prickly pear: pads, flowers

sagebrush: leaves, stems

skunkbush: leaves, stems

yucca: roots, leaves

Near Wetlands, Riverbanks, Lakesides, or Bogs

alder: bark, twigs, catkins

angelica: leaves, stems, roots

cottonwood: bark, twigs, buds

horsetail: aerial portions

pedicularis: leaves

skullcap: leaves, flowers, stems

stinging nettle: leaves, roots

sweet grass: blades

veronica: leaves, flowers, stems

wild asparagus: roots

wild mint: leaves, flowers, stems

willow: bark, twigs, leaves

willowherb: leaves, flowers

yerba mansa: leaves, roots

Woodlands or Partially Shaded Places

alumroot: leaves, roots

arnica: leaves, flowers, flowerbuds

aspen: bark, twigs

blueberry: leaves

chickweed: leaves, flowers, stems

cleavers: leaves

cranesbill: leaves, roots

Douglas fir: needles, resin, twigs

elderberry: flowers

fir: needles, resin, twigs

hawthorn: flowers, twigs, thorns

osha: leaves, roots

pine: needles, resin, twigs, pollen

redroot: roots, bark, twigs

rose: flowers, flowerbuds, leaves

Siberian elm: bark, leaves

Solomon's plume: roots

spikenard: roots

spruce: needles, resin, twigs

starry Solomon's seal: roots

sweet root: leaves, roots

uva-ursi: leaves

usnea: all

violet: leaves, flowers

wild cherry: bark, twigs, flowers

SUMMER

The summer's heat comes in quickly and lasts only for a few short, sweet months at higher elevations. Plants are at their prime—in bloom, fully vital, and heavily scented. Monsoon season sweeps across the mountain west, bringing much needed moisture in midsummer, just when the plants have had it with the high heat of June. The humid and wet relief brings in a new bounty of plant life—mushrooms and the fruiting season. Take advantage of the long days of summer and plant yourself in the woods.

Where to find summer plants

Open Meadows, Disturbed Soils, or Forest Edges

alfalfa: leaves, flowers

amaranth: leaves

apple: leaves, fruit

beebalm: leaves, flowers

bistort: roots

black walnut: green hulls

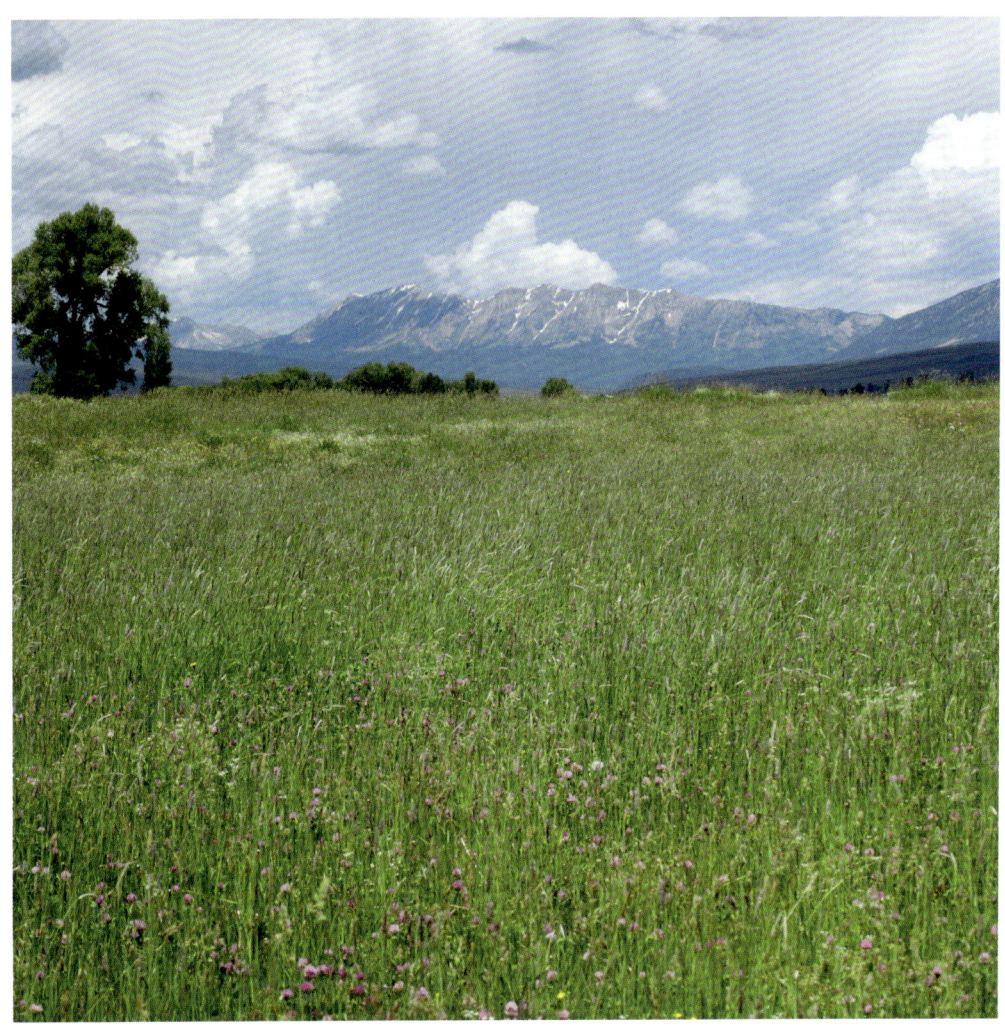

A field full of red clover and wild caraway blossoms in the heat of summer.

bluebells: leaves, flowers
burdock: leaves
catnip: leaves, stems, flowers
chicory: flowers, roots
crabapple: leaves, fruit
dandelion: leaves, flowers
dock: leaves
estafiate: leaves, stems, flowers
fireweed: leaves, flowers, flowerbuds
goldenrod: leaves, flowers, flowerbuds
grindelia: leaves, flowers, flowerbuds
horehound: leaves, flowers, stems

hyssop: leaves, flowers
linden: flowers
mallow: leaves, flowers, seedpods
motherwort: leaves, flowers, stems
mullein: leaves, flowers
northern bedstraw: leaves, flowers, stems
peach: leaves, twigs, fruit, pits
pearly everlasting: leaves, flowers
pineapple weed: leaves, flowers
plantain: leaves, flowers, seeds
purslane: leaves, stems, flowers
raspberry: leaves, fruit, stems

red clover: leaves, flowers
Saint John's wort: leaves, flowers, flowerbuds
shepherd's purse: leaves, flowers, stems, seedpods
sweet clover: leaves, flowers
valerian: leaves, flowers, stems
vervain: leaves, flowers
wild caraway: leaves, flowers, seeds
wild hops: strobiles, leaves
wild lettuce: leaves, stems
wild strawberry: leaves, flowers, fruit
wormwood: leaves, flowers, stems
yarrow: leaves, flowers, stems

Desert, Among Sagebrush, or Rocky Soil

chaparral: leaves
cota: leaves, flowers, stems
globemallow: leaves, flowers, seedpods
juniper: leaves, twigs
Mormon tea: stems
Oregon grape: leaves, roots
piñon: needles, resin, twigs
prickly pear: pads
sagebrush: leaves, flowers, stems
skunkbush: leaves, stems, fruit
snakeweed: leaves, stems, flowers
yucca: leaves

Near Wetlands, Riverbanks, Lakesides, or Bogs

angelica: leaves, flowers, stems, seeds
horsetail: aerial parts
pedicularis: leaves, flowers
skullcap: leaves, flowers, stems
stinging nettle: leaves, seeds
sweet grass: blades
veronica: leaves, flowers, stems
wild mint: leaves, flowers, stems
willowherb: leaves, flowers
yerba mansa: leaves, roots

Woodlands or Partially Shaded Places

alumroot: leaves, roots
arnica: leaves, flowers

blueberry: leaves, fruit
chickweed: leaves, stems, flowers
cleavers: leaves, stems, flowers
cranesbill: leaves, flowers
Douglas fir: needles, resin, twigs
elderberry: fruit
fir: needles, resin, twigs
osha: leaves, flowers, seeds
pine: needles, resin, twigs
rose: leaves, flowers, flowerbuds
Siberian elm: bark, leaves
spruce: needles, resin, twigs
sumac: fruit
sweet root: seedpods, leaves
usnea: all
uva-ursi: leaves
violet: leaves, flowers
wild cherry: fruit, stems

FALL

The autumnal harvest season brings in fruit, seeds, berries, roots, and new growth of leaves before plants go dormant for winter. The air has chilled and frost begins to set in, making some fruits more ripe for the picking. Hawthorn, rosehips, and mountain ash berries are all worth waiting for; don't harvest them until the chilling nights sweeten the fruit. This is the last opportunity to dig up roots before the ground freezes. Some years winter comes early and the snow-covered ground is impenetrable come November; other years, you can gather roots in the mountains until Thanksgiving.

Where to find fall plants

Open Meadows, Disturbed Soils, or Forest Edges

amaranth: seeds
apple: bark, twigs, fruit
black walnut: black hulls

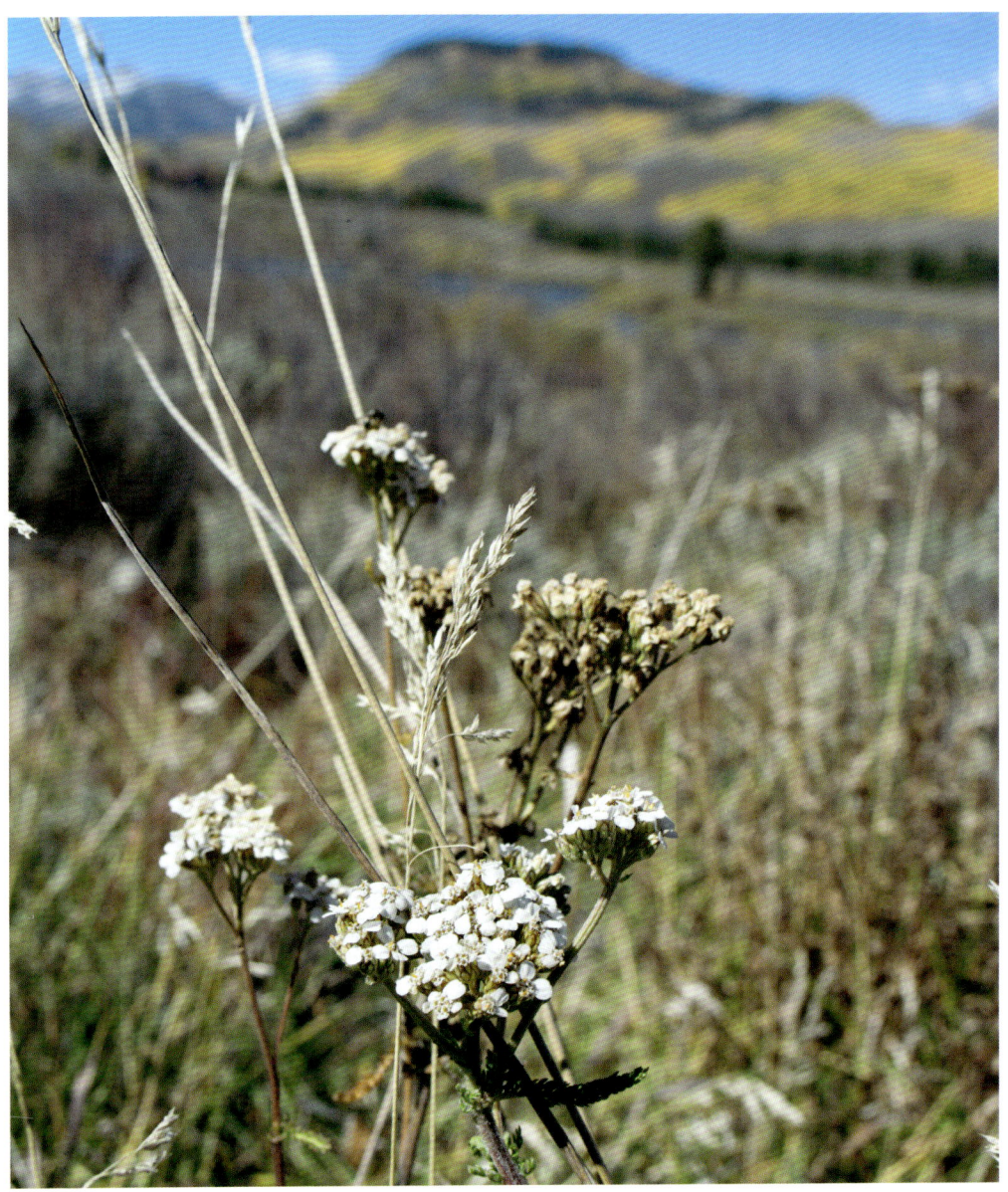

One of the last remaining yarrow blossoms contributing subtly to autumn's tonal display.

burdock: seeds, roots

chicory: roots

crabapple: bark, twigs, fruit

dandelion: leaves, roots

dock: leaves, roots

estafiate: leaves, stems

goldenrod: leaves, flowers

grindelia: leaves, flowers

mallow: leaves, seedpods, roots

motherwort: leaves

mullein: leaves, roots

peach: twigs

plantain: leaves

raspberry: roots

shepherd's purse: leaves
sweet clover: leaves, flowers
teasel: roots
valerian: roots
vervain: leaves, flowers
wild caraway: leaves, seeds
wild lettuce: leaves
wild licorice: roots
wild strawberry: leaves
wormwood: leaves
yarrow: leaves

Desert, Among Sagebrush, or Rocky Soil

chaparral: leaves
cota: leaves, flowers
juniper: leaves, twigs, fruit
Mormon tea: stems
oak: bark, twigs
Oregon grape: leaves, roots
piñon: needles, resin, twigs
prickly pear: pads, fruit
sagebrush: leaves, stems, fruit
skunkbush: leaves, twigs, fruit
snakeweed: leaves, flowers, stems
yucca: roots, leaves

Near Wetlands, Riverbanks, Lakesides, or Bogs

alder: bark, twigs, strobiles
angelica: leaves, seeds, roots
horsetail: aerial parts
pedicularis: leaves
stinging nettle: leaves, seeds, roots
wild asparagus: roots
willow: bark, twigs
yerba mansa: leaves, roots

Woodlands or Partially Shaded Places

alumroot: roots
aspen: bark, twigs
chickweed: leaves, stems, flowers
cottonwood: bark, twigs
cranesbill: roots

Douglas fir: needles, resin, twigs
elderberry: fruit
fir: needles, resin, twigs
hawthorn: fruit, twigs
mountain ash: fruit
osha: leaves, seeds, roots
pine: needles, resin, twigs
redroot: roots, bark, twigs
rose: fruit
Siberian elm: bark, leaves
Solomon's plume: roots
spikenard: roots
spruce: needles, resin, twigs
starry Solomon's seal: roots
sumac: fruit
sweet root: roots
usnea: all
uva-ursi: leaves
wild cherry: bark, twigs, fruit, stems

WINTER

Its snowy glory notwithstanding, winter can be the darkest and most cruel time of year. For the most part, plants are buried and the harvest slows. Many people find winter to be a time of deep reflection or notice it can come with hints of depression. Treat yourself well, get outside, pull in the blue sky, and breathe in deep cooling breaths.

The trees and some shrubs keep vibrant during these cold months, offering their new or old growths of medicine. Among the forms of dried fruits, rosehips can be gathered deep into winter as long as the red hips are still somewhat gummy in texture. The cottonwood and aspen trees are loaded with resinous buds that will turn to either leaves or catkins come spring. These sticky buds are among my most prized wildcrafted medicine of the entire year. The forever-green needles of the conifers will always be there when we need them, but they can be most useful in the winter when coughs settle deep into our

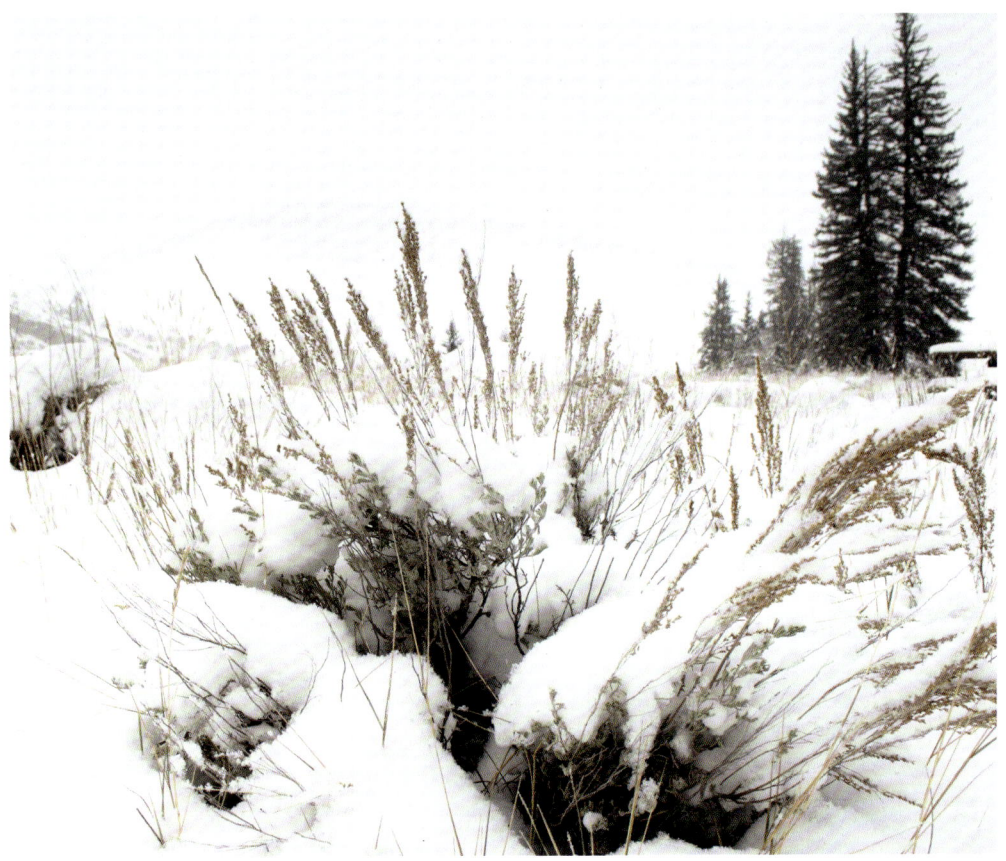

The leaves of sagebrush can still be picked from beneath the snow. Though less aromatic, they remain useful in medicine-making.

lungs. Junipers provide the last clinging blue cones (or, as we call them, "berries") that can be gathered. Usnea, the lichen known as old man's beard, is another winter's delight. No need to pick it straight from the evergreens it grows on—it can be harvested from the top of the fallen snow.

Where to find winter plants

Desert, Among Sagebrush, or Rocky Soil

chaparral: leaves
juniper: leaves, twigs, fruit
Mormon tea: stems
oak: bark, twigs
piñon: needles, resin, twigs
sagebrush: leaves, stems
skunkbush: stems, fruit

Near Wetlands, Riverbanks, Lakesides, or Bogs

alder: bark, twigs, catkins, strobiles
willow: bark, twigs

Woodlands or Partially Shaded Places

aspen: bark, twigs, buds
cottonwood: bark, twigs, buds
Douglas fir: needles, resin, twigs
fir: needles, resin, twigs
Siberian elm: bark, leaves
spruce: needles, resin, twigs
usnea: all
wild cherry: bark, twigs

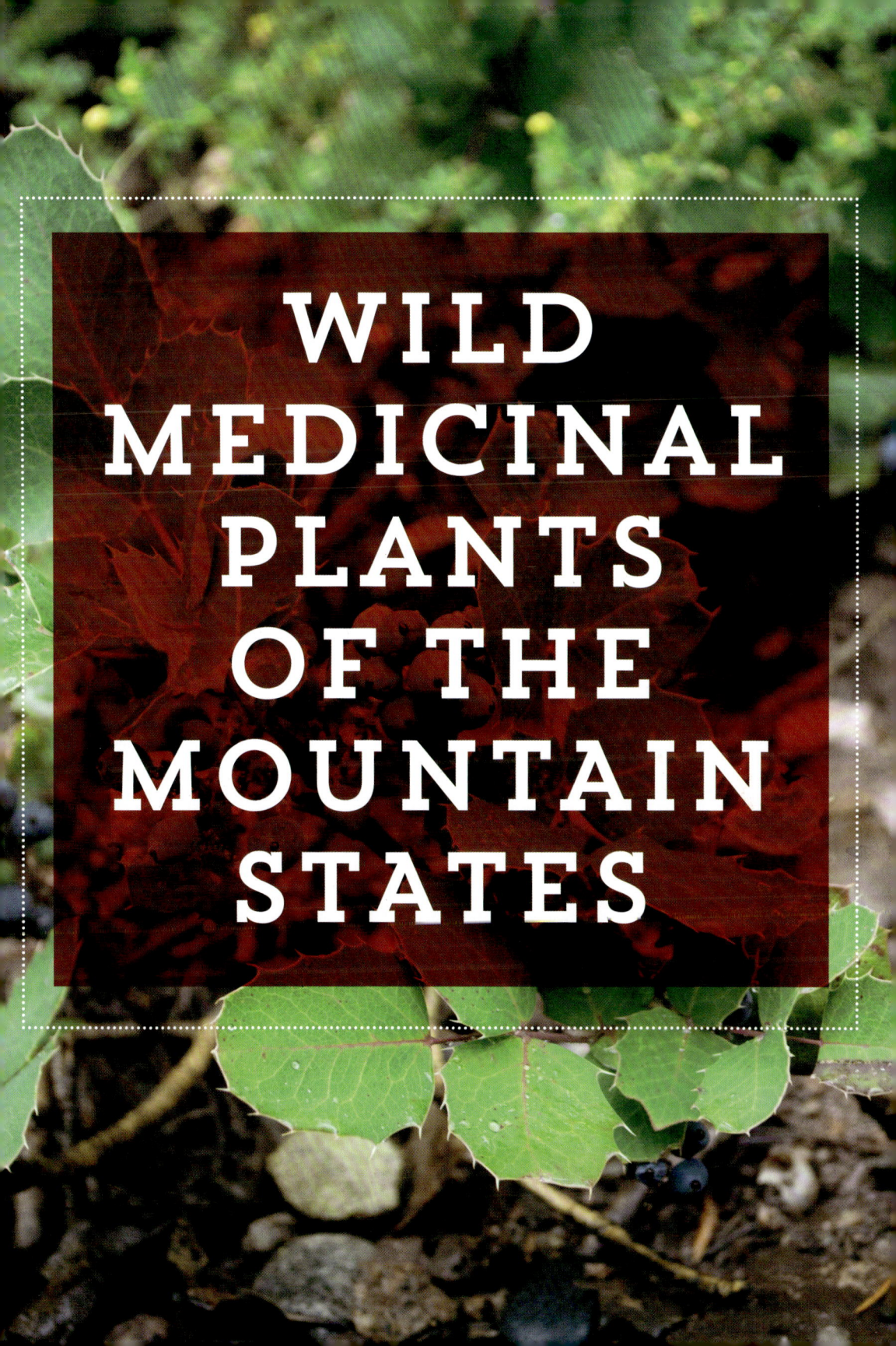

WILD MEDICINAL PLANTS OF THE MOUNTAIN STATES

alder

Alnus species
PARTS USED bark, twigs, leaves, catkins, strobiles

The bitter principles of alder offer valuable medicine that can be useful in salves, tinctures, or teas.

How to identify

Alder can be found near flowing water, growing as a large shrub or small tree with many trunks. *Alnus rubra* and *A. viridis* subsp. *sinuata* grow in the north and west of our region, but *A. incana* (mountain alder) is by far our most abundant species. All can be distinguished from other trees by their male catkins, which are long, slender, and pliable, turning into tiny pollen-producing flowers come spring. The female catkins (technically, strobiles) are green cone-like structures that become hard and woody after pollination.

Alder looks very similar to birch and can be partly distinguished by its less pointed leaves and its shorter, thicker lenticels in the mature bark. Alder's woody cones persist after pollination, whereas the female catkins of birch disintegrate once the seeds have released, and are rarely left over after a season.

The bark on alder is brown and smooth with a little sheen. Leaves are lobed and toothed around the margins, growing alternately from the branches. As a deciduous tree, alder will shed its green leaves come autumn, leaving behind the distinct ornaments of the catkins and cones that are visible to hikers or drivers-by.

Where, when, and how to wildcraft

The alder catkins, bark, and twigs can be gathered in winter but seem to be most potent in early spring. Gather the catkins before they begin to pollinate, and the cones while they are still green in fall.

Move throughout stands of trees along the water's edge as you gather, pruning only a little from each tree. Clipping branch ends can give you useful little twigs that hold both catkins and cones. If you clip bigger branches, the bark can be peeled with a knife or pounded with a rock to loosen it from the heartwood. The best time to gather bark is in spring and fall, when it's running rich with sap, and the bark separates more easily.

Medicinal uses

Alder twigs, bark, catkins, and cones are used for their bitter principles and their perceived ability to fight infections. Alder catkins, bark, and twigs also have a pain-relieving quality to them, which is always welcome to a sore throat. The bitter components help to astringe the GI tract, allowing better absorption of nutrients for those that tend to have a leaky gut or sluggish digestion. Alder also assists the lymphatic system, which is a vital component in the functioning of the immune system.

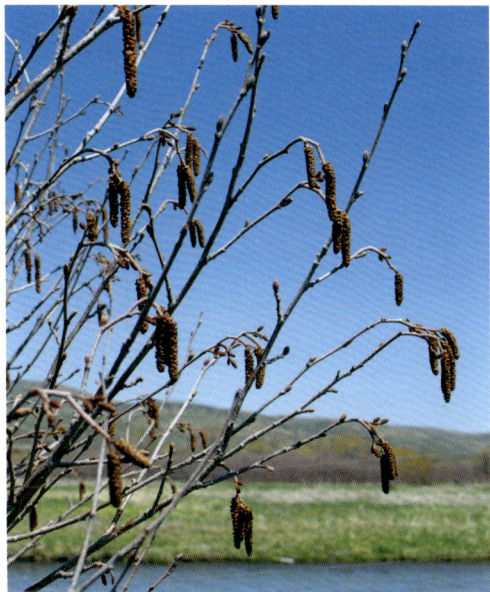

The catkins of *Alnus incana* adorn the tree like tiny ornaments.

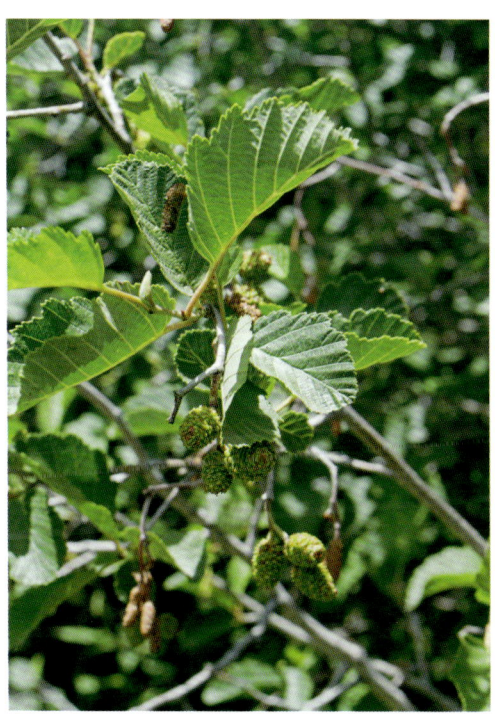

Green cone-like strobiles of alder.

Alder infused in oils helps with relieving the pain or soreness of trauma or overexertion related to exercise.

Sitz baths can be useful in calming the inflammations of hemorrhoids or genitourinary infections.

Future harvest

The harvest of alder trees needs to be done very respectfully, as the trees are great bank stabilizers and help critical riparian areas to function properly.

alfalfa

Medicago sativa
lucerne
PARTS USED leaves, flowers

This fine nutrient-rich herb shouldn't be limited to grazing cattle. If alfalfa helps their milk production, imagine what it can do for nursing mothers.

How to identify

A perennial herb of the pea family, alfalfa has the iconic clover pattern of leaves: each leaf is trifoliate, with three leaflets. The leaflets are oblong with tiny serrations around the apex, only slightly hairy on the underside and smooth on the top. Leaflets of sweet clover, a close lookalike before flowering, are serrated around the entire margin. Flowers grow in a clustered raceme, with many usually purple flowers, but flower color can vary from white to light blue to shades of purple. The seed-pods are a tight coil shape and hold many tiny yellow-tan seeds.

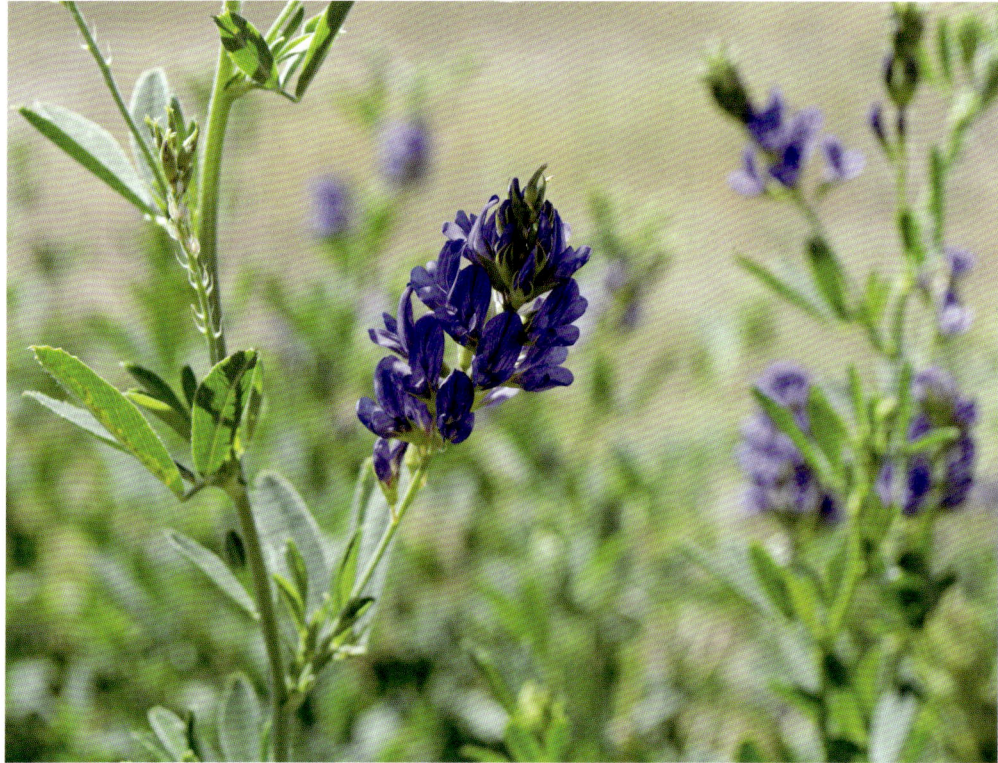

Flowers of alfalfa can range from a deep bluish purple to a white-lilac color.

Where, when, and how to wildcraft

Find alfalfa growing in any kind of disturbed soil, whether it is pastureland or construction sites. Make sure you are gathering in a clean spot, free of pollutants or heavy metals, as this plant pulls heavily from the soil. It prefers nutrient-rich soil. Alfalfa can be found in the foothills and mountains, flowering in summer. Gather young leaves and flowers in spring through summer.

Harvesting a large quantity of alfalfa can be quite easy, and it tastes much more flavorful when gathered in the wild. Gather leaves while they are vibrantly green and young. Wait until after the passing of several dry, sunny days in a row if you intend to dry the plant for future use. Cut the lively, flowering top half of the plant.

Medicinal uses

I consider alfalfa to be almost more food than medicine. It is loaded with vitamins, along with amino acids, minerals, and trace elements. One of my favorite nourishing brews to sip is a blend of alfalfa, stinging nettle, wild raspberry leaves, rosehips, wild mint, cleavers, red clover, and pineapple weed. This mineral- and vitamin-rich infusion can be consumed daily.

I also utilize this common weed, fresh or dried, in things like medicinal broths and stocks, combining it with marrow-filled bones and vegetables—but the bones can simply be left out. Also, a completely herb-based broth mixes alfalfa with chickweed, stinging nettle, horsetail, red clover, and wild caraway seeds. Slip this into soups, sauces, and rice for a disguised medicinal boost.

Another medicinal-culinary twist would be to mix any of those same herbs into a vinegar, as mineral- and vitamin-rich herbs extract best in vinegar-based liquids. Honey can be added at the beginning or end to make an oxymel. Raw honey provides another medicinal component that can herbally enrich the extraction further, as well as sweetening your potion. This oxymel can be used as a tonic; sip ½–1 ounce per day.

Oil infused with alfalfa can help treat skin conditions and dryness.

Future harvest

No worries for the future when harvesting alfalfa—it is usually a weed escaped from the pasture. Something to consider is that many genetically modified species of alfalfa have now escaped into the wild and are growing among the feral *Medicago sativa* of the mountain west.

HERBAL PREPARATIONS

Tea
Hot infusion
1 ounce fresh or dried leaves and flowers
1 quart water
Drink 1–3 times per day.

Vinegar
1 part freshly chopped leaves and flowers
4 parts vinegar
Take 1 tablespoon 1–3 times per day.

Oil
Infuse with fresh or dried leaves and flowers.

alumroot

Heuchera species
mountain saxifrage
PARTS USED roots, leaves

*The most important astringent in my insect-bite-soothing oil, alumroot
decreases the redness and itchy inflammation associated with stings and bites.*

How to identify

It isn't the flowers of alumroot that catch
your eye, but most likely the scalloped and
kidney-shaped red leaves changing color in
the autumn. The tall slender stalks can reach
2 feet in height and are adorned with tiny,
delicate, whitish green flowers. Roots are
scaly with old growth and dark brown with a
creamy pink interior. They can be large and
gnarled or stunted from growing in rocky soil.

Where, when, and how to wildcraft

Find alumroot in shady, rich soils of dry,
craggy alpine outcroppings or growing down
moist sloping hillsides facing either north or
south. It grows on mountain peaks over 9000
feet in Colorado and Nevada and under 5000
feet in Montana and Wyoming. Find it growing
near raspberry brambles in the canyons or
alongside valerian in the rolling mountain
meadows.

   Dig the root in the spring or fall, and cut
off the leaves and flowerstalk. Before processing the root, scrub off the external dead
growth. Cut up the root and use it fresh in
oils and tinctures. To dry the leaves and root,
chop while fresh, and let dry on a rack.

Medicinal uses

One of the most astringent plants in the
mountain west, alumroot can be infused into

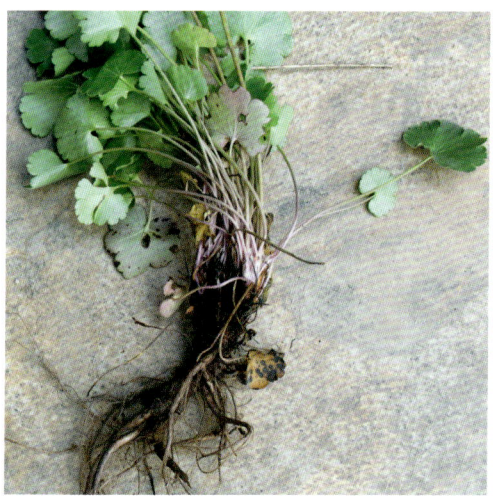
Freshly dug roots of *Heuchera parvifolia*.

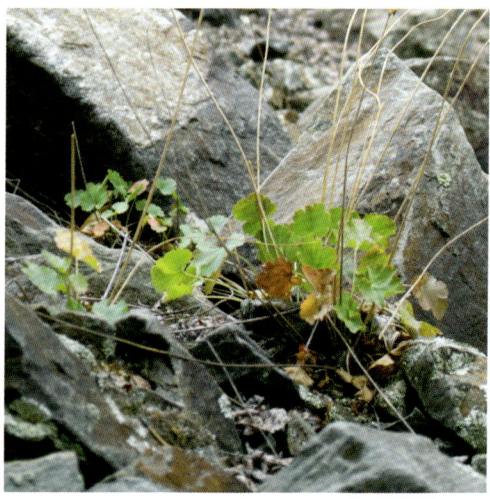
Find alumroot in rocky outcroppings.

oils, tinctures, or teas. The root holds the most astringency and can be used against diarrhea and other gastrointestinal upsets.

A tea or decoction of the roots creates a gargle for a sore throat or a rinse for a mouth beset with stubborn canker sores. Try adding Oregon grape roots and the bark of alder or cottonwood, plus a generous pinch of plantain after the decoction comes off the heat. Let this steep for another 10 minutes, while cooling enough to use. A tincture of this herb combination would make a helpful spray for the mouth and throat.

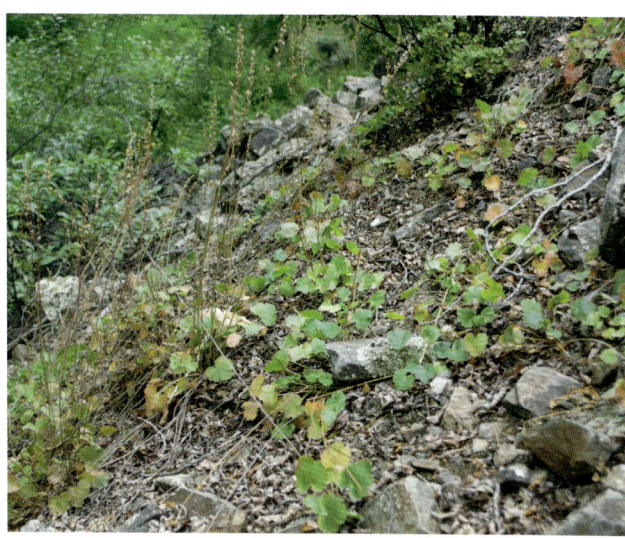

A hillside covered in alumroot. Always harvest this often rare-to-find plant with extra care.

The fresh root may also be chewed or sucked on for mouth irritations, or for making a spit poultice for small wounds. A decoction of the fresh root has many uses, as a tea sipped to ease internal intestinal discomfort, as an enema or sitz bath to relieve hemorrhoids, or as a mouth rinse or gargle.

Alumroot can be infused into oil and used topically on bug bites, stings, or even the most daunting hemorrhoids. For an anti-itch oil, combine alumroot with rose petals, uva-ursi, and plantain. I find this formula works best when fresh plant material is used for the oil infusion.

In first aid, the powdered root can be beneficial as an astringent wound-healer that will stop bleeding in minor wounds, cuts, and scrapes. It is not advised for use on large or open wounds.

Future harvest
Heuchera rubescens, which has reddish or pink flowers, is a protected plant in Colorado.

HERBAL PREPARATIONS

Tea
Cold infusion
1 tablespoon fresh or dried chopped leaves
 and root
1 cup water
Decoction
2–4 ounces fresh or dried chopped root
1 quart water
Drink hot or cold 3–4 times a day.

Tincture
1 part fresh leaves and root
2 parts menstruum (75% alcohol, 25%
 distilled water)
or
1 part dried leaves and root
5 parts menstruum (60% alcohol, 40%
 distilled water)
Take 5–10 drops 3 times a day.

Oil
Infuse with fresh or dried leaves and root.

amaranth

Amaranthus species
pigweed
PARTS USED leaves, seeds

Harvest this pesky weed with impunity and utilize its leaves and seeds
for their nutritional and medicinal benefits.

How to identify

Amaranths can reach 6 feet tall or more, depending on the quality of soil in which they grow; plants of the mountain west tend

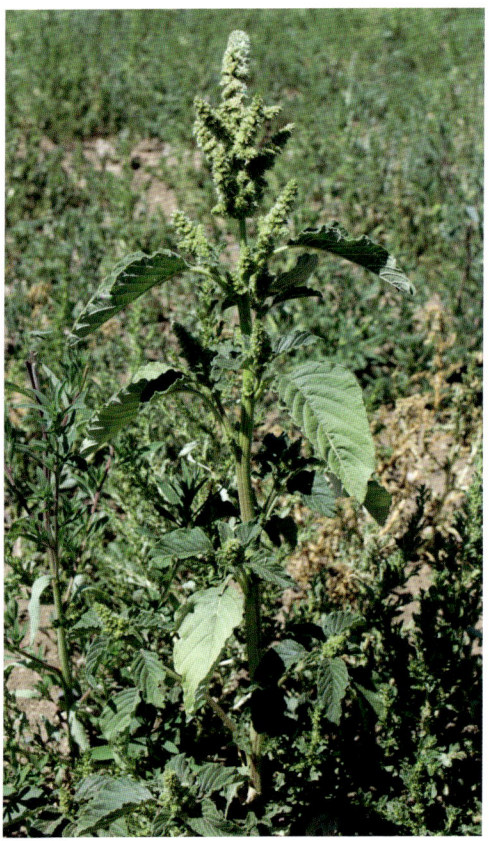

Find amaranth growing among many other weeds in abandoned lots or sunny fields.

to be shorter when growing in dry, compact, or rocky soil. Wide-based lanceolate or ovate leaves grow alternately up a green stalk that turns red as the plant ages. Green flowers are small, lack petals, and grow in a cone-like raceme. Seeds are smooth, shiny, and black, held in place by bristly brown bracts. The most common species in the mountain west are *Amaranthus retroflexus* and *A. powellii*.

Where, when, and how to wildcraft

Head for a sunny spot. Cut the stalks of amaranth while the leaves are still a lively green and the stalk has begun to take on a reddish tint. Seeds can be harvested in late summer, early fall, or even through the winter.

Cut the upper foot of a flowering amaranth stalk, loaded with leaves, or pick individual leaves from many plants. Bundle a few stalks together and hang them upside down to dry. Strip off the dried leaves and store in a sealed container. Cut or break off the loaded seedheads of amaranth and beat the seeds off into a bucket, using your fingers to work them out. The seeds will then need to be winnowed, which releases the chaff from around the small seeds.

Medicinal uses

Amaranth pops up all over the mountain west. Instead of just pulling it out of the

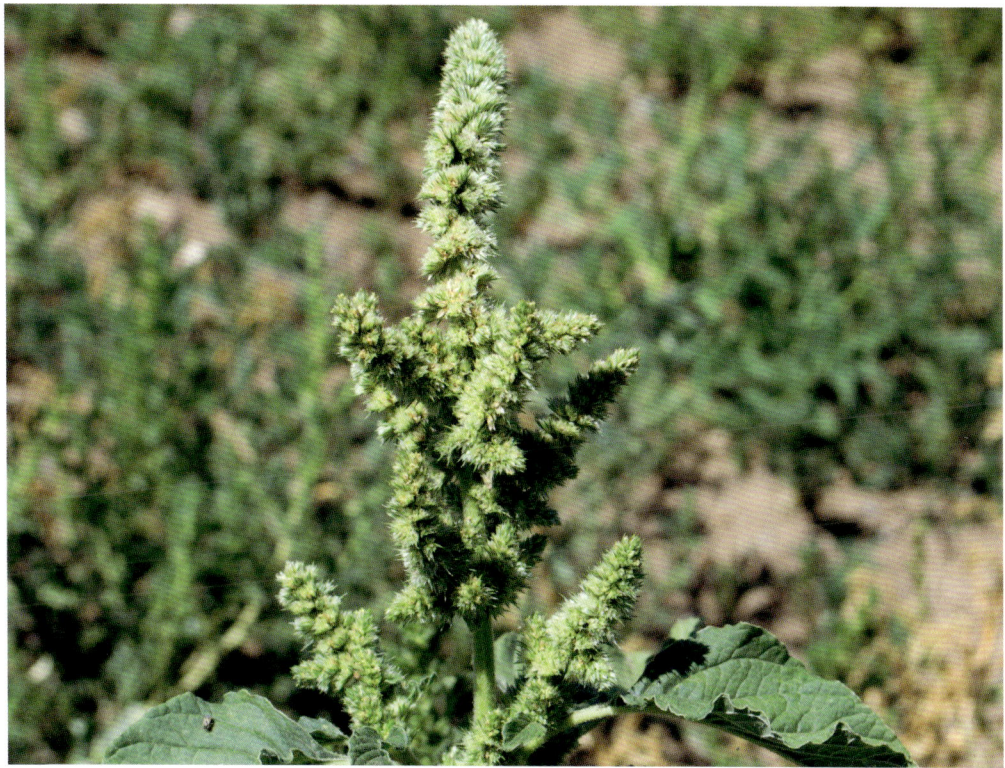
Gather the leaves of amaranth while vibrantly green, and the flowerheads once they start to brown.

ground, add it to vinegars and teas for its nutritive assets. It has a mild astringent property that can soothe inflamed mucous membranes, especially in cases of a raw stomach, swollen gums, or a sore throat. In an oil infusion, this astringency can be beneficial for cuts and scrapes.

The small black seeds will become somewhat demulcent when soaked in water for a few hours or overnight, like those of plantain or flax. This can be a soothing drink for a digestive tract healing from ulcers, colitis, or leaky gut.

Future harvest

Have at it. Amaranth is known to pop up just about anywhere the sun is shining, especially in disturbed areas, and can be counted on to reseed itself year after year.

HERBAL PREPARATIONS

Tea
Hot infusion
1 tablespoon fresh or dried leaves
1 cup water
Cold infusion
1 tablespoon seeds
1 cup water
Drink as needed.

Vinegar
1 part fresh leaves
3 parts vinegar
Take 1 tablespoon 1–3 times a day.

Oil
Infuse with fresh or dried leaves.

angelica

Angelica species
archangel, wild celery
PARTS USED roots, leaves, stems, flowers, seeds

Aromatic and spicy, angelica is useful for a host of complaints. Take it internally for an upset tummy or rub it on as an infused oil to soothe a chest cold.

How to identify
First of all, be 100% certain with your identification of any and all plants in the carrot or parsley family (Apiaceae). This family contains some of the most toxic plants in North America: water hemlock (*Cicuta* species) and poison hemlock (*Conium maculatum*) can be fatal if ingested in even minuscule quantities (see caution).

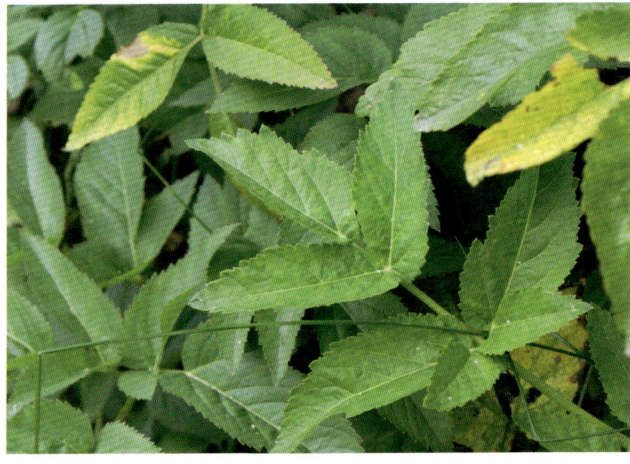

Angelica leaves are ovate and much wider than the thin lanceolate leaves of its poisonous cousin water hemlock. Notice too that the primary veins of angelica end at the tips of the serrations of the leaves.

Angelica has a showy umbel that resembles a firework, with many rounded clusters of white, light pink, or yellow flowers radiating from one point at the top of the stalk. Leaves are usually bipinnately divided into leaflets. The margins of the ovate leaflets are serrated. Leaf stems (petioles) have sheaths that hug the main stalk. Stalks of angelica are a shade of purple or red and are always hollow. The roots are white or creamy and heavily scented with a spicy celery aroma. Most angelica roots are solid throughout, whereas water hemlock and poison hemlock tend to have hollow areas within their roots. Angelica seeds are aromatic, dorsally flattened, and ribbed.

Where, when, and how to wildcraft
Angelica prefers cool, moist mountain soil and can be found lining irrigation ditches or near riverbanks. Gather the more fragrant leaves and stalks in summer of the plants' second year. Seeds can be collected in late summer or fall. Harvest roots in spring or fall.

To dry, hang the stalks bundled together with the leaves on them. Gather the seeds once they are fully ripened, and make sure to dry them thoroughly before storage. Rub the seeds off the umbel before storing. Roots can be dug, given a good washing, chopped, and

From Syrup to Candies

Syrup is a sugary sweet creation you can make with just about any herb. Used alone or blended in combination with tinctures, syrups can be used to create cough syrups and are an easy way to administer herbs to youngsters.

Begin by washing your freshly gathered herb, chop, and fill a pot about a third full. Cover the herbs in water so they are submerged by a few inches. Bring the water to a simmer while mashing or stirring, and continue simmering for 5 minutes. Turn off the heat and let the pot sit for another 5–10 minutes. Strain out the cooked plant matter, pouring the liquid into a clean pot. Then add ½–1 cup of sugar per cup of infused herbal water. The more bitter the herb, the more sugar you will want to use. Heat over medium-high heat, stirring continuously until the sugar is melted. Bring it almost to a boil, and turn down to simmer for a few minutes longer while still stirring. Pour into a clean glass jar. Let cool. Store the syrup in the refrigerator for up to 2 months maximum. Add 25% of an alcohol extraction to make the syrup more shelf stable.

Medicines can also be used in candied herb form. For example, if you had intentions to candy roots (osha), stems (angelica), or conifer tips (Douglas fir), you can easily do so while making herbal syrup. Right after your sugar has melted, add more freshly cut herbs to the syrup on the stove. Heat for 3 minutes on a low simmer, then using a slotted spoon strain out the pieces from the syrup. Place the pieces onto parchment paper laid out on a cooking tray. Place the tray into the oven preheated to its lowest temperature. Let the pieces of candied herb dry for an hour to several hours until they firm up.

Leaves (mint) and flowers (violets) can also be candied, though traditionally these are made by painting a coating of egg white onto the fresh herbs and then dipping them in super-fine sugar. The leaves or flowers are then placed on parchment paper for a day to dry out.

Once dried, store the candies in a bag or jar. Store in the freezer for the longest shelf life.

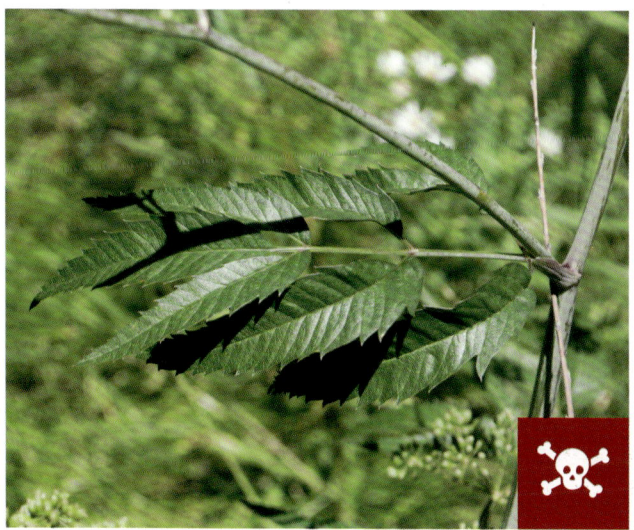

Don't eat me! For comparison's sake, here are the lanceolate and serrated leaves of angelica's poisonous lookalike, water hemlock (*Cicuta* species).

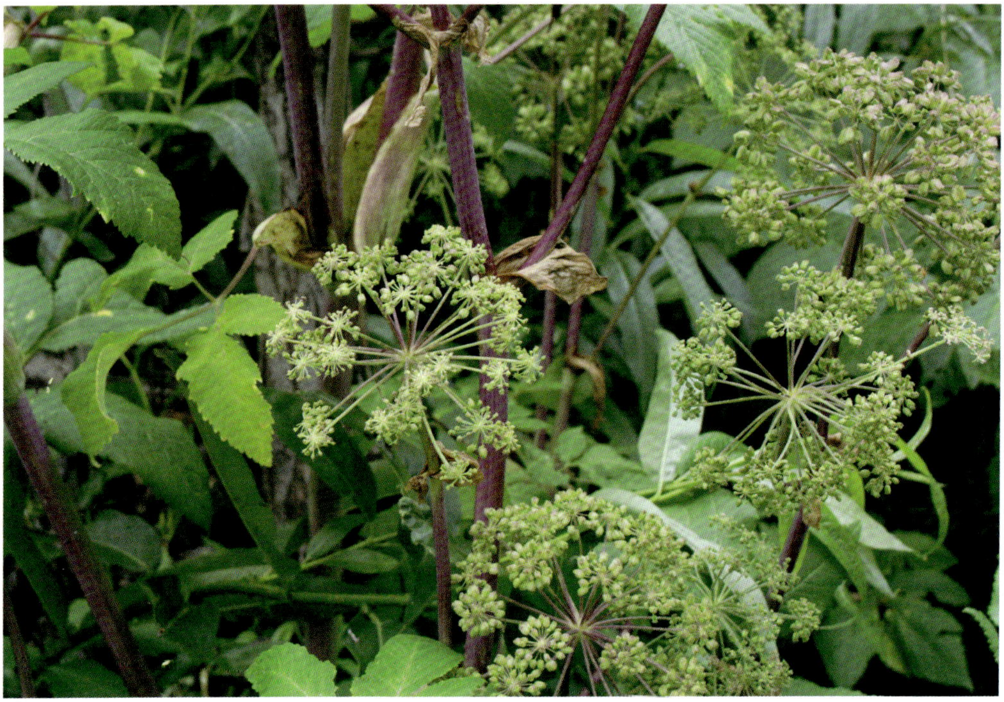

Aromatic seeds of angelica can be gathered for medicine-making. The seeds of both angelica and water hemlock are ovate, but angelica's seeds are ribbed and winged—water hemlock seeds are only ribbed.

dried on a rack or using the lowest temperature in the oven or dehydrator.

Medicinal uses

Angelica is warming and stimulating, while having an aromatic, bitter flavor. It does well in formulas for digestion, menstrual cramps, and illness.

Make a tincture of fresh roots and seeds to ease stomach cramping, nausea, and gastrointestinal irritability. The roots and seeds can be antispasmodic for menstrual cramps, encouraging the flow and regulating menstruation.

Roots in a tea or tincture help stoke a fever to the point of perspiration, while calming the nervous system, uplifting spirits, and helping to fight viruses. Angelica is similar to osha in this way. It helps soothe respiratory congestion in the lungs, too.

Sore, achy body parts would appreciate a rubbing oil made from fresh or dried angelica plant parts. This makes a good chest rub, as well.

You can chop the leaf stems and main stalks of angelica and candy them for a stored medicinal treat.

⚠ Caution

Angelica is not for use in pregnancy.

It is critical to differentiate angelica from water hemlock and poison hemlock. Angelica species tend to have fatter, more ovate leaflets. Water hemlock has thinner, more lanceolate leaves. Poison hemlock has more dissected, fern-shaped leaves, with a purple-spotted stem. Many botanists advise looking at the primary lateral leaf veins. If the veins end in between serrations, it could be one of the poisonous hemlocks; if the primary lateral veins end at the tips of the serrations, "all is hip," as the saying goes, and the plant is considered safe. I have seen variations to this with *Cicuta* species, however, so use this only as one of several identification tools.

The seeds of both angelica and water hemlock are ovate, but angelica's seeds are ribbed and winged—water hemlock seeds are only ribbed. The roots of water hemlock and poison hemlock, if cut longitudinally, will usually show air pockets, but certain *Angelica* species sometimes show them as well. Finally, angelica roots are aromatic; however, if you have just been digging angelica roots, any root will smell of it, and poison hemlock too has been noted to have a celery-like scent.

Future harvest

Angelica grows abundantly throughout our region. If collecting seeds, leave at least one umbel in the stand full of seeds.

HERBAL PREPARATIONS

Tea
Hot infusion
1 tablespoon fresh or dried seeds, leaves, flowers, or stems
1 cup water
Decoction
4 tablespoons fresh or dried seeds or root
1 quart water
Drink 1 cup 3 times a day.

Tincture
1 part fresh seeds, stems, flowers, or root
2 parts menstruum (80% alcohol, 20% distilled water)
or
1 part dried seeds or root
5 parts menstruum (60% alcohol, 40% distilled water)
Mix 20–40 drops in half a glass of water and sip slowly over an hour 3 times a day.

Oil
Infuse with fresh or dried leaves, seeds, stems, or root.

apple

Malus species
wild apple
PARTS USED bark, twigs, leaves, flowers, fruit

Wild apples are more than a major fruit-forage score. Each apple tree
also holds a plenitude of useful medicine in its bark, twigs, leaves, and flowers.

How to identify

Wild apple trees can reach heights of 40 feet but are usually much smaller, hosting clusters of fragrant pink or white blooms every spring. Each flower is 1–2 inches wide and consists of five petals. The smooth bark is bronze or gray. Oval leaves grow alternately and have small serrations along the edges. Fruits can be big or small, though smaller varieties are usually called crabapples. The fruits of feral apples are at least 2 inches in diameter and range in color from yellow-green to orange and red.

Where, when, and how to wildcraft

Apples linger around old homesteads and turn up around campgrounds and along roadsides and trails. Some could have been planted with intention; others may have sprouted up from tossed apple cores and fallen seeds. Find apple trees in fertile soils and among other trees in partial shade. This is not a tree you will find at high elevation: it grows mostly below 7000 feet.

Aromatic flowers blossom in spring and can be gathered

Wild apples aren't just for eating—there is valuable medicine in all parts of the tree.

along with the attached twigs and bark, which you can chop up for medicine-making. Fruit begins to ripen in August and continues to produce until October, when you will find the last apples fallen on the ground. Fruits can be plucked and tasted for their potent astringency, bitterness, and crispness, properties that blend well in tinctures and teas.

Medicinal uses

The astringency of apple bark, twigs, leaves, and wild fruit can be quite helpful for gastric irritations or loose stools. It can help quell heartburn or acid reflux. When combined with a demulcent herb like mallow, Siberian elm, or plantain, it can really help soothe and heal the tissues of the esophagus. The bitter taste of apple and its cooling and anti-inflammatory qualities are useful in bitter formulations, easing digestion by increasing secretions. The anti-inflammatory properties of apple combine well with the astringency for soothing red and painful sore throats. Crushed fresh apple leaves make a useful poultice for insect bites and stings or minor wounds. The leaves and flowers can be extracted into oil for astringent-requiring remedies.

Dehydrate apple slices after you have squeezed lemon over them and sprinkled them in cinnamon. Store these for jazzing up wintertime tea blends or simply stopping diarrhea. On the other hand, a fresh ripe apple or its juice can help clear constipation.

Apple cider vinegar is a staple in my medicine-making, and I am fortunate enough to have an organic local orchard that supplies our needed quantities. This shelf-stable menstruum will last for decades and is the preferred way to extract essential nutrients and minerals from herbs. On its own, apple cider vinegar is medicinal in many ways and can help soothe an upset stomach.

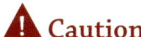 **Caution**

Apple leaves, seeds, and bark contain a small amount of cyanogenic glycosides, which can convert into a potentially toxic substance in the human body. Although apple is regarded as completely safe to use, large quantities of seeds eaten at one time could be fatal.

Future harvest

There are plenty to go around, but just in case you fall in love with a particularly sweet-fruited tree, a sprouted apple seed does not represent the apple it came from. Apples do not come true from seed, meaning, there really is no telling what kind of apple tree will spring up if planted.

HERBAL PREPARATIONS

Tea
Hot infusion
3 tablespoons fresh or dried flowers and
   leaves, or dried fruit
1 cup water
Decoction
1 ounce fresh or dried twigs and bark
1 quart water
Drink as needed.

Tincture
1 part fresh twigs, bark, flowers, or fruit
2 parts menstruum (75% alcohol, 25%
   distilled water)
or
1 part dried twigs, bark, flowers, or fruit
5 parts menstruum (60% alcohol, 40%
   distilled water)
Take 30–60 drops 3 times a day.

Oil
Infuse with fresh or dried flowers or leaves.

Arnica species

PARTS USED leaves, flowers, flowerbuds

The warming and circulating energetics of arnica make it the perfect wild herb for mountain extremists who may be a little overzealous or uncoordinated in their endeavors.

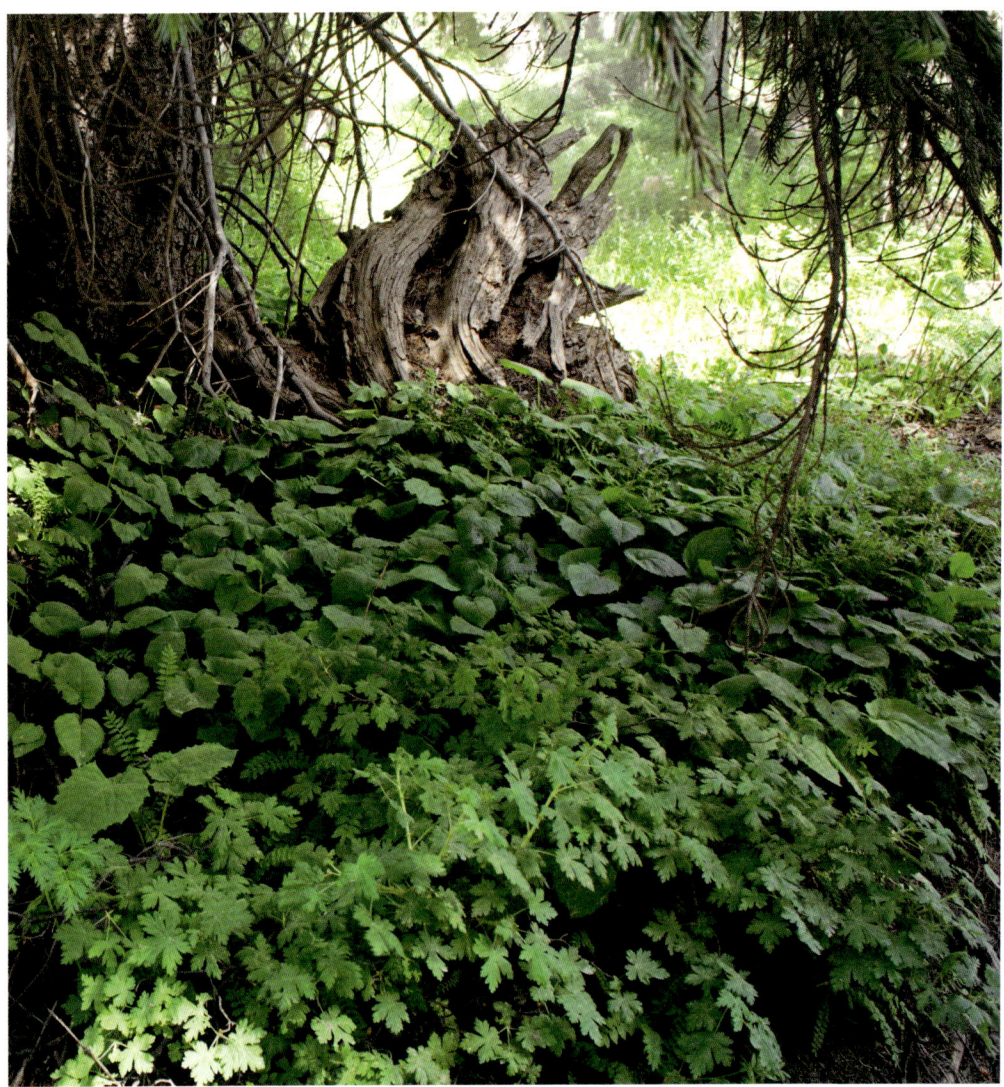

It is perfectly sensible to visit stands of arnica even when plants are not in flower. The leaves are just as powerful and may even offer more medicine than the flowers.

How to identify

The bright yellow flowers of arnica have a daisy-like appearance. *Arnica cordifolia*, the primary species used for medicine, has heart-shaped basal leaves. The few leaves that grow along the stem tend to be more of a lance shape, and are arranged oppositely. If you happen to pick a flower or get close enough for a sniff, you will discover a sweet pine-citrus-balsam scent.

About a dozen different species of *Arnica* occur in the mountain states. I find *A. cordifolia* to be the most aromatic and therefore potentially useful, harboring the most medicinal properties.

Where, when, and how to wildcraft

Arnica sprawls on the fertile and rocky floors of mountain canyons, nestling throughout mixed conifer and aspen forest. Find it in high alpine meadows and mixed forests between 3500 and 10,000 feet in elevation. *Arnica cordifolia*'s heart-shaped leaves may be matted along the forest floor with only a few flowers blooming at a time. *Arnica longifolia* can be found in the high alpine.

Begin gathering the leaves of arnica in early summer, and find flowers budding and in bloom beginning in May and continuing until September. The leaves of arnica hold great medicinal properties—you need gather only one leaf per plant. Gather a bounty of the flowers and buds when there are many to be seen.

Be mindful of where and how you walk when tending to an arnica patch. This is a delicately growing plant with shallow roots that can be negatively impacted by trampling feet or erosion.

The flowers and leaves may be used fresh, wilted, or dried. Arnica flowers fluff out and seed into pappus when dried, but don't fret, this is still valuable medicine. It is better to

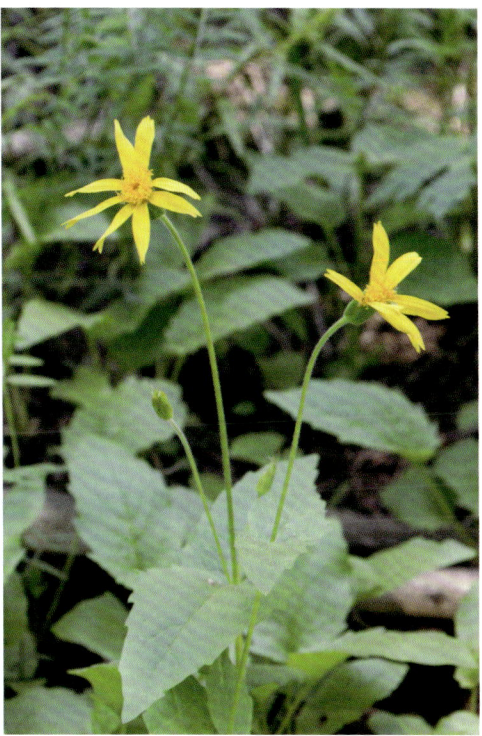

Arnica cordifolia has the loveliest scent when the heart-shaped leaves or flowers are crushed.

gather mostly leaves if you are harvesting arnica to dry it for later medicine-making. Always be sure to dry your arnica indoors, away from sunlight.

Medicinal uses

The medicinal magic of arnica can be quite profound. This is an herb that should not be taken internally without the guidance of a trained herbalist.

The fresh or dried flowers and leaves of arnica are best infused in oil for rubs and salves or extracted in alcohol for external use as a liniment. The primary use of arnica is for inflammation and soreness after overexertion. The best way to use arnica is right after an injury occurs and you anticipate bruising. The energetic properties are warming and circulating to the area of application. It is especially useful when heat helps the injury feel better.

Arnica oil, the most commonly used form, can be overly expensive to buy at a store. Better to prepare your own! Once you have, you can mix it with other medicinal oils such as yarrow and sweet clover for an exquisite massage oil.

A liniment of arnica is another topical format. It can be diluted with 1–2 parts water and applied as needed, or applied undiluted straight on the area. Do watch if irritation occurs, then dilute next time. A standard infusion may be applied externally as well, using the steeped plant matter as a poultice covered by a tea-soaked cloth.

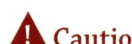 Caution

Do not consume arnica as an infusion. Consult a trained herbalist before consuming it in any form. Arnica can cause upset stomach, especially in children and elders, and is not for large or daily doses. Like other sunflower family members, arnica contains constituents that can cause allergic reactions in sensitive individuals. Do not use liniment or oil on open wounds or cuts.

Future harvest

Do be gentle with arnica, as its roots and rhizomes are not that deep. Pulling too hard can easily uproot the plants. Take only a few flowers so that the plant can reproduce.

aspen

Populus tremuloides
quaking aspen, trembling aspen
PARTS USED bark, twigs, buds

*The interwovenness of an aspen grove is a reminder of the interconnectedness
of all earthly creatures. Be a supporting, interconnected tree in your own life.*

How to identify
People who move here from eastern North America often mistake aspen for birch, but unlike birch bark, aspen bark does not peel off spontaneously. Aspen trees are in the willow family (Salicaceae). Branches form slightly resinous buds in the winter that will turn into the quaking leaves and fuzzy catkins. Leaves are ovate to heart-shaped with serrated margins and a lighter colored underside. They sit on a long, flattened petiole, which is the reason leaves tremble, with a fluttering sound, in the wind. Aspen trees are 30–70 feet tall and grow in groves, each having either male or female trees. Each grove is one giant organism that is connected through the underground root system of its trees. When one aspen falls, it directly impacts the roots and health of its neighbor.

Where, when, and how to wildcraft
While aspens are found all over the mountain west, most grow

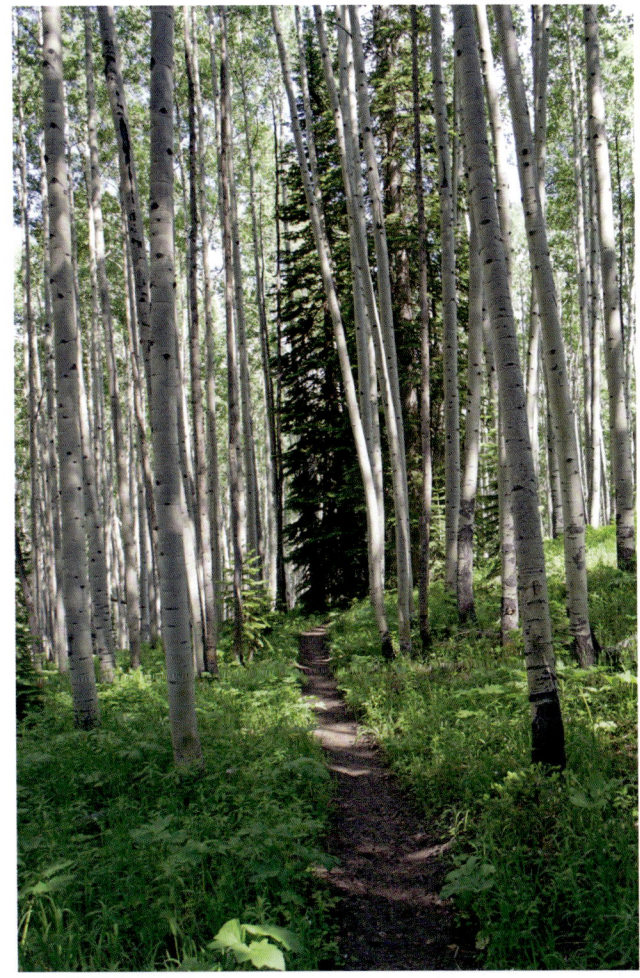

Walking through the woods can provide you with many freshly fallen aspen twigs and may even lead you to tasty samplings of identifiable plants that might inspire your formulating.

Peeling Bark

Though it can sometimes be done in fall, bark peeling is easiest of all in spring, when the running sap makes separating the layers of bark most manageable. The living inside bark is what we are after for flavoring bitters, providing medicinal benefits, and to strip when drying for tea. If the outer bark and fully barked twigs are all you can obtain, these are also useful. A few of the most common trees that provide great medicine are willow, aspen, Siberian elm, cottonwood, alder, and cherry.

I rarely take from live trees, as it's so easy to find branches other ways. Find large wind-fallen branches or beaver-dropped trees, or contact a local tree trimmer with the specifics of the tree you would like to collect.

Start by making a longitudinal cut with a knife down your twig, just deep enough to hit the heartwood. Choose twigs that are about ½ inch or thicker in diameter. In the sap-running months, the bark will separate easily from the wood. Alternatively, take a rock and pound the branches until the bark begins to separate from the heartwood. Peel off the outer bark for immediate use or drying.

I don't even bother stripping the bark from small young twigs. I simply clip them into small pieces and toss them in with my peeled barks. Chop the bark finer if needed, and spread it to dry on a mesh screen or in a dehydrator. Dry thoroughly before storing in a glass jar.

at elevations under 10,000 feet. Find them in mixed conifer forests, on sloping hillsides, and in mountain valleys.

Gather the buds during the winter months. Look to find windfallen branches or trees, or trim young twigs from trees while they host the buds. Strip buds off the twigs and use both in concoctions.

Collect bark during the spring and fall when the tree is flowing with sap, making the bark easy to peel off the heartwood. This is important, as the inner bark is what holds the more sweet and bitter properties. Sample the bittersweet-tasting cambium of spring branches while peeling bark. The inner bark can also be peeled off any recently fallen timber any time of year, for making fresh extractions or drying for tea.

Medicinal uses

The almost vanilla-like aromatics of aspen bark have a cooling bitterness, while the buds provide a more warming bitter property. Both aspects of the plant make it a suitable herb to use in alcohol-extracted bitter formulations. Extractions of the buds can be beneficial when the cold season arrives in the arid west, helping sufferers to expectorate stuck mucus.

Like other trees in its family, such as the willows or cottonwoods, aspen also has pain-relieving benefits. The pain-relieving properties of trees of the Salicaceae are thought to come from the cooling and astringent aspects of the bark, which can aid in bringing down fever and fight inflammation. These qualities extract best from aspen buds gathered in winter or bark peeled in spring and fall.

Peeled bark can be used in formulations needing an astringent and can mend the digestive tract during a bout of diarrhea. It can be included in sitz bath blends with herbs such as plantain, strawberry leaves, yarrow, and pineapple weed.

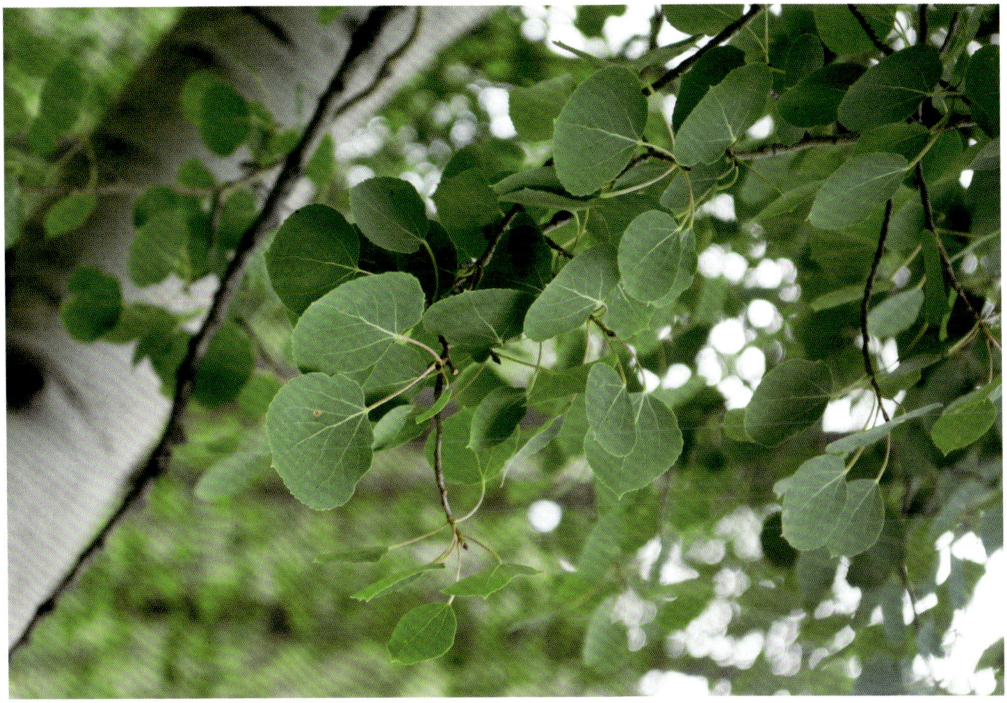

The long petioles of the flat, rounded leaves of aspen allow them to quake and tremble in the slightest breeze.

⚠ Caution

Large doses of aspen tincture or tea can be overdrying and cause headaches or mild nausea. Do not use aspen buds if you are allergic to aspirin.

Future harvest

Taking only fallen branches or trimming branches from live trees shouldn't affect the longevity of an aspen. However, taking bark from a live tree can threaten its integrity.

HERBAL PREPARATIONS

Tea
Decoction
1 ounce fresh or dried peeled bark
1 quart water
Drink 1 cup 3 times a day.

Tincture
1 part fresh buds, freshly peeled bark, or twigs
2 parts menstruum (90% alcohol, 10% distilled water)
Take 10–20 drops 3 times a day.

Oil
Infuse with fresh buds or twigs.

balsamroot

Balsamorhiza sagittata
arrow-leaf balsamroot
PARTS USED roots, leaves, flowers

If balsamroot dwells in your area, you may be familiar with the late spring
sight of hills lighting up in yellow. This is the prime time to gather the resinous root.

How to identify
Flowers of balsamroot are bright yellow and have the characteristic formation of the Asteraceae—ray flowers radiating from the central disc flowers. Balsamroot leaves are a silvery green, and their undersides are even lighter in color. The leaves stand out against the arid landscapes balsamroot likes to inhabit. The arrowhead-shaped leaves grow densely from the large taproot. Roots are thick, resinous, and corky-looking.

Where, when, and how to wildcraft
Find balsamroot on rocky, dry, exposed hillsides at middle elevations, between 5000 and 9000 feet. Gather the taproot before or while the plant is flowering. This is when the roots are most resinous and aromatic, best

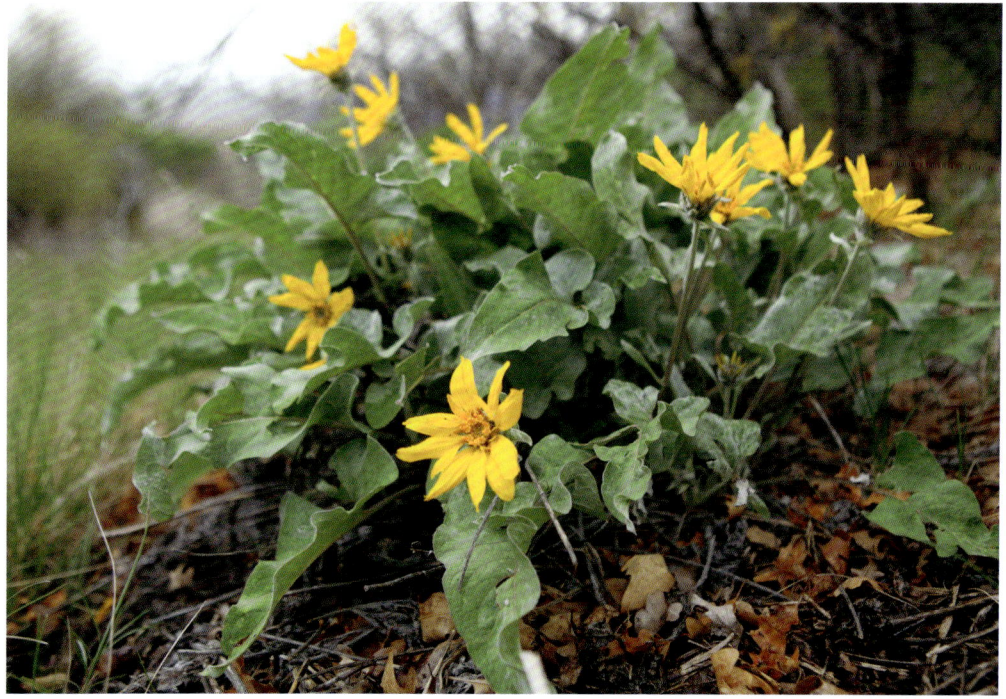

The perfect time to harvest the root is while the flowers of balsamroot are vibrantly blooming.

for fresh plant tincturing. Gathering after the plant dies back tends to yield a dried-up root that lacks some aromatics but still holds viable medicine.

To unearth balsamroot, try using a shovel, as a digging trowel may not be sufficient. Loosen the dirt by digging in a circle around the plant. Roots clean up well, as they are generally in drier soil that will crumble off while washing. The late summer roots can be chopped up and dried for use in decoctions, or try keeping a piece in your mouth, sucking it like a lozenge for sore throats or coughs.

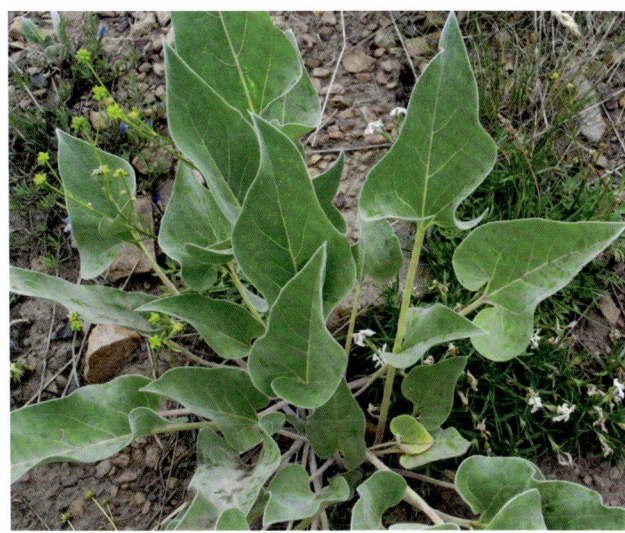

The leaves of *Balsamorhiza sagittata* are shaped like an arrowhead.

Medicinal uses

The aromatics of the roots and flowers can be distilled into essential oil. Flowers and leaves of balsamroot can be infused in oils for chest rubs. Dried or fresh roots, which assist in loosening stuck mucus, can be infused into honey and taken for coughs, colds, and other ills of winter. Balsamroot honey has a warming quality to it and can be a great addition to tea when feeling feverish. The dried roots can be used as a smudge.

Caution

As part of the family Asteraceae, balsamroot should be used with caution if you have a known allergy to the sunflower and its relatives.

Future harvest

Balsamroot is a hardy plant that takes harvesting well and regrows from roots left behind in the ground. Nevertheless, please be light-handed with your harvesting.

HERBAL PREPARATIONS

Tea
Hot infusion
3 tablespoons fresh or dried leaves and
    flowers
1 cup water
Decoction
3 tablespoons fresh or dried root
1 quart water
Drink 1–2 cups 3 times a day.

Tincture
1 part fresh root; try adding leaves and
    flowers
2 parts menstruum (75% alcohol, 25%
    distilled water)
or
1 part dried root, leaves, or flowers
5 parts menstruum (60% alcohol, 40%
    distilled water)
Take 20–40 drops 3 times a day.

Oil
*Infuse with fresh or dried flowers, leaves,
or root.*

beebalm

Monarda species
wild bergamot, oregano de la Sierra, mountain monarda, sweet leaf
PARTS USED leaves, flowers

Beebalm's firework flowers match its spicy and stimulating medicine in intensity.

How to identify

Beebalm is a mint-family plant with a square stem and highly aromatic, opposite leaves. Flowers radiate in clusters from the central stem and vary in color by species. Blooms of *Monarda fistulosa* are rose-pink or slightly purple; those of *M. pectinata* (pony beebalm) are sometimes white or pink. The lanceolate leaves are slightly toothed and have a soft fuzzy feel from tiny hairs.

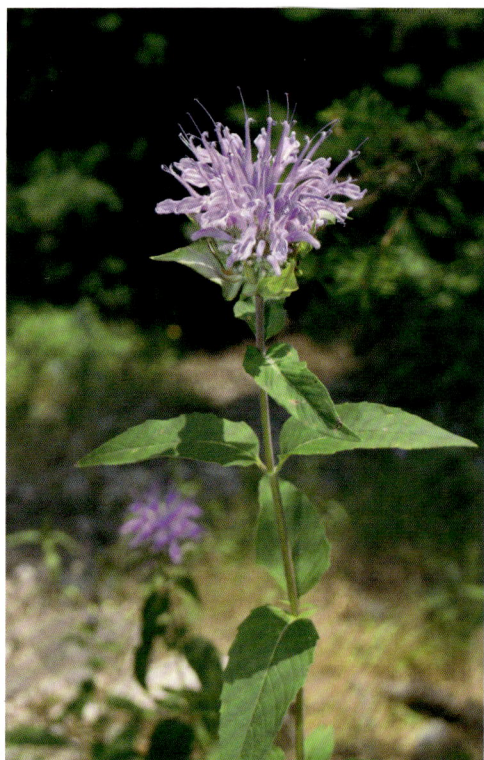

Harvest when the flowers are laden with aromatics and vibrant in color.

Where, when, and how to wildcraft

Beebalm is generally not found higher than 8500 feet. It dwells in colonies, so you rarely see a single plant. It grows predominantly throughout the eastern foothills of the Rockies in sunny meadows and canyon bottoms, near dry or running creek beds.

In early spring the young leaves can be gathered for medicinal uses. In midsummer you will find plants in full blossom and highly aromatic. The heat of the sun makes the aromatic oils more potent, making this the best time to gather. Gather leaves and flowers from various plants or, if you are in a large enough stand, cut the top portion of the plant, which yields an ample amount of leaves and flowers.

Medicinal uses

Beebalm is a warming, aromatic herb with flavors of lemon and oregano. As a tea it can be very strong and spicy if steeped for too long. Try infusing honey with the fresh flowers and leaves.

Beebalm's medicine as tea or tincture helps push fevers outward, bringing the heat to the surface of the body; be prepared to break into a sweat. It can be very stimulating

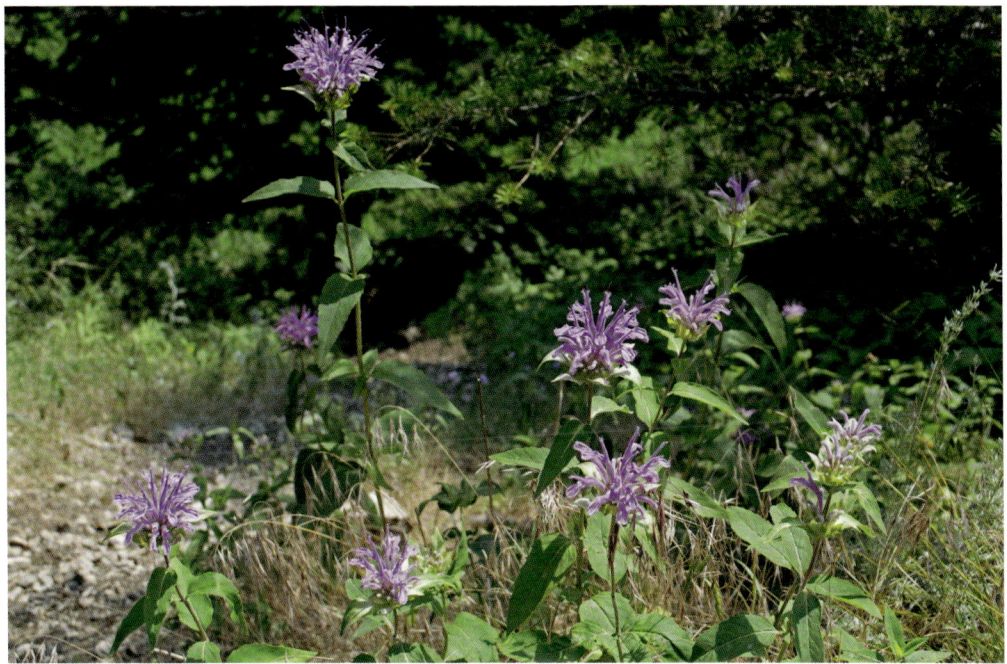

Clip the stalks that are abundant in leaves, and always leave some flowerheads behind for spreading seeds.

due to its spicy aromatics; this can be helpful in dispersing the action of other herbs throughout the body. Whatever the mix, it can be a powerful addition, bringing warm circulation to an area and acting as an antifungal or antimicrobial agent. It presents itself well in combination with garlic, cottonwood buds, and mullein flowers for a superb ear oil, suitable for children. In topical oil-based preparations, like salves, it can relieve fungal infections.

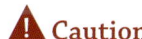 Caution

Do not use in pregnancy.

Future harvest

Beebalm does not grow densely throughout the mountain west; only in certain places does it really take off. Be gentle with your gathering if you are not in an area where it is common.

HERBAL PREPARATIONS

Tea
Hot infusion
1–2 tablespoons fresh or dried leaves and
    flowers
1 cup water
Drink 1 cup 3 times a day.

Tincture
1 part freshly chopped leaves and flowers
2 parts menstruum (75% alcohol, 25%
    distilled water)
or
1 part dried leaves and flowers
4 parts menstruum (60% alcohol, 40%
    distilled water)
Take 10–20 drops 3 times a day.

Oil
Infuse with fresh or dried leaves and flowers.

Bistorta bistortoides
knotweed, smartweed, smokeweed
PARTS USED roots

The root of bistort can be dug for first-aid applications while out in the wilderness, or for easing digestive troubles closer to home.

How to identify

Bistort is in the buckwheat family (Polygonaceae). Flowers, mostly white but sometimes light pink, cluster together in a cylindrical spike. Bistort can be so common in alpine meadows that it can look like a soft blanket of snow in midsummer. It grows about a foot taller than most other tundra plants, making it easy to spot. Most leaves are basal; only a few are carried on the jointed stalk. Leaves are elliptic, oblong, or lanceolate, and alternate. Roots of bistort are small but dense with tiny thread-like rootlets coming off the sides.

Where, when, and how to wildcraft

Bistort can be found blooming in high alpine meadows, above treeline or below, in late summer. It prefers the moist climate created by clouds that linger over the mountains. The roots can be dug while the plant is easy to identify but are best toward the end of its life cycle in fall; note where you find the flowers and return later, if you can.

Dig up the root, ensuring you are not decimating one area, and spread out your harvest. Chop up roots, dry them, and grind them into powder before storage.

Medicinal uses

Bistort is a strongly astringent plant. Simmer the roots in decoctions used for external wound washes. Internally, a small amount of tea or a dropperful of tincture has potential to bring relief to issues that need a dose of astringency, such as leaky gut or diarrhea. When used as a mouthwash, it has been said

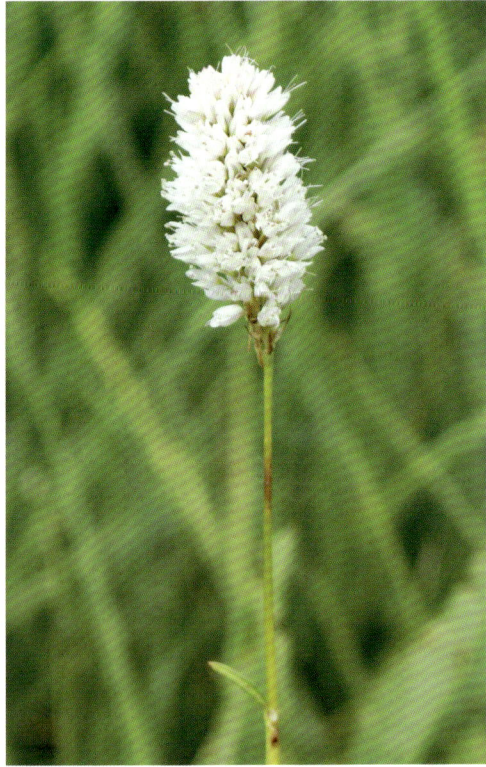

The Dr. Seuss–like puffball flower of *Bistorta bistortoides* dots mountain meadows through to the end of summer.

to alleviate sore throats, canker sores, and tender gums.

Dried bistort root powder is good for weepy or infected wounds. Combine it with other powdered antimicrobial herbs such as yerba mansa, Oregon grape, or osha. You can make a hot poultice by mixing boiled water into the powdered or fresh mashed root. Try adding fresh plantain to the poultice and apply to abscesses or boils.

Caution
Bistort contains tannins, which can be irritating to the stomach if too much is drunk.

Future harvest
Since we are going for a root harvest, be gentle with how you dig for this small plant. Spread your forage out over a vast mountain meadow.

HERBAL PREPARATIONS

Tea
Decoction
1 tablespoon fresh or dried root
1 quart water
Use as an external wash or take small sips.

Tincture
1 part fresh root
2 parts menstruum (75% alcohol, 25% distilled water)
or
1 part dried root
5 parts menstruum (60% alcohol, 40% distilled water)
Take 10–20 drops 3 times a day.

Oil
Infuse with fresh or dried root.

black walnut

Juglans nigra
eastern black walnut
PARTS USED fruit

A rich brown tincture of black walnut is very strong medicine for both internal and external infections. A little bit goes a long way.

How to identify

Black walnut trees have fairly straight trunks with deeply furrowed bark varying from light to dark gray. Alternate leaves are composed of 15 to 23 leaflets that are pinnately divided, with a single leaflet at the end. The male flowers are long green catkins that droop from the branches in spring. Female flowers form in clusters of two to five at the ends of branches. The female flowers turn into the round green fruits. Leaves and the green hulls of the fruit are highly aromatic and smell of citrus with a hint of pine. In autumn, when the fruits ripen, the hull will soften and turn to a yellow-brown, then finally go black.

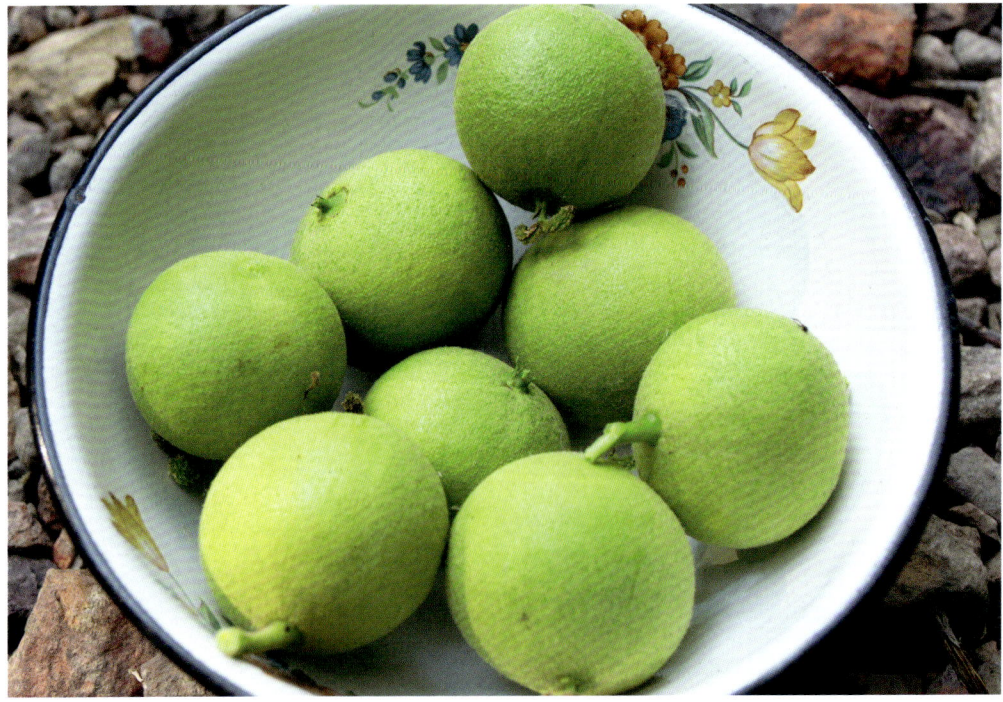

When the green hulls of black walnut are young enough, they can be sliced up and added to oil infusions or alcoholic macerations.

Where, when, and how to wildcraft

Although not native to the mountain west, black walnut is definitely a commonly found tree in cities of lower elevation. Find black walnut trees in fertile soils of farmlands or in neighborhood yards below 6000 feet. It's usually the case that you'll need to ask permission, because the tree is in someone's yard. I have had only positive responses of "What is that tree? It makes a huge mess! Take as much as you'd like." Pluck the young green hulls in midsummer, while they are soft enough to cut into quarters. The browning hulls can be gathered in late summer or early fall, or once fallen and hulls have turned black.

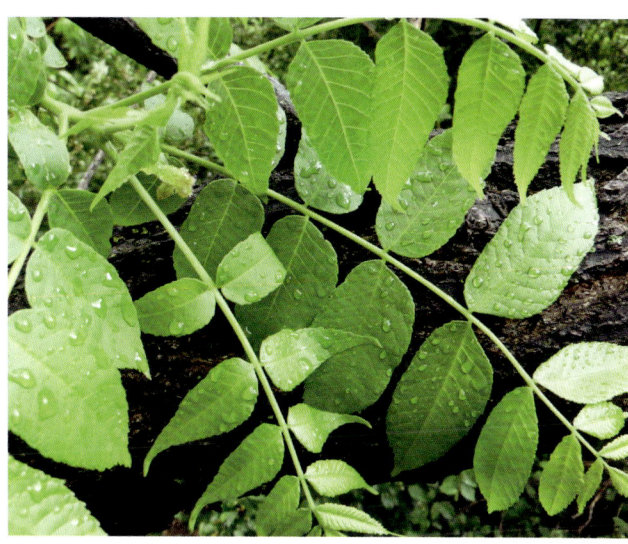

The ever-so-slightly alternate leaves of *Juglans nigra*.

Medicinal uses

Numerous traditional methods of using black walnut call for either all fresh green hulls or freshly fallen hulls that are starting to turn brown. Black walnut has a long-standing history of use as an antiparasitic when taken as a tincture in small doses. Topical applications of infused oil, liniment, or decoction can help to alleviate and clear fungal infections like athlete's foot. An alcoholic extraction in combination with beebalm and Oregon grape can assist quite well in treating bacterial overgrowth, whether used internally or externally. It can be painted on a nursing mother's nipples in the case of thrush, but must be wiped off before an infant begins to nurse again.

Small doses are heavily suggested for black walnut, as larger doses (as in 3 dropsperful 3 times a day) can act as a laxative. A small dose (5–10 drops 3 times a day) can be restorative for the gastrointestinal system, especially if the person is having issues with malabsorption.

⚠ Caution

Do not use in pregnancy or internally while nursing.

Future harvest

Gathering the hulls, fresh or blackened, poses no threat to the survival of black walnut trees.

HERBAL PREPARATIONS

Tea
Sitz bath decoction
2–4 ounces fresh or dried green hulls
1 gallon water

Tincture
1 part fresh green hulls turning brown
2 parts menstruum (80% alcohol, 20% distilled water)
Use small doses, just 5–10 drops no more than 3 times a day.

Oil
Infuse with fresh green hulls.

Mertensia species
mountain bluebells, chiming bluebells
PARTS USED leaves, flowers

With properties quite similar to but milder than those of comfrey,
bluebells finds its way into many of my skincare formulas.

How to identify

A variety of bluebells is commonly found throughout the mountain west. Plants can be dwarfed in size and scattered through mountain meadows or quite tall and growing in large bountiful stands. Leaves are ovate to lanceolate, and either hairy or smooth. They can be noticeably veined and grow alternately up the flowering stalk. Nodding light pink, purple, or blue tubular flowers blossom in branched clusters.

Where, when, and how to wildcraft

Many blooming bluebells can be found spread through fields or in tall stands, on the edges of forest floors, mountain meadows, and alpine streams, soaking up the spring moisture from rain showers and snowmelt runoffs. Gather the leaves and flowers from spring to summer when they are young and vibrant. I like to utilize the top leaves and flower blossoms.

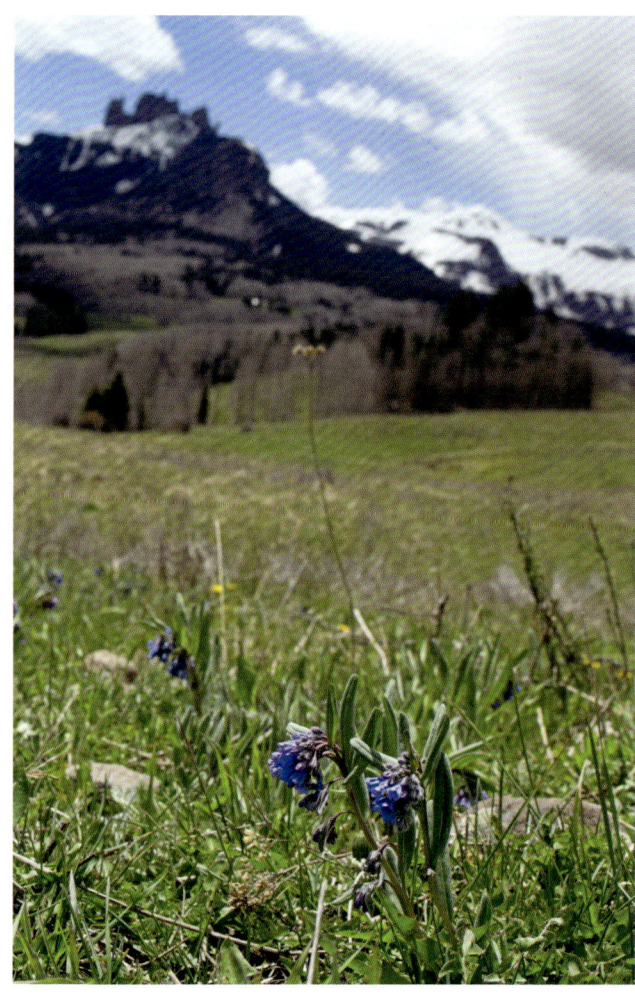

Gathering bluebells high in the mountains can lead you to the most breathtaking places.

Pluck flowering tops here and there, never decimating one area of growth.

Medicinal uses

I use bluebells in my skin-healing formulas as I would comfrey: in face serums and salves, in oil blends, or as a liniment. As a face serum, bluebells helps to treat the dry, wind-scoured face of the mountain woman. It blends well with Saint John's wort (*Hypericum* species),

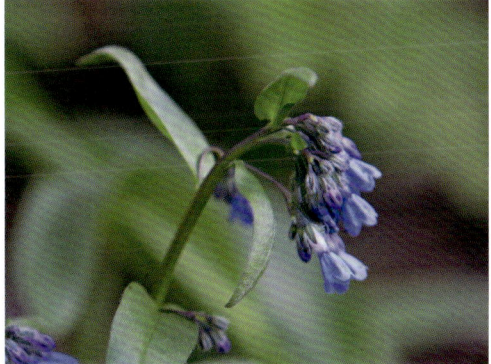

The bell-shaped flowers of *Mertensia* species can vary from light pink to shades of purple and blue.

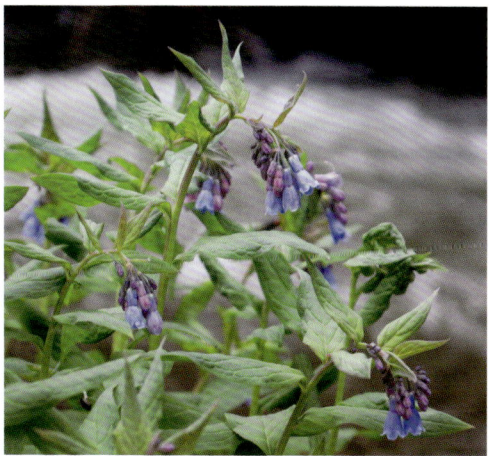

The flowers of *Mertensia ciliata*, the largest of our local bluebells, bear a distinct resemblance to those of its relative, comfrey (*Symphytum officinale*).

gumweed (*Grindelia* species), and cottonwood buds (*Populus* species) for an easing salve that soothes skin irritations and discomforts. As an oil, soak, or liniment it can be a great healing agent for seriously sprained or broken bones. A tea can be drunk to soothe coughing fits; use only while sick.

Caution

All species of bluebells contain small amounts of alkaloids, but this is not a problem if you are only using preparations for topical applications. Avoid drinking too much tea on a regular basis. Bluebells is considered a safe plant to eat.

Future harvest

Although abundant where they grow, graze these native plants with care. There is no need to uproot the plant or cut down a whole stand. Pick a few leaves and flowers from each plant.

HERBAL PREPARATIONS

Tea
Hot infusion
3 tablespoons fresh or dried leaves and
    flowers
1 cup water
Drink 1 cup per day.

Tincture
1 part fresh leaves and flowers
2 parts menstruum (75% alcohol, 25%
    distilled water)
or
1 part dried leaves and flowers
5 parts menstruum (60% alcohol, 40%
    distilled water)
Take 10–20 drops 3 times a day.

Oil
Infuse with fresh or dried leaves and flowers.

blueberry

Vaccinium species
bilberry, huckleberry, whortleberry
PARTS USED leaves, fruit

People are surprised by the blueberries that grow here in the mountains, expecting the bushes to be much larger than the short, often-missed groundcover of our hills.

How to identify

These shrubs can be tiny, as shrubs go, standing not more than a few feet from the ground and usually sprawling along a hillside or sparse forest. Leaves grow alternately along a woody stem. The flowers, shaped like a bell, are usually whitish pink, and they have an inferior ovary that swells into a purple, red, or blue berry. At the tip of the berries is a star-like mark from the sepal, where the flower once was.

Where, when, and how to wildcraft

Berries begin to ripen in July, depending on your elevation and location, and harvesting can last until late August. Vacciniums like to grow in acidic soils, so you will find them in or near conifer forests. Blueberries can feel elusive in some parts of the mountain west. Usually this is because you have not visited the right place or you forgot to look low enough. Blueberries can be found in Colorado, Wyoming, western Utah, and rarely Nevada. They are primarily found in the Pacific Northwest, Alberta, Idaho, and western Montana. Montana even has a huckleberry industry—everything from milkshakes to preserves.

Down on hands and knees may be the easiest way to get acquainted with blueberries. The berries may be abundant, and you

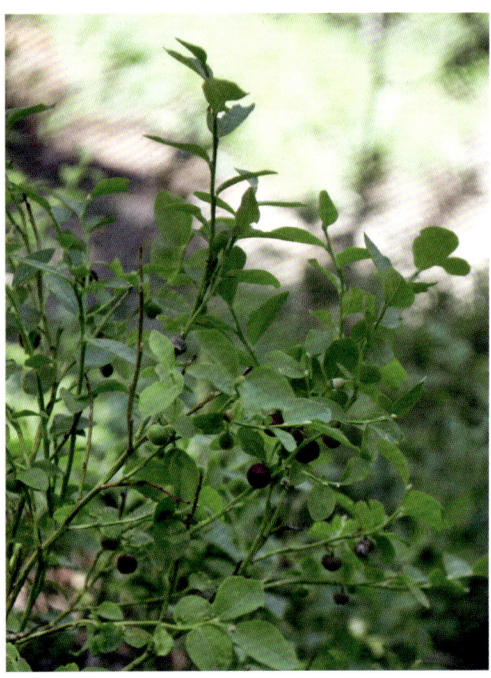

Taste your leaves for vibrancy and flavor before harvesting from a stand of blueberries—the aspect they face on a mountain and the soil they dwell in matter.

would not even know it just looking from above. When the shrubs are loaded with ripe berries, you can sweep your hand through the plant and comb out the fruits. These morsels are small and take dedicated time to harvest in quantity. Berries can be dried or frozen fresh.

Freezing Berries

To get the most out of your berry harvest, you must gather enough to freeze. There is a trick to freezing berries; it's not just a matter of tossing a bag of fruit in the freezer. First, place the berries on a tray lined with parchment paper, spreading them out so they are not touching one another. Freeze berries on the tray. Once they are frozen, place berries in a bag or container. By separating them first, you are now able to grab a handful of berries and do not have to saw into a massive brick of frozen fruit. Many berries, such as chokecherries and elderberries, can be frozen while still on the stem. This makes removing the berries from the stem a lot easier, and keeps berries whole rather than smooshing them while fresh. Use the smooshed fresh ones to make a new batch of tincture or honey.

When gathering a harvest of blueberry leaves, clip the stems while in flower when the leaves are vibrant green. Dry the leaves on the stem, and then garble them off.

Medicinal uses

The leaves and fruit of *Vaccinium* species are slightly astringent. Both leaf and berry together are beneficial in soothing and combating a urinary tract infection, acting as an antiseptic and diuretic. There is some compelling evidence that the leaves of *Vaccinium* species can help to lower blood sugar.

The fruit is high in antioxidants and, when from the wild, carries the most scrumptious flavor in the mountains. Use it for flavoring cordials, elixirs, tinctures, honeys, syrups, and vinegars, and dry, for tea blends. The nourishing berry helps to strengthen and heal the eyes when there is poor vision or common eye irritations. It has an affinity to the circulatory system, improving circulation, toning the blood vessels, and protecting them from disease.

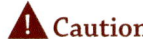 Caution

Extended long-term use of the leaves has been shown to cause gastric upset.

Future harvest

Be conscious of the fact that many critters, big and small, rely on berries for food. I am sure blueberry is a favorite with bears and grouse. Enjoy what you like, but leave some berries behind. Do not take whole plants, ever. Please be mindful that some species are rare and threatened.

HERBAL PREPARATIONS

Tea
Hot infusion
1 ounce fresh or dried leaves
1 quart water
or
1-3 tablespoons fresh or dried berries
1 cup water
Drink 3 times a day.

Tincture
1 part fresh leaves or berries
2 parts menstruum (75% alcohol, 25% distilled water)
or
1 part dried leaves or berries
5 parts menstruum (60% alcohol, 40% distilled water)
Take 30–60 drops 3 times a day.

burdock

Arctium species

gobō

PARTS USED roots, leaves, seeds

Burdock supports the skin and liver incredibly well. It can be used externally or internally, and even ranks as a vegetable foodstuff, raw or cooked.

How to identify

Big, soft, basal leaves mark the first year of this hardy biennial. Leaves are bright green on top, lighter in color on the underside, and are covered in velvety fuzz. The basal rosette of leaves can grow to about 18 inches across. Second-year plants send up large, leafy flowering stalks. The thistle-ish flowers are a magenta puff of disc-shaped florets surrounded by spiky green bracts. These hooked bracts are what turn into the brown clinging seedpods, or burrs, which host a few hundred seeds each. Burdock roots grow deep, averaging depths of around 2 feet; brown outer flesh, which can hold a lot of dirt, covers the dense, creamy white interior.

Where, when, and how to wildcraft

Burdock can be found throughout the mountain west, mostly growing where humans have settled, near ranches, farms, or old homesteads. Being a lover of disturbed soils, this biennial frequents places where soil is not compacted, such as a tilled garden or worked-over farmland. Roots should be gathered in the fall of the first year or while the plant puts forth its young shoots the following spring, but before the plant puts up a flowering stalk. Gather the seeds after the plant has died back and the flowers have lost the last of their purple pigment.

The taproot of burdock can grow enormously deep. I have to admit, I am rarely able to get the entire root out of the ground when harvesting. I like to grow burdock in the garden, which gives me the advantage of prepping the soil, keeping it sort of loose, so the root will be easier to harvest come fall. If the brown outer flesh of the root is caked with too much dirt, even after a good rinse, simply peel it off with a peeler or knife.

The brown burr heads of burdock can be collected by the handful, as they cling

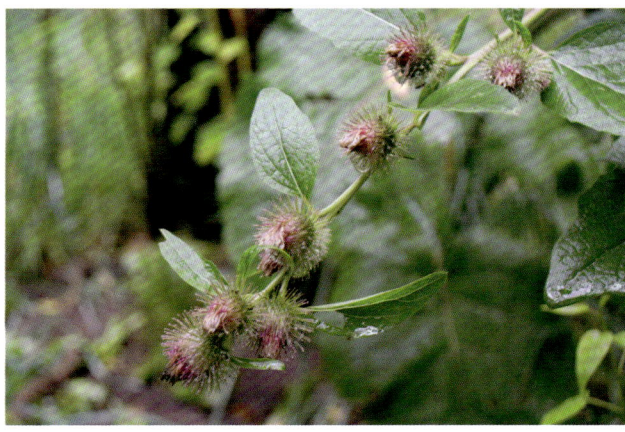

The burrs can be picked as the flowers of burdock are starting to brown.

together in clumps. Lay the clump on a flat surface and use a rolling pin to gently break the seedheads apart, separating out the chaff. Take small amounts between your fingertips and winnow the chaff away above a bowl, letting the seeds drop in.

Medicinal uses

Burdock is one of the weedy food-like medicines we have abundantly in the mountain west. The roots may be a pain to dig, and the seeds a hassle to get out of the prickly chaff, but burdock is worth getting to know as an alterative and blood purifier. Burdock always makes it into my stocks and broths along with dandelion, seaweed, and medicinal mushrooms like reishi and shiitake, giving that extra support to my system.

Burdock root helps treat the skin when eruptions are happening, used internally as a tincture along with Oregon grape, dandelion, or milk thistle. Being an alterative it helps the liver process toxins more efficiently and can help to alleviate acne due to hormonal imbalance. It works well against chronic psoriasis or eczema, taken internally or used externally in oils, salves, or baths. Try an acne serum by combining the infused oil of burdock leaves and roots along with plantain.

The seeds can be decocted or tinctured and used as a diuretic for water retention or supporting kidney function.

⚠ Caution

Steer clear if you have a known allergy to plants of the sunflower family (Asteraceae). An allergy may show as itchiness or stomach irritation. Sometimes the use of burdock to ease skin conditions such as acne and eczema can worsen the ailment before it makes it better. Avoid burdock if you are taking prescription medications that metabolize through the liver.

Future harvest

There is little to no concern in harvesting *Arctium* species in the mountain west. In some places burdock is not so common, but growing it in the garden is quite easy: taking seeds from a plant and spreading them in tilled soil should do the trick.

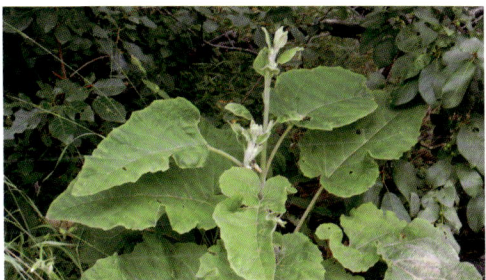

Dig *Arctium* species before they get to this near-flowering stage. Instead, try to collect it in its first year's spring or fall, or in the spring of the second year before it has flowered.

HERBAL PREPARATIONS

Tea
Hot or cold infusion
1–3 teaspoons fresh or dried root
1 cup water
Decoction
1 ounce fresh or dried root or seeds
1 quart water
Drink 1–2 cups 3 times a day.

Tincture
1 part fresh root
2 parts menstruum (80% alcohol, 20% distilled water)
or
1 part dried root or seeds
5 parts menstruum (60% alcohol, 40% distilled water)
Take 20–40 drops 3 times a day.

Oil
Infuse with fresh or dried root and leaves.

Nepeta cataria

PARTS USED leaves, stems, flowers

Catnip drives some felines mad with passion. But for us? It calms the mind and dampens the fluttering butterflies of a nervous or upset stomach.

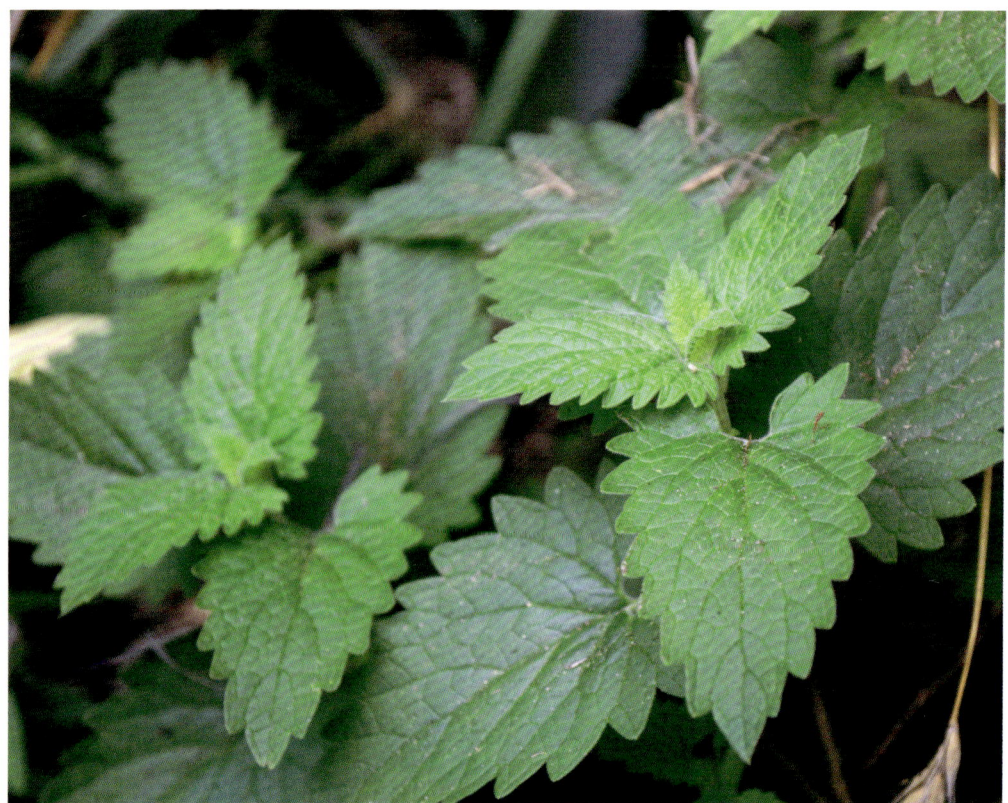

The young leaves of catnip can be gathered for tea- or tincture-making.

How to identify

Crunch the leaves of catnip and inhale the smell that makes cats wild. It has a minty, almost musty, sweet odor. The leaves are soft to the touch with tiny little hairs that cover the entire plant. Leaves are serrated around the margins and triangular in shape. Being in the mint family, catnip has a square stem and opposite leaves. Flowers are white and pink with purple highlights. The two-lipped flowers grow in spike-like terminal clusters.

Where, when, and how to wildcraft

Find catnip growing in disturbed areas, like alleyways, parks, or unkempt landscaping. Start harvesting the leaves in the spring and continue while the plant is flowering through late summer.

Medicinal uses

This is a calming herb suitable for the youngest beings, especially when dealing with the tremendously painful experience of teething; when a bout of a feverish virus makes them uncomfortable; or when restlessness or being too wound up has them staying up late. Catnip has a soft yet very effective sedative quality, making it a wonderful addition to sleepytime formulas.

Catnip also supports adults and adolescents quite well, providing relief in the face of intense social situations. A cup of the tea can help you relax after you've had to be around a bunch of people. If there is a problem in life that is giving you butterflies in the stomach, catnip can be your little assistant, calming the intensity of the anxiety.

Catnip also works on a deeper tissue level, giving the musculoskeletal system a wave of tension release. This can be from spasms or cramping anywhere in the body, including gastrointestinal issues, menstrual cramps, a disruptive spastic cough, or a kink in the neck. It can be used as an oil, tincture, or tea for these maladies.

Used with bitters or indigestion formulations, it can help to dispel hiccups, or gas, when combined with a carminative herb such as wild caraway or fresh sweet root seeds.

Along with other vitamins and minerals, catnip has a fair amount of potassium, which adds to its beneficial effects during and after experiencing fevers.

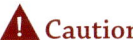 **Caution**

It is advised to do without catnip in a delicate pregnancy, as it can slightly increase uterine stimulation.

Future harvest

As with many mints, catnip grows on its own terms and will often respond to harvesting with increased growth. That being said, don't kill the plant for harvest. Gently take from it and let it continue growing with wild abandon.

HERBAL PREPARATIONS

Tea
Hot infusion
1–3 tablespoons fresh or dried leaves, flowers, and stems
1 cup water
Drink as needed.

Tincture
1 part fresh leaves, flowers, and stems
2 parts menstruum (75% alcohol, 25% distilled water)
or
1 part dried leaves, flowers, and stems
5 parts menstruum (60% alcohol, 40% distilled water)
Take 30–60 drops 3 times a day.

Oil
Infuse with fresh or dried leaves, flowers, and stems.

chaparral

Larrea tridentata
creosote bush, greasewood
PARTS USED leaves

When the rains come, pouring down onto the desert, a fragrant mix of artemisias fills the air. But soaring above even their potent scents is the distinctive aroma of chaparral.

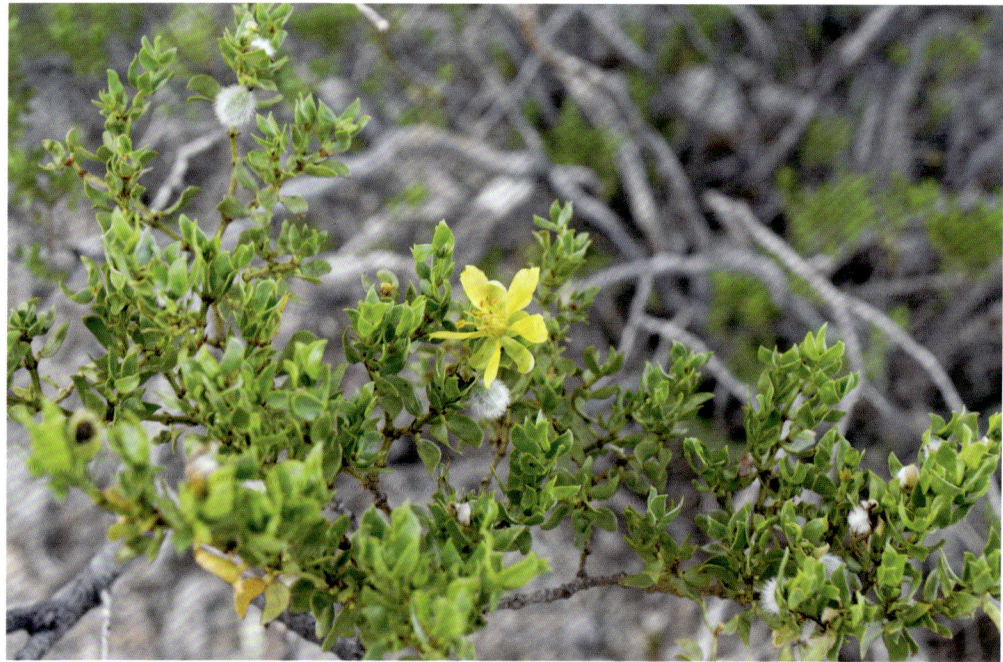

Fuzzy pods, a yellow flower, and the many little strangely aromatic leaves of chaparral.

How to identify

Chaparral is a woody shrub that grows in the desert west. It has star-shaped yellow flowers that bloom from early spring until late summer and that tend to be more abundant during wet years. The seeds are fuzzy round pods. The leaves are small, curled, resinous, and shiny green. Green branches are held upright, giving the plant its bushy appearance.

Where, when, and how to wildcraft

Chaparral is an herb that does not grow in the northern Rockies states, but I use it often enough to drive south or west to find it. Chaparral can be found growing in the southwestern corner of Utah and the southern half of Nevada. Discover it growing in the desert as a shrubby tree—when you find it inhabiting an area, you will find plenty of it. The leaves are the sought-after part, and you can simply walk around pruning little branches off numerous different plants. Tincture or infused oil can be made from the fresh leaves, or dry the whole twigs and crumble the leaves off later.

Medicinal uses

Chaparral is very important in the healing traditions of the desert west. As a first-aid herb, it is antimicrobial and is best used as tincture or oil.

When applied topically as an oil, chaparral is very beneficial at treating fungal itchiness, eczema, and psoriasis. It also has the ability to combat viruses such as herpes and HPV and so can be a useful component in treatments (including soaks or washes) for cold sores and genital warts.

In small doses, such as 5 drops of tincture several times a day, chaparral can work with inflammation associated with imbalance of the flora in the intestinal tract. It has the most unique intensely bitter taste, which is hard to take down as a tea, and as a tincture I always prefer to mix it in water. It retains its ability to combat herpes and HPV when taken internally.

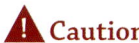 **Caution**

Not for use while pregnant or nursing. Prolonged use of chaparral has resulted in hepatotoxicity in several reported case studies.

Future harvest

Be sure to prune the shrubs with clippers rather than breaking off whole branches; this will prevent weakening of the plant.

HERBAL PREPARATIONS

Tea
Sitz bath infusion
3 ounces fresh or dried leaves
1 gallon water

Tincture
1 part fresh leaves
2 parts menstruum (75% alcohol, 25% distilled water)
or
1 part dried leaves
2 parts menstruum (60% alcohol, 40% distilled water)
Take 5–10 drops 3 times a day.

Oil
Infuse with fresh or dried leaves.

---

chickweed

Stellaria species
PARTS USED leaves, stems, flowers

Like so many medicinal herbs, this voracious little weed,
chock-full of nutrients, is most vital and vibrant when used fresh.

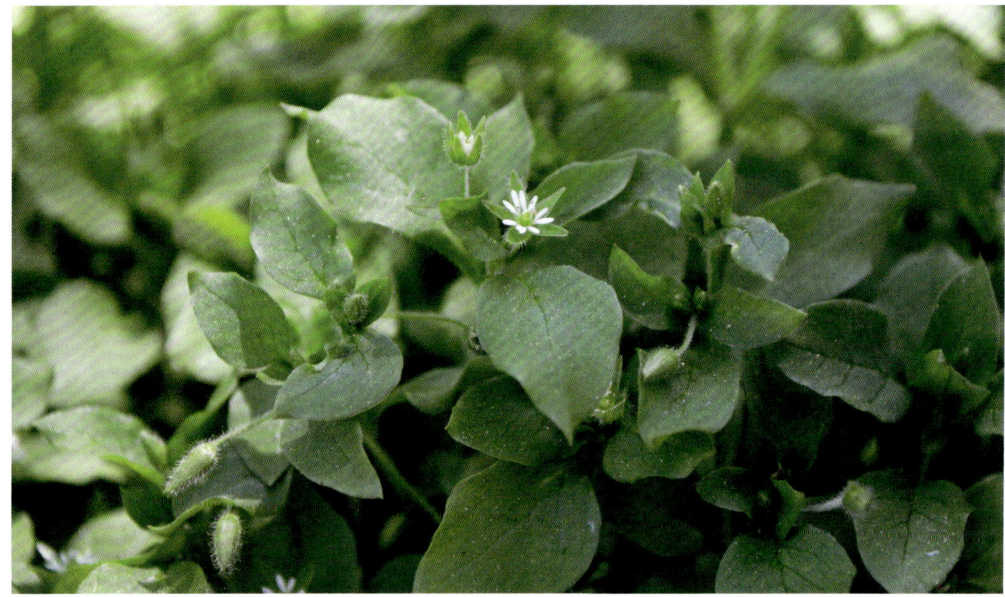

Harvest chickweed while it is bright green in the late spring or early summer, or you can wait for it to shoot up again with the cooler temperatures of autumn.

How to identify

Chickweed has small white flowers and opposite, succulent leaves, but the line of fine hairs along the central stem is what distinguishes chickweed from other similar-looking plants. Plants trail low, their stems forming branched mats that root back to the ground. Flowers, singly or in a small cluster, are carried on the tip of each stem. At first glance, flowers may look like they have ten petals, but there are only five—each petal has a very deep indentation.

Where, when, and how to wildcraft

Chickweed prefers a cool climate, particularly flourishing in spring and sometimes fall, which keeps it vibrant and crisp for harvesting. Find it growing in the shaded corners of yards, disturbed soils, and sheltered, somewhat moist areas. Come the heat of the summer, as the plant dies back after flowering, it will wither or become dry and stout. Otherwise, this little weed is harvestable almost all year long. It seems to just keep growing, providing new shoots in late fall and possibly even in the winter under conifers or if the snow on a south-facing aspect is melted. Chickweed is best gathered just before or right as it flowers in spring.

This plant will rarely be found alone. It grows in patches, making it easy to harvest. The whole plant is edible and provides medicinal nourishment. Try to snap off only the top few inches, but it is okay if you accidentally pull up the whole plant—it's easy to do. Rinse your harvest well, removing any dirt, and lay it on a towel. Roll the damp chickweed up in the towel and place it in the refrigerator for a few days to a week. Or, dry the aerial portions of the plant on drying racks.

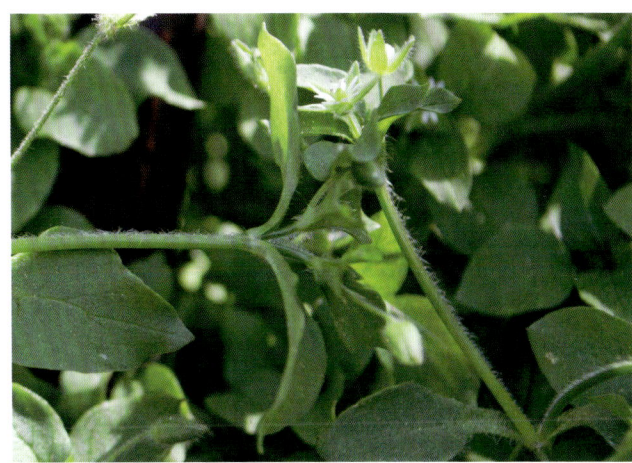

A key identifying characteristic of common chickweed (*Stellaria media*) is the line of hairs that grows up the stem.

Medicinal uses

Chickweed is a cooling herb that can bring relief to warm and irritated skin conditions. It works well on sunburns, rashes, and bug bites. The leaves, stems, and flowers can be used to create oils and salves for healing wounds and rubbing on insect stings or nips. A poultice or an infusion can be made for washing and treating skin irritations.

Because of the high mineral and nutrient content in chickweed, it is a great herb to infuse in vinegar in order to get out all the goodness it has to offer. A hot infusion of fresh chickweed is ideal, but the stored dried herb can be used too, though it may lose some of its vitality. Blend chickweed with other freshly harvested spring clippings. Try juicing your chickweed greens or adding them to smoothies for a nutritional boost.

Future harvest

Chickweed is a delicate little plant that has a huge determination to live. You won't impact it by harvesting it in quantities.

HERBAL PREPARATIONS

Tea
Hot infusion
1-3 tablespoons fresh or dried leaves, stems, and flowers
1 cup water
Drink 1-3 times a day.

Vinegar
1 part fresh leaves, stems, and flowers
2 parts vinegar
Take 1 tablespoon 1-3 times a day.

Oil
Infuse with fresh or dried leaves, stems, and flowers.

chicory

Cichorium intybus

PARTS USED roots, flowers

Roasted roots of chicory are bitter in a way reminiscent of coffee,
making it a robust herb to add to decoctions when a rich flavor is desired.

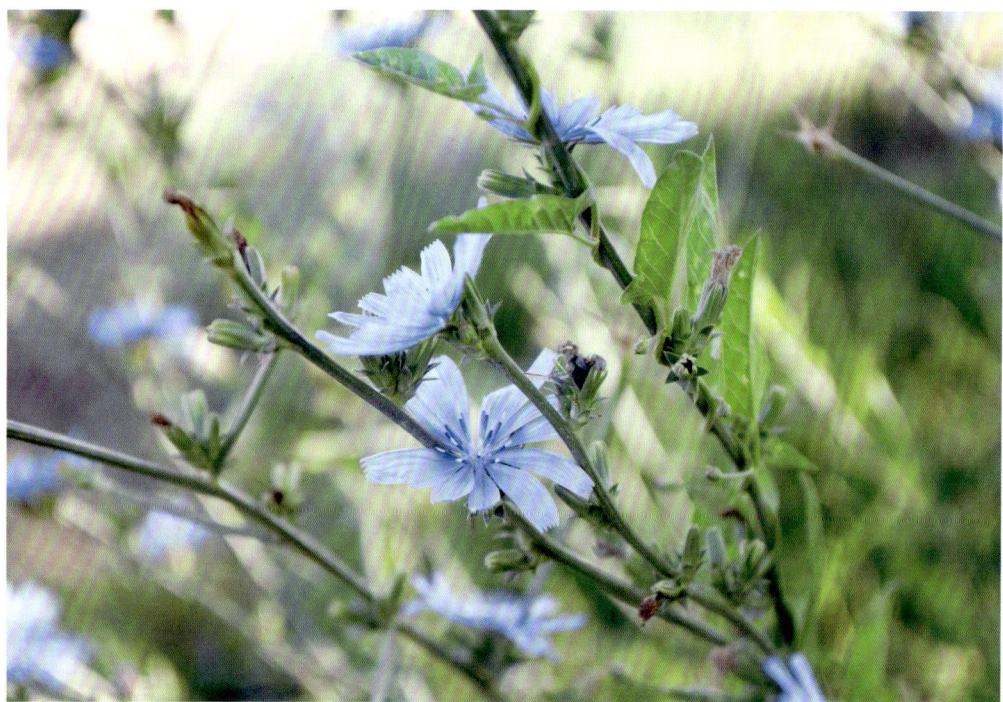

Each chicory flower blooms for only a day.

How to identify

The blue flowers of chicory dot the shoulders of dirt roads and highways all over the mountain west. Each flower blooms for only one day. Chicory is biennial, meaning it lives for two years, producing only the rosette of basal leaves the first year and flowers in its second year. Chicory can reach heights of 5 feet and has a scraggly look with its somewhat woody, jointed stem. Leaves and flowers grow sporadically along the branched stems. When any part of the plant is broken, it exudes milky sap.

Young basal leaves look similar to dandelion leaves; however, the jagged leaf edges of chicory point both outward and upward, not toward the leaf base like those of dandelions do. Young leaves could also be confused with another edible plant, wild lettuce; however, chicory lacks the prickles on the underside of the central leaf vein.

Where, when, and how to wildcraft

Chicory grows abundantly in some places and is rarely seen in other areas of the west. It likes to grow below 7500 feet and is usually found in the lowlands between mountain ranges, along roadsides or in sunny pastures.

Gather the creamy-colored taproot of first-year chicory plants in the fall and second-year plants in the spring, before they have flowered. Roots are impressively large and take some digging to uncover.

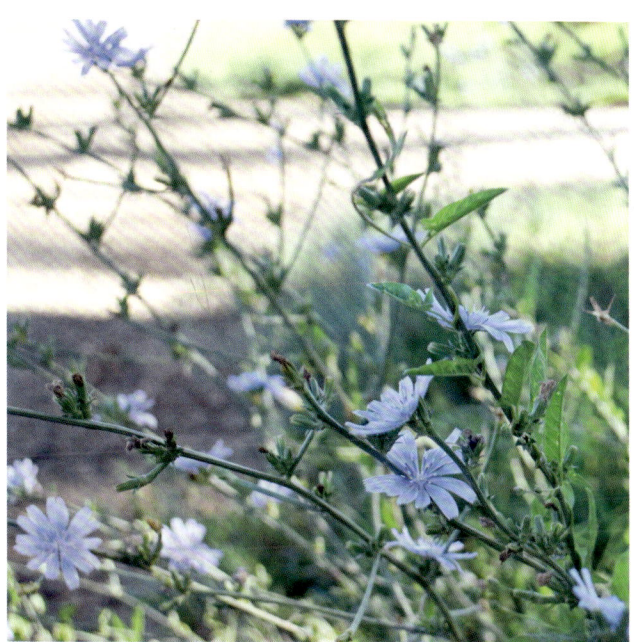

Dry chicory flowers and add them later to your roasted-root tea blend for a little pop of color.

Medicinal uses

The best way to have the bitter roots of chicory is to roast them before decocting, which brings out a flavor reminiscent of coffee. Add a splash of coconut milk or cream and you will have yourself a morning latte that is a gentle diuretic, cleansing to the kidneys and bladder.

A useful alterative root blend is chicory, dandelion, and burdock, which is nourishing to the liver and blood, as well as being hugely tasty. Chicory roots fresh or roasted can be used in bitters tinctures to help aid digestion.

⚠ Caution

Chicory is in the Asteraceae, and some people may have allergic reactions to this plant family.

Future harvest

Chicory reseeds itself quite well, which is why you can find this nonnative plant on noxious weed lists. Feel free to harvest roots at will.

HERBAL PREPARATIONS

Tea
Decoction
1 ounce fresh, roasted, or dried chopped root
1 quart water
Drink 1 cup 3 times a day.

Tincture
1 part fresh root
2 parts menstruum (75% alcohol, 25% distilled water)
or
1 part dried root
5 parts menstruum (60% alcohol, 40% distilled water)
Take 20–40 drops 3 times a day.

cleavers

Galium species
bedstraw
PARTS USED leaves, stems, flowers

*While walking in the woods, snip yourself a bundle
of cleavers—fresh preparations are always the best.*

How to identify

Cleavers is best recognized by the whorled
leaf pattern that runs up the square stem.
The leaves grow in whorls of four to eight
and are oblanceolate in shape. *Galium
boreale*, one of our more common mountain cleavers, has whorls of four. Stems are
leggy and branched; they sprawl across the
ground rather than standing up. Both leaves
and stems have tiny hooked hairs, by which
means the plant is able to creep over other
plants. Flowers are tiny; white, yellow, or
green in color; have four petals; and blossom in late spring. *Galium aparine* has fuzzy,
sticky burrs or seedpods that easily stick to
socks and shoelaces. Other native species
can also be found, usually growing more
sparsely in the mountains, and do not have
the same hairy stickiness.

Where, when, and how to wildcraft

Find vibrant green cleavers on mountainous
forest floors beneath the tall osha and sweet
root. Or locate it in lower-elevation shady
places, near chickweed or violets. The higher
you are in elevation, the later you will be able
to gather fresh leaves. Find it thriving from
spring until late summer—if in the shade.

Almost all parts of cleavers will stick
to you. The plant and the seeds have fine

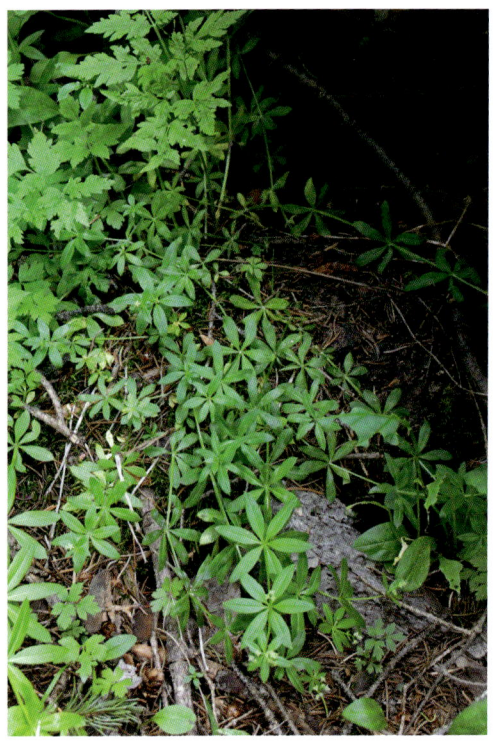

Long strands of cleavers can be found clinging
to the forest floors.

hooked hairs that grab hold of fabric. Cleavers also pulls easily from the ground, which
makes you take more than you really need.
With a pair of scissors, or pincher fingers,
take only the top young whorls from the
plant. If you happen to uproot the entire
plant, it's okay: utilize it all.

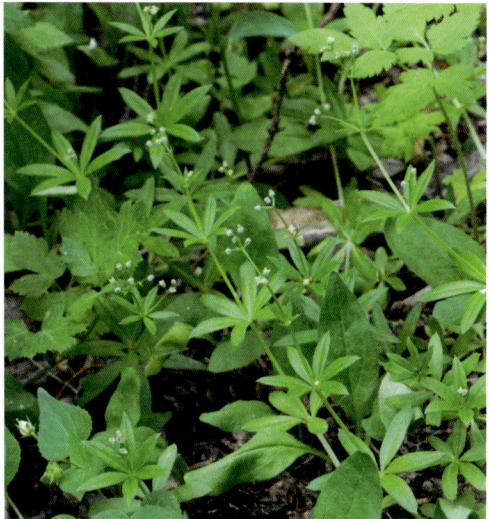

The white flowers of *Galium* turn to clinging burrs which may reveal that you have been to a patch of cleavers without even knowing it.

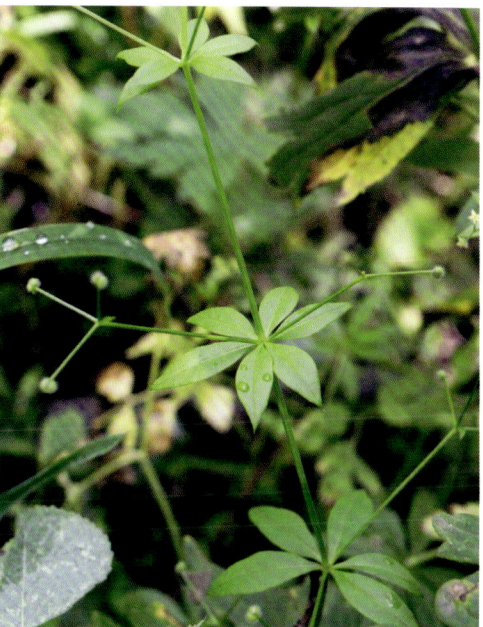

Cleavers provides a perfect example of the whorled leaf pattern.

Medicinal uses

Cleavers is high in nutrients and can be juiced or infused into vinegars, alcohol, water, or even oil. It has cooling energetics and a drying action. It has an affinity for soothing bladder and kidney issues. It is also supportive to the functions of our lymphatic system, helping to relieve swollen glands. Cleavers can be useful in healing internal wounds like ulcers of the mouth or stomach.

Externally, it also has properties that will help with the redness and inflammation of wounds and skin infections such as cysts or boils. Infused into oils, the leaves and stems of cleavers can be beneficial for skin issues like eczema or psoriasis and regenerating the skin.

Future harvest

Cleavers is usually found growing in thick stretches, making it easy to harvest an ample amount of tops without causing a shortage of growth. The clinging burrs are spread easily by passing animals or hikers.

HERBAL PREPARATIONS

Tea
Hot infusion
1 tablespoon fresh or dried leaves, stems, and flowers
1 cup water
Drink as needed.

Tincture
1 part fresh leaves, stems, and flowers
2 parts menstruum (75% alcohol, 25% distilled water)
Take 30–60 drops 3 times a day.

Vinegar
1 part fresh leaves, stems, and flowers
4 parts vinegar
Take 1 tablespoon 1–3 times a day.

Oil
Infuse with fresh or dried leaves, stems, and flowers.

Thelesperma species

Navajo tea, Hopi tea, green thread

PARTS USED leaves, stems, flowers

Tie up the stems and flowers of cota while basking in the desert sun.
There is something purely medicinal about just touching plants.

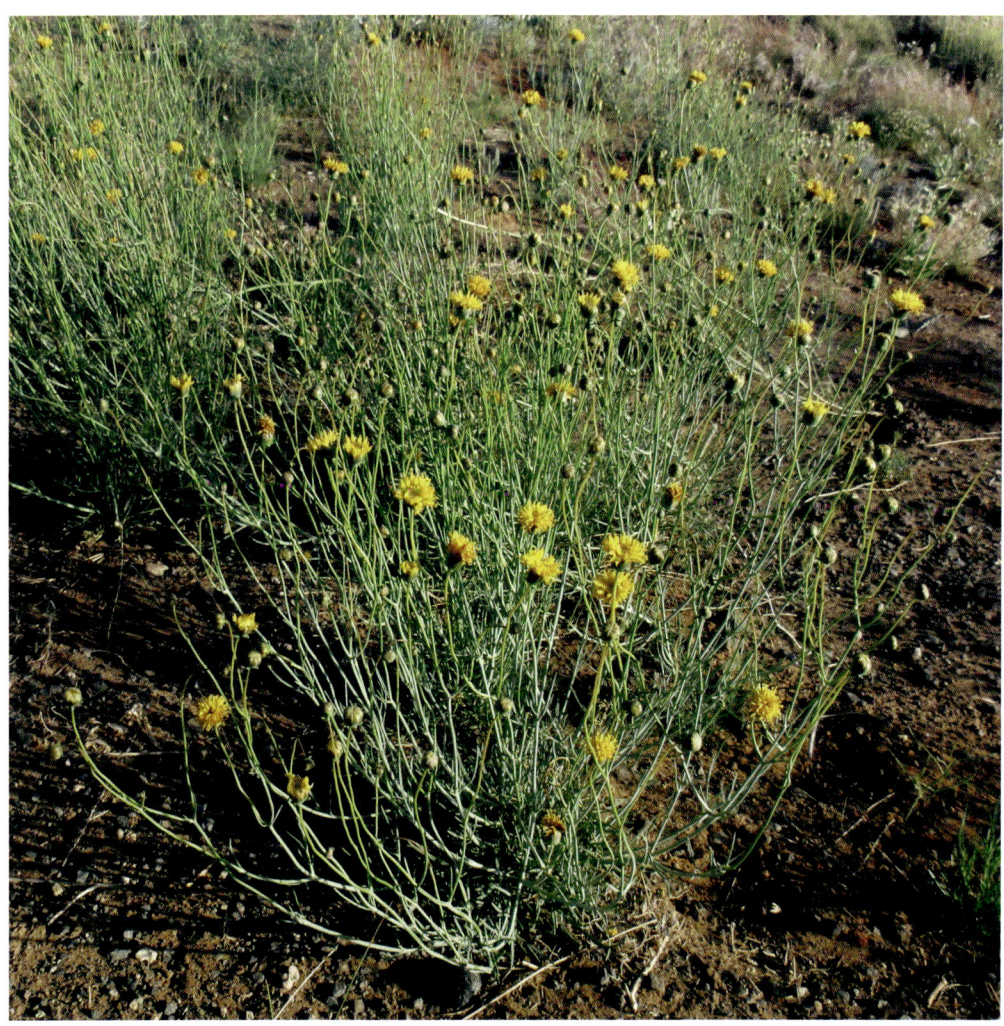

The thin, thread-like stems of cota can be snipped at the base and dried along with the entire plant, for a refreshing infusion.

How to identify

Slender green stems arise from a small beige taproot. The entire plant has a glaucous coating, which makes it look somewhat blue-green. Thin, thread-like leaves grow from the base and sporadically along the stem. There may be a dozen stems or a single stem growing from the root, but only one flower sits atop each stalk. Flowers are yellow; some species, for example, *Thelesperma filifolium*, have both ray and disc flowers, while others such as *T. megapotamicum* have only disc flowers.

Where, when, and how to wildcraft

Cota is found in Colorado and Utah—primarily in the Four Corners area—Nevada, Wyoming, and in parts of Montana. Plants inhabit dry soils or open meadows at elevations between 3500 and 8000 feet.

Gather the stems, complete with leaves, as the flowerbuds are beginning to blossom, and when the plant is most fragrant. The stems and flowers make a beautiful bundle for tea. Cut stems about 3 inches above the ground. Then make a simple bundle by folding three to five flowering stems over again and again, until the bundle is about palm size. Fasten the bundle with string, or carefully use another piece of cota stem to wrap it all up.

Medicinal uses

Cota is one of the great-tasting wild teas of the desert west. It has a soft, sweet taste that can aid as a gentle diuretic, providing relief to irritated urethras or helping with mild water retention. The energetics of cota are cooling, which makes it a pleasant drink on a hot summer's day, or for the overheated and exhausted individual.

Caution

Cota is in the Asteraceae, and some people may have allergic reactions to this plant family.

Future harvest

First, make sure not to pull this plant out by its roots. Second, be sure to leave adequate foliage and at least three plants in a stand. This keeps it healthy for the following year.

HERBAL PREPARATIONS

Tea
Hot infusion
1 dried bundle
1 quart water
or
1–2 tablespoons fresh or dried leaves,
    stems, and flowers
1 cup water
Drink 1–2 cups 3 times a day.

---

cottonwood

Populus species
poplar
PARTS USED bark, twigs, buds

Cottonwood groves are wintertime treasure troves, filled with sticky, resinous, medicinal buds. I can never gather enough!

How to identify

Cottonwood trees have scaly or rough, gray-brown bark with deep furrows. They average 50–100 feet in height. Branches may look bare in the winter, but they hold aromatic buds that exude a sweet balsam-scented resin. Leaves are alternate and ovate, lanceolate, or heart-shaped with toothed edges. All *Populus* species are dioecious, meaning the tree is either male or female; the main difference between catkins is the male catkins shed pollen while the female catkins produce the seeds. We have some pretty outstanding buds to select from. *Populus angustifolia*, *P. deltoides*, and *P. balsamifera* are a few of the species local to the mountain states, all of which have highly aromatic buds. In spring, people sometimes curse the seeds of the cottonwood as they clog gutters and obscure windshields; I prefer to think of the cottony seed appendages as fairy fluff.

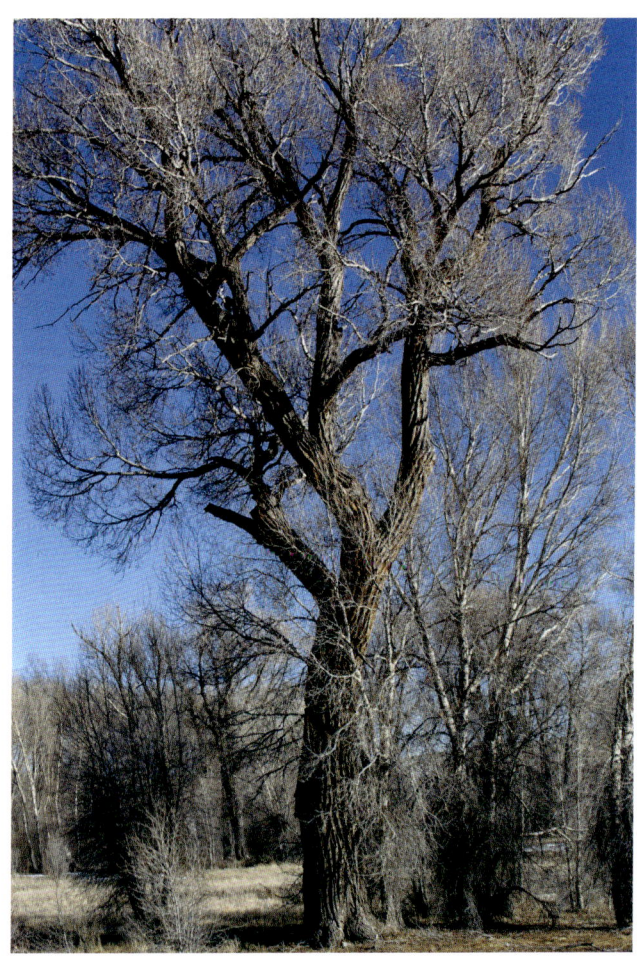

Branches wave in the wind all winter long, and I watch in anticipation, knowing that branches full of resinous buds will fall, sooner or later.

Where, when, and how to wildcraft

Cottonwood trees dominate the riverbanks, irrigated fields, and floodplains of the west. Gather their riches of buds and bark in winter and spring. Look for them at their most resinous, which can be at the start of winter. I usually begin to gather the buds when the winds come in early spring, but before they begin to sprout.

Wind, beavers, and tree trimmers are my favorite allies when it comes to gathering cottonwood limbs and buds. Find a beaver-fallen tree or a spot where many branches have freshly fallen. Sit there and pick through the twigs to collect just the buds. Stay long enough to garble, quietly in nature, if you have the time to surrender yourself—if you don't, make the time. You can also take the branches home for a more thorough collection and for utilizing the twigs and bark.

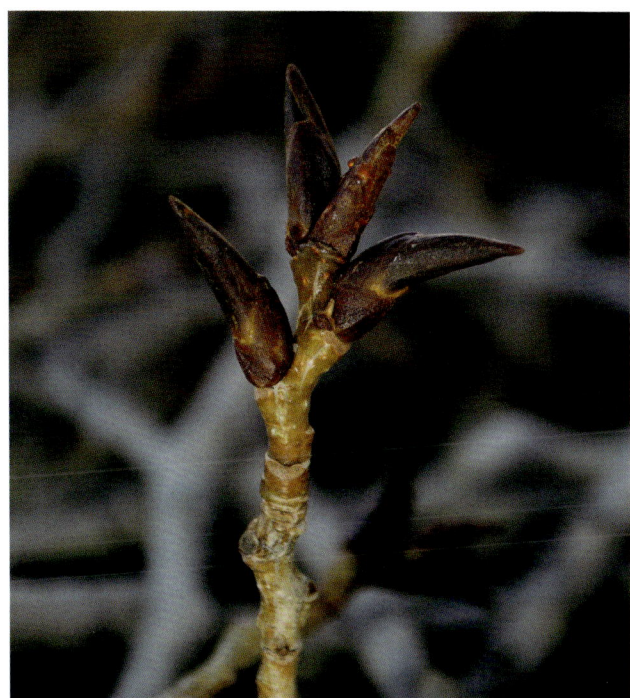

Notice the resins of the cottonwood bud; this is one of my most prized and cherished medicinals.

Medicinal uses

I cannot speak highly enough of cottonwood bud–infused oil. I run out of it every year, though each year I make twice the amount as the previous year. The oil provides one of the best topical pain relievers I have ever seen. It has the ability to decrease inflammation and relieve chronic pain whether in the form of an oil, salve, or cream. It is also superior at healing skin ailments like rashes, dry and cracked skin, and itchy spots. Try it in lip balm and massage oil. Rubbed on the chest, cottonwood buds provide a warming anodyne effect that also aids in loosening mucus in the lungs. Oil infused with cottonwood buds also has a great preserving quality to it and can help lengthen the shelf life of handmade products.

Cottonwood bark also carries pain-relieving qualities. Try it in a sitz bath along with grindelia, plantain, yarrow, bluebell, and raspberry leaf. Make a decocted cleansing soak for scrapes and cuts. Try blending the bark with plantain and yarrow for a soothing and healing tea.

Cottonwood buds or bark in a tinctured bitters formula can be very stimulating to the appetite, while increasing the secretions of bile that help with digestion. This same bitters formula can also work well for sore throats and coughs. The buds have drying and warming actions useful when fevers are present accompanied by a sore throat. The drying properties may decrease mucus drip that is irritating the throat, while the anti-inflammatory properties help soothe painfully red membranes. For a fever, cottonwood acts as a diaphoretic, increasing the body temperature slightly to help fight an infection. Diaphoretic herbs can help to warm your body temperature, sparking a sweat which then acts to cool you down.

Cottonwood honey is great for coughs and for clearing out the winter gunk from our lungs—all that dust, fireplace smoke, and stagnant air we've been breathing.

Caution

Do not use cottonwood buds if you are allergic to aspirin.

Future harvest

Please do not go chopping limbs off trees for any reason, unless you are pruning your own. Cottonwood branches come down very easily and unexpectedly; there are plenty of fresh downed branches to be found.

Malus species
PARTS USED bark, twigs, leaves, flowers, fruit

*Spring and fall take on a whole new meaning once you fall in love
with crabapple's medicine of fragrant flowers and astringently bitter fruits.*

How to identify

There is no greater scent than when all the crabapple trees go into bloom each spring. Sweeter than roses, the floral fragrance lingers through neighborhood streets. Crabapples look very similar to apple trees, with rough brown bark and white to fuchsia blossoms. They differ in that their fruits are smaller, less than 2 inches in diameter, and they vary in color from yellow-green to pink-red to magenta-orange. The trees are stout with dense branches bearing leaves that are ovate and slightly serrated or scalloped.

Where, when, and how to wildcraft

Crabapples are drought-tolerant trees that handle extremely cold temperatures quite well. They grow in backyards and old town sites, near old buildings and farmhouses. I've noticed some trees take a year off, producing fruit only every other year, possibly having to do with environmental factors such as early frost, moisture, and nutrient availability. More rain during the summer makes for juicier apples; drought years usually mean mealy fruit.

The flowers, twigs, bark, and leaves can be gathered in the spring. Crabapples are ready for picking in September and into October. Frost sweetens them, making them soft and more suitable for harvesting. Get a bushel basket and start picking. My favorites to

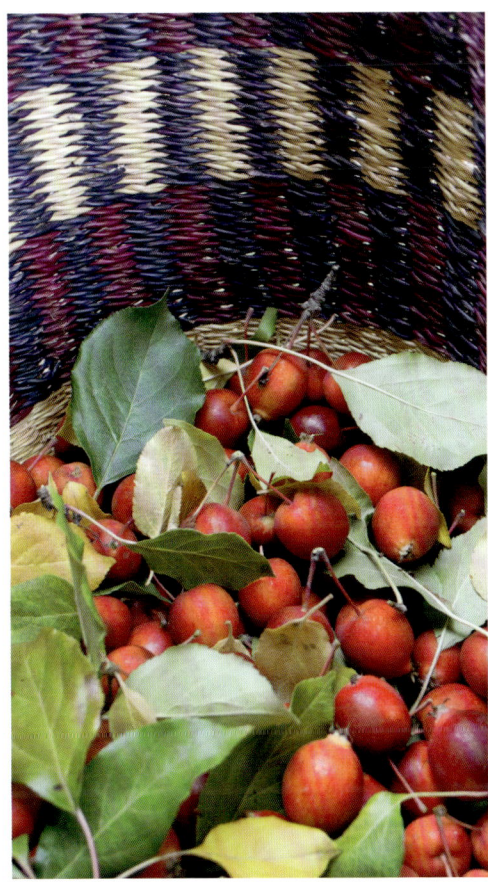

A basket full of ripe crabapples bound for a bitters formula.

gather are the deep red ones that are larger in size or the miniature Braeburn-looking crabapples; these varieties are juicy and slightly sweet but sour.

Medicinal uses

Very similar to those of apple, the medicinal properties of crabapple are influenced by its bitter astringency. The flowers, bark, twigs, and leaves can all be used in the same way as those of apple, though I find some crabapples to have more aromatic flowers and more tart fruits.

I like to make a tincture of the sweet-smelling flowers in the spring. I will then sometimes add the chopped fruits to the mixture when they are ripened in the fall, straining them out within a few weeks.

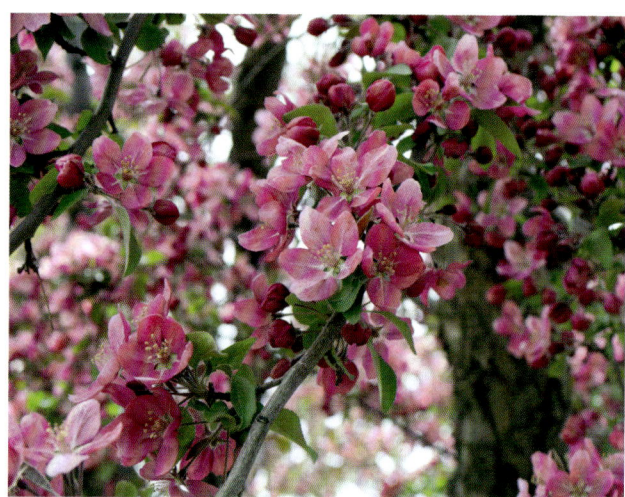

Fragrant blossoms of crabapple trees make a lovely elixir.

The blossoms also make a wonderful elixir: separately infuse both honey and alcohol with fresh flowers, then combine after straining. Use a 1:5 ratio of honey to alcohol. This can be a powerful aid for people experiencing heartache.

The fresh fruit eaten or tinctured can be an aid for constipation, functioning as a slight laxative. The fresh leaves crushed or infused into oil can be used as relief for insect bites and minor wounds. Use the flowers and leaves in oil infusions that can be made into salves or ointments requiring astringency.

⚠ Caution

Crabapple leaves, seeds, and bark contain a small amount of cyanogenic glycosides, which can convert into a potentially toxic substance in the human body. Although crabapple is regarded as completely safe to use, large quantities of seeds eaten at one time could be fatal.

Future harvest

Most trees have more fruit than their branches can hold or the birds can eat.

HERBAL PREPARATIONS

Tea
Hot infusion
3 tablespoons fresh or dried flowers and
    leaves, or dried fruit
1 cup water
Drink as needed.

Decoction
1 ounce fresh or dried twigs and bark
1 quart water
Drink 1 cup 3 times a day.

Tincture
1 part fresh twigs, bark, flowers, or fruit
2 parts menstruum (80% alcohol, 20%
    distilled water)
or
1 part dried twigs, bark, flowers, or fruit
5 parts menstruum (60% alcohol, 40%
    distilled water)
Take 30–60 drops 3 times a day.

Oil
Infuse with fresh or dried flowers or leaves.

cranesbill

Geranium species
wild geranium

PARTS USED roots, leaves, flowers

Crush a few leaves and take in a deep breath of cranesbill's fragrant leaves.

How to identify
The flowers of cranesbill species vary from hues of white to magenta, with some having purple veins through the petals. Many flowering stems grow from one plant, with their many leaves carried on long petioles. The leaves of most cranesbills are palmately lobed with three to five lobes. They can be fuzzy or smooth and likewise vary in their degree of resinousness. Seeds form a thin beak-like bundle, inspiring the common name.

Where, when, and how to wildcraft
Cranesbill grows in open meadows of the foothills or in the shade of damp forests at higher elevation. Gather the roots in the spring or fall. The leaves and flowers should be gathered on a warm dry day in summer while blossoming.

Medicinal uses
Many species of *Geranium* inhabit the United States and all can be used interchangeably, though the strength of the medicinal properties will vary from species to species.

The whole cranesbill plant can be used fresh or dried in a decoction for a soak. These soaks can be useful for postpartum hemorrhoids or for sore, blistered feet. Harvest *Plantago* species and cranesbill during a backpacking trip if your feet are starting to feel the painful effects of ill-fitting shoes. Simmer the herbs in a pot of water over a stove or

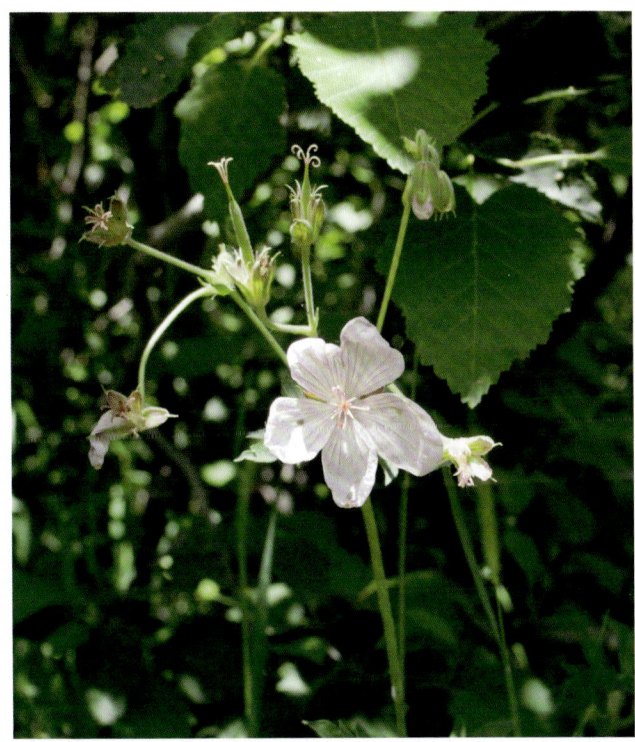

The colors of the flowers may vary from plant to plant, but all the seeds take the shape of a crane's bill.

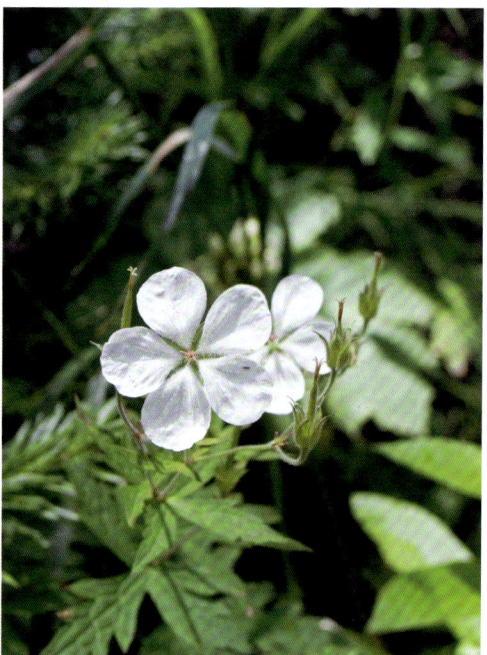

Notice the highly lobed leaves of *Geranium* species.

campfire, and let the soak cool enough to put your feet in.

The super-astringent roots of cranesbill can be useful for bouts of diarrhea, when taken as a tea, tincture, or fresh chew. A chew of the fresh roots also aids mouth sores or can be formed into a poultice and applied to wounds or insect bites. The roots may also be infused into oil for these applications.

Future harvest

When harvesting the root of geranium be very mindful of the surrounding soil and how many plants you disrupt on your endeavor.

HERBAL PREPARATIONS

Tea

Hot infusion
1–3 tablespoons fresh or dried leaves and
   flowers
1 cup water
Drink 1 cup 3 times a day.

Sitz bath decoction
4 tablespoons fresh or dried root
1 quart water

Tincture

1 part fresh leaves, flowers, and root
2 parts menstruum (75% alcohol, 25% distilled water)
or
1 part dried leaves, flowers, and root
5 parts menstruum (60% alcohol, 40% distilled water)
Take 10–20 drops 3 times a day.

Oil

Infuse with fresh or dried leaves, roots, and flowers.

dandelion

Taraxacum species

PARTS USED roots, leaves, flowers

Dandelion, that arch-nemesis of the weekend lawn warrior, belongs anywhere but the compost pile or trash bin.

How to identify

Bright yellow flowerheads crop up all over in the springtime, and most of them belong to the beloved dandelion. It looks as though a single flowerhead, held by a green bract, sits atop the scape, but in fact the bloom consists of hundreds of tiny ray flowers. When broken, the wide and hollow stem (or scape) flows white latex. The leaves are always basal and lobed, having uneven edges like those of a key or the teeth of a lion—hence the common name, a corruption of the French, *dent de lion*. All leaves form a thick rosette around a taproot that is usually a pale cream color. Several flower stems will arise out of a single rosette. Pappus is the white fluff we see once dandelions, turned from suns to moons, have gone to seed.

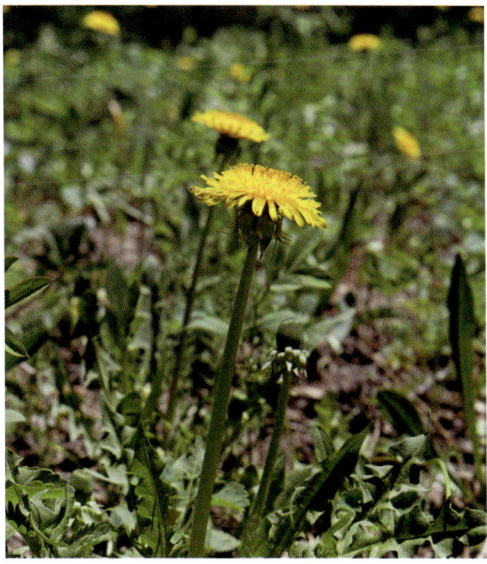

All parts of dandelion can be collected and utilized as superb medicine or food.

Where, when, and how to wildcraft

Finding a clean place to gather dandelions is important. Most gardeners will gladly have you come weed their beds, but make sure they are not using chemicals or hosting dogs. In the mountains, however, dandelions abound! There is always an abundance of dandelions to be found in pristine conditions where foot traffic is minimal.

The leaves are the first offering put forth each spring. Gather a few leaves from each plant or dig up the whole plant to use the root as well, though the root is best dug before flowers blossom in spring or after they die back in summer or fall. Once the flowers bloom, harvest by taking either just the head or the entire scape as well.

Medicinal uses

Dandelion root and leaf is another useful bitter herb for stimulating the flow of bile and digestive secretions. It has a positive effect on the microflora of the gut, helping to feed the good biotics that live there. Dandelion improves the function of the liver and acts as an alterative, helping to excrete toxins from the body. The root is also a strong diuretic, aiding bladder infections by flushing out pathogens, thus providing a better habitat for good flora.

The flowers infused in oil make emollient massage oils that help to hydrate the skin, soothe breasts inflamed from nursing or hormonal shifts during the lunar cycle, or calm inflamed lymph nodes, helping them to better process any stagnation. All therapists of the bodywork industry should make this massage oil. It provides relief to sore and achy joints, muscles, and connective tissues.

Caution

Dandelion is in the Asteraceae, and some people may have allergic reactions to this plant family.

Future harvest

Dandelion is a voracious little weed, and it sure does grow everywhere, with a healthy disregard for trampling and overgrazing. Harvest to your heart's content.

Alterative

Herbs that are alterative help the body clear and eliminate congestion held within body systems. Herbs can be alteratives for any system of the body, for example, the bladder (dandelion), lymphatics (redroot), skin (burdock), or gastrointestinal tract (dock). Keeping systems clear makes them run more efficiently, making us more vital.

HERBAL PREPARATIONS

Tea
Hot infusion
3 tablespoons fresh or dried leaves, or fresh roasted dried root
1 cup water
Decoction
1 ounce fresh, dried, or roasted root
1 quart water
Drink 1–2 cups 3 times a day.

Tincture
1 part fresh root or leaves
2 parts menstruum (75% alcohol, 25% distilled water)
or
1 part dried root or leaves
5 parts menstruum (60% alcohol, 40% distilled water)
Take 30–60 drops 3 times a day.

Oil
Infuse with freshly wilted flowers.

Rumex species

cañaigre

PARTS USED roots, leaves

Docks are a common sight in the west. The browned seedheads
in the fall will tell you exactly where to dig their astringent root.

How to identify

Docks can be spotted from afar by the tall,
dark brown stalks and seedheads of the previous year. Plants can grow quite large, reaching
3–5 feet tall. Leaves are long, thick, and lanceolate; they form a basal rosette in spring.
The stalk is jointed, and smaller leaves grow
alternately along it, with clasping leaf bases.
The small flowers are green, red, or brown,
and turn into winged seeds. Roots can be
quite large and are cream or yellow in color.

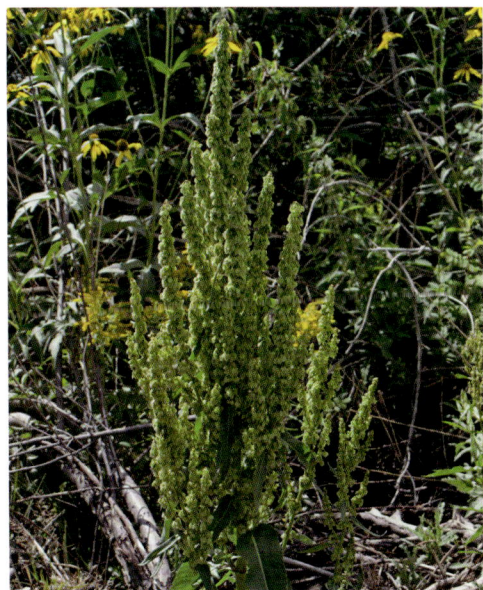

Taste a piece of dock root to experience the tart
astringency of *Rumex* species.

Rumex crispus (crispy dock, yellow dock)
has curly or wavy edges and is one of the
more medicinally notorious species. *Rumex
occidentalis* (western dock) is abundant
throughout the west and has large leaves that
have a minimal astringency.

Where, when, and how to wildcraft

Find dock growing in sunny fields, canyons,
vacant lots, on hillsides, close to ditches, or
at the edges of forests. Gather the young
leaves in the spring or in the summer as they
toughen up and turn more tart. Snap or trim
the leaves from the base. The younger leaves
growing along the stalk can be harvested
anytime. Roots can be gathered in the fall or
spring. Dig them after the plant has gone to
seed or when the leaves are sprouting in the
spring; clean well and chop into small pieces
for drying.

Medicinal uses

Yellow dock derives its name from the yellow root. It is used as an alterative for liver
problems or skin eruptions, such as boils
or acne.

Docks are useful as a bitter herb that helps
to stimulate the flow of bile. Dock can be
combined in formulas to help aid digestion
of fatty foods. Do note that it can also act
as a mild laxative. This makes it useful for

constipation, where it can help to soothe the accompanying intestinal inflammation and irritation. Make a decoction to sip or take small frequent doses of the tincture, such as 5–30 drops every hour. Start small—everyone reacts differently to the laxative effect of this plant!

Yellow dock can be helpful in absorbing iron from the diet, making it potentially useful when anemia is present. The way the plant does this is not fully understood, though it has been hypothesized that the mineral content and bitter properties play a large role. It combines well with other herbs like dandelion root, alfalfa, and stinging nettle in either a vinegar extraction or decoction, which can be sipped as a mineral-rich tea. Add a dollop of molasses to enrich it even further.

Dock leaves are a remedy to make the sting of stinging nettle subside. Simply crush the fresh leaf and rub its juices on the affected spot. The leaves and root can also be extracted into oils and used in salves for troubled skin that is itchy, infected, or has sores. It can be combined with burdock root or leaf to help tame acne breakouts, either applied topically in an oil or taken internally as a tincture or tea.

Caution

The aerial parts of dock are especially high in oxalic acid, which, if consumed in large quantities, can cause gastric upset or greatly affect people who suffer from kidney disease and stones.

Future harvest

Dock has a tendency to grow back even after you take a large chunk of root from the plant. Harvesting the roots, especially of the more weedy species, shouldn't harm the stand.

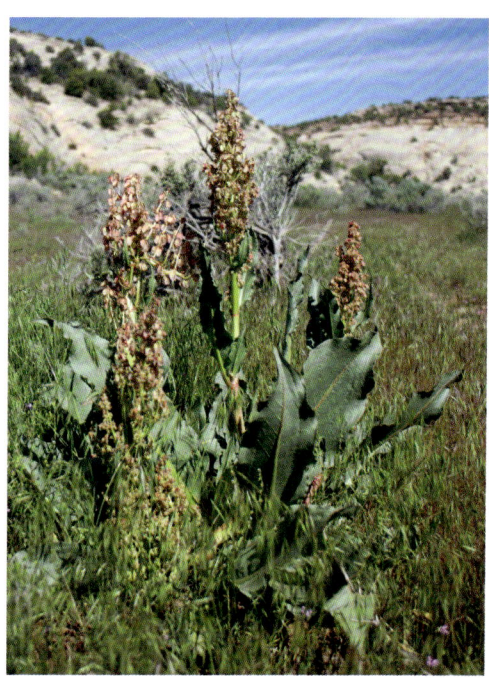

Find docks in varying locations throughout the west, from the desert to wet meadows to the alpine.

HERBAL PREPARATIONS

Tea
Decoction
3–4 tablespoons fresh or dried root
1 quart water
Sip slowly throughout the day for relief of constipation.

Tincture
1 part fresh root
2 parts menstruum (75% alcohol, 25% distilled water)
or
1 part dried root
5 parts menstruum (60% alcohol, 40% distilled water)
Take 10–20 drops 3 times a day or as needed.

Oil
Infuse with fresh or dried leaves and root.

Douglas fir

Pseudotsuga menziesii

PARTS USED twigs, needles, resin

The taste of fresh Douglas fir is that of a tart grapefruit peel.
Turn to it to formulate more palatable tinctures.

How to identify

Douglas fir trees are great evergreen conifers averaging 100 feet tall when mature. The bark is gray, becoming thicker and darker with age. Smooth bark of young trees will eventually turn rough and crack as the tree gets older. Soft, flat, blue-green needles grow in an alternating spiral along the branch. Douglas firs differ from "true" fir trees in that their cones hang from the branches; these cones can also be found on the ground. *Abies* species, which are the true firs, have cones that sit erect on the branches and disintegrate while there. Cones of a Douglas fir are 2–3 inches long and light brown. Three-pronged bracts are situated between the scales of the cone and have a distinctive upward bend.

Where, when, and how to wildcraft

Find Douglas fir on mountain slopes at elevations of 6000–9500 feet from Colorado north and west all the way to the Pacific coast of northern California, Oregon, Washington, and into Canada. The needles of any conifer can be gathered year-round, though I find the young, spring tips of Douglas fir and spruces to be the best. The tips are the new growth at the ends of branches. Find a forest full of Douglas fir and meander among trees, plucking only a few tips from each.

The resins are best gathered while soft and gooey, when they are flowing up or down the tree in spring and fall. Resins can be collected gently in the winter months—find them dripping off the tree from old wounds—but do not reopen a scar on the tree.

If you are wildcrafting or harvesting a fresh Christmas tree, consider using the

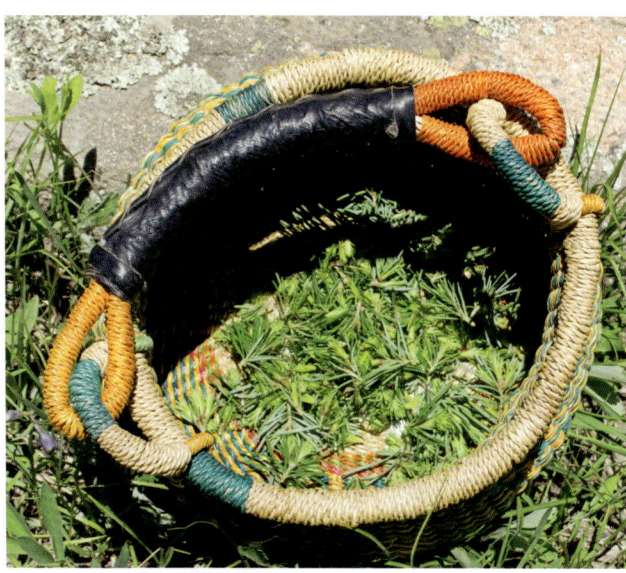

Warm late spring days in the mountains are made for picking conifer tips; one of my favorites is *Pseudotsuga menziesii*.

entire tree for medicine-making. The twigs can be clipped off, needles can be stripped, or bark can be peeled to use as another addition to tea-blending or tincture-making.

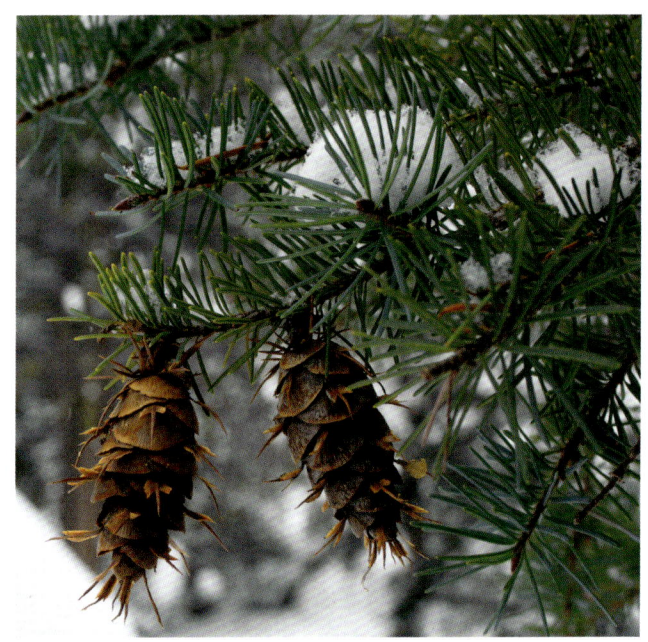

Medicinal uses

The fragrance and taste of Douglas fir tips is reminiscent of grapefruit peels. The aromatics accompany infused oil combinations for skincare, like beard oils; try doing a double or triple infusion. In a tincture formula, the needles can bring a bright essence of uplifting citrus notes.

A hot tea can be perfect at the onset of a cold or flu, as Douglas fir is a warming decongestant. It can be handy in nasal steams to help unstick the gunk in the sinuses and relieve congested lungs.

Three-pronged, tail-like bracts, poking out from between the scales, are a distinguishing feature of Douglas fir cones.

 Caution

Douglas fir is not for internal use during pregnancy without consulting a physician. When taken internally, resins of plant can be irritating to kidneys.

Future harvest

Prune the tree lightly and you will do no harm to its longevity. Pick resin that is either fallen to the ground or thick on the tree. Do not saw or chop around the resin chunks; these act as scabs to the tree and are protecting it from bugs and pathogens. Pick built-up, protruding chunks of resin, but never pick the scab clean.

HERBAL PREPARATIONS

Tea
Hot infusion
1 ounce fresh or dried needles and twigs
1 quart water
Drink 1–2 cups 3 times a day.

Tincture
1 part fresh needles, resin, or twigs
2 parts menstruum (75% alcohol, 25% distilled water)
Take 20–40 drops 3 times a day.

Oil
Infuse with fresh needles, resin, or twigs.

elderberry

Sambucus species

PARTS USED flowers, fruit

When anyone in the house starts to feel even the least bit off-kilter,
my first reach into the medicine cabinet is for elderberry elixir or tea.

How to identify

The leaves of elderberry trees are pinnate with an odd number of leaflets, commonly three to nine, resulting in a leaflet at the tip of the leaf. Compound leaves are paired opposite one another along a pithy stem. They are serrated and are mostly lanceolate in shape but can be ovate. The leaves have a musky, unpleasant odor when rubbed; the leaves of the only lookalike, mountain ash, do not. Branches are arranged opposite along the stem throughout the shrub. Flowers are white with five petals and five stamens. The inflorescence can be branched with flat-topped clusters, or flowers can form a pyramidal shape.

Where, when, and how to wildcraft

Find elderberry trees throughout the Front Range of the Rockies, north to Alberta and Saskatchewan and westward, growing in mixed forests, along hillsides, and in meadows. They prefer partial shade and damp soils. Species bearing black or blue berries—the ones worth harvesting—are found throughout this mountainous region, just not as densely or commonly as *Sambucus racemosa* (red elderberry). Many ornamental elderberry trees grace neighborhoods, parks, or other landscaped areas. Make sure to harvest in areas that are free from being sprayed. Gather the flowers in late spring or early summer.

Flowers of all *Sambucus* species can be used interchangeably for topical use, but the flowers of some species, such as *S. racemosa*, can be mildly nauseating internally. Also, the red berries of *S. racemosa* are mildly toxic and should not be used for any medicine-making.

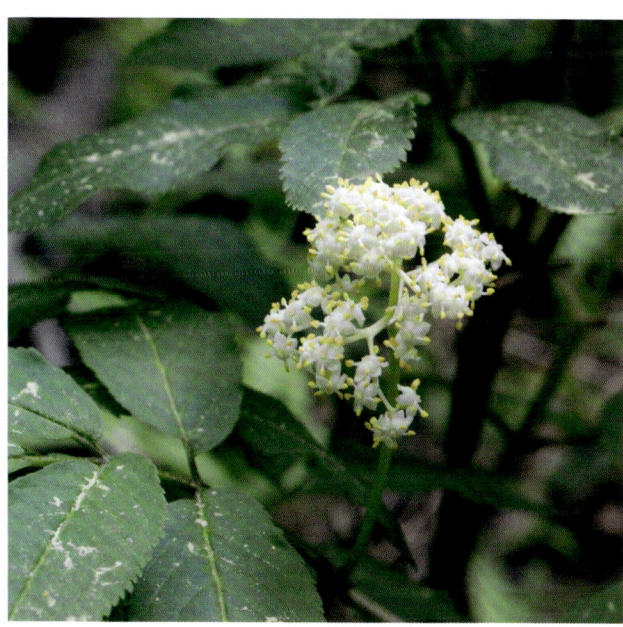

Sambucus racemosa, blooming in early summer.

All elderberry fruits of all species contain seeds that are toxic if they are not cooked or dried. If tempted in the field, spit them out, and don't chew the seeds if you want to taste.

The main flower stems of elderberry are also toxic, and most of the smaller flower stems (pedicels) should be removed before processing the flowers or berries. Harvest flowers by clipping the flower stem under the first branch of the inflorescence. Dry the flowers while they are on the pedicels, but once dried, garble through the big stems, removing the individual flowers. Berries can be frozen fresh or dried in a dehydrator or in the oven at its lowest temperature.

Medicinal uses

Dried elderberries, beebalm, and pine needles with a dollop of osha honey make a suitable tea to drink when the weather is cold and damp and viruses are running rampant. Elderberry elixir, tincture, syrup, and honey are all fantastic ways to get the medicinal components extracted from the fruit. Take 20–30 drops every hour when you are beginning to feel sickness creeping into your body. The flowers are diaphoretic and can be combined with herbs such as wild mint, yarrow, valerian flowers, or beebalm for feverish children.

The flowers of the elderberry have a long history of being used in skincare products to maintain a clear complexion. Flowers can be infused in oil for facial serums—a beloved combination is elderflower and rosehip seed oil. Infuse elderflowers in witch hazel for a few weeks and strain though a fine filter for a fabulous tonifying facial spritz;

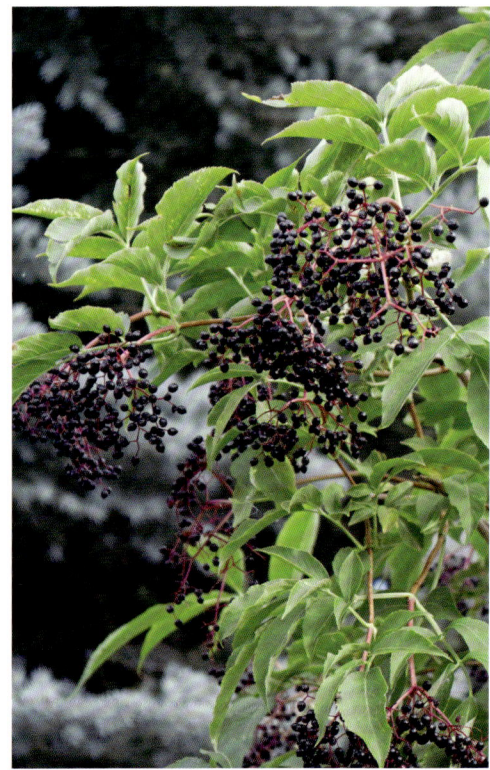

Sambucus nigra occurs both in the wild and planted as an ornamental throughout the west.

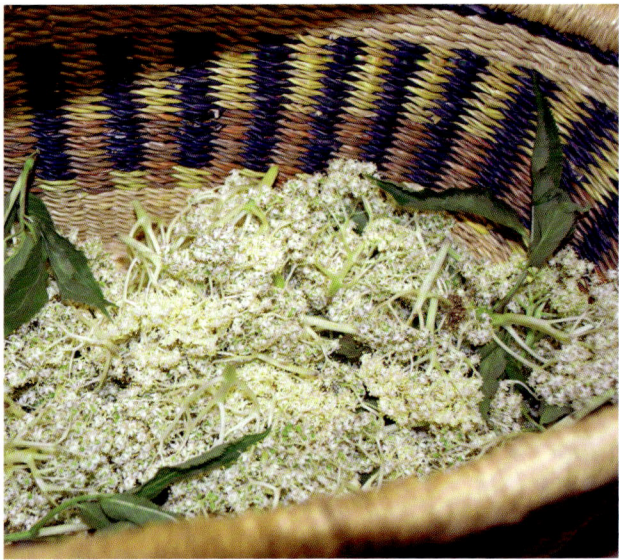

A basket filled with elderberry flowers; the flowers of all species are white and have many topical uses.

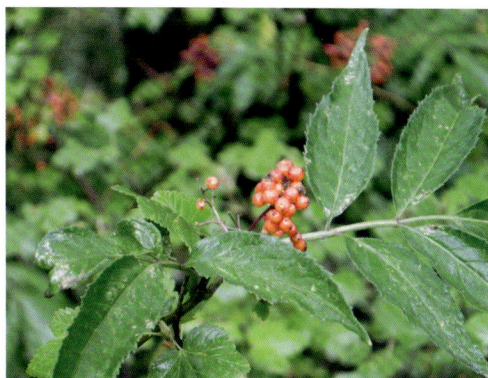

The red berries of *Sambucus racemosa* are mildly toxic. I don't use them for medicine or making cosmetics.

add hydrosols such as rose or juniper for more skin-nourishing and -revitalizing benefits. Berries, once dried and ground, can be infused into oil for their purplish red coloring stain that can look gorgeous in balms for cheeks and lips.

⚠ Caution
Seeds and stems are toxic and should not be ingested while fresh. The flowers of *Sambucus racemosa* (red elderberry) have been known to induce slight nausea. Red elderberries should only be consumed after being cooked, and the berries of all other species should be dried before use.

Future harvest
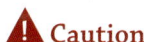 Harvesting modest amounts of the flowers or fruits should pose no threat to the longevity of the elder tree.

HERBAL PREPARATIONS

Tea
Cold infusion
1 tablespoon fresh or dried flowers
1 cup water
Hot infusion
1–3 tablespoons dried berries or fresh or dried flowers
1 cup water
Decoction
1 ounce dried berries
1 quart water
Drink 1–2 cups 3 times a day.

Tincture
1 part dried berries
2 parts menstruum (75% alcohol, 25% distilled water)
Take 30–60 drops 3 times a day.

or
1 part fresh flowers
4 parts menstruum (60% alcohol, 40% distilled water)
Take 20–40 drops 3 times a day.

or
1 part dried flowers or berries
5 parts menstruum (60% alcohol, 40% distilled water)
Take 30–60 drops 3 times a day.

Oil
Infuse with fresh or dried flowers or dried berries.

Artemisia ludoviciana

white sagebrush, silver wormwood, western mugwort, prairie sage

PARTS USED leaves, stems, flowers

When gathering any artemisia, I always roll a piece between my fingers to release the aromatics and tuck it behind my ear, taking the scent with me for the rest of the day.

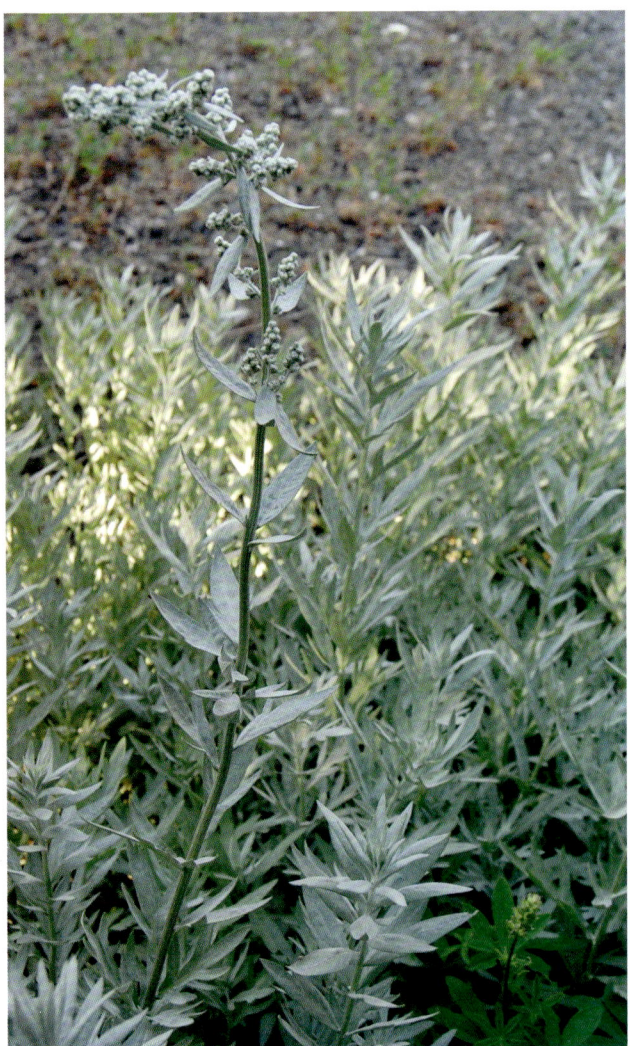

Estafiate beginning to bloom.

How to identify

Estafiate is a perennial that grows alone, in gatherings, or in thickets on thinly supported stems. The stems can grow tall, to about 6 feet in places, but generally average not much more than 2 feet. The many-branched stalks are covered in deeply clefted and irregularly shaped leaves, growing alternately. The leaves are layered with a soft down and appear to be a silverish green. The flowers are a soft green, in little rounded heads composed mainly of disc flowers. Nodding groups of flowers grow at the top of the plant in a spaced-out inflorescence.

Where, when, and how to wildcraft

Find estafiate growing all over the mountain west, in the arid lowlands, riparian meadows, or along mountainsides at 9000 feet. Where it grows it grows aplenty, and a large quantity can be harvested in a short amount of time. Simply clip the top half of the plant, leaving behind a lot of leaves for regrowth. It begins to flower in summer and can be gathered at any point after the leaves are showing. Collect the flowering stems and bundle them while fresh; secure the bundle with thin twine and let it dry.

Medicinal uses

One of the more palatable artemisias to use for bitter formulations, estafiate can be a digestive aid and has a delicate wormwood flavor. As estafiate is warming and stimulating, it is a good asset to fevers that are not producing a sweat; drink a cup of tea or take a few drops of tincture every half hour until its diaphoretic action kicks in and sweating takes place. Estafiate helps to stimulate the uterus, which can be beneficial for crampy menses; however, for the same reason, it must not be used internally during pregnancy.

A steam inhalation of estafiate can clear coughs—add usnea and conifer twigs such as pine or spruce for additional expectoration and antimicrobial benefits. An oil infusion or topical liniment can be useful for fungal infections, or add it to wound-healing salves.

Bundles of estafiate can be soaked in a large pot of simmering water for use as a bath soak. Burning bundles as a traditional smudge results in a dense, mildly aromatic smoke—hold it under an injury to relieve the pain. Try throwing some on a fire after a long backpacking trip, and let your bare feet sit over the smoking herb. It may give you better feeling feet for the next day's adventure.

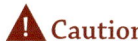 **Caution**

Not for use internally during pregnancy.

Future harvest

Estafiate grows abundantly all over our region. Still, take care not to rip the plant out of the ground. Only the aerial portions need to be gathered.

HERBAL PREPARATIONS

Tea
Hot or cold infusion
1–3 tablespoons fresh or dried leaves, stems, and flowers
1 cup water
Cold, drink before or after meals. Hot, sip slowly to support a fever and use as a diaphoretic.

Tincture
1 part fresh leaves, stems, and flowers
2 parts menstruum (75% alcohol, 25% distilled water)
or
1 part dried leaves, stems, and flowers
5 parts menstruum (60% alcohol, 40% distilled water)
Take 10–20 drops 3 times a day.

Oil
Infuse with fresh or dried leaves, stems, and flowers.

Abies species

PARTS USED twigs, needles, resin

It's a natural high to walk among the mighty firs of the alpine.
Their uplifting, mentholated aromatics make enchanting blends,
whether in teas, tinctures, honeys, or oils.

How to identify

One of the first ways to identify firs is by their cones, which grow in the upper branches, so you will have to look high up in the tree to notice them. They sit on top of the branches and can resemble mushrooms once the scales of the cone have fallen away. The cones point toward the sky as opposed to hanging down from the branches, the way they do in spruce. Cones disintegrate while on the tree; if you happen to find one on the ground, an animal probably knocked it down.

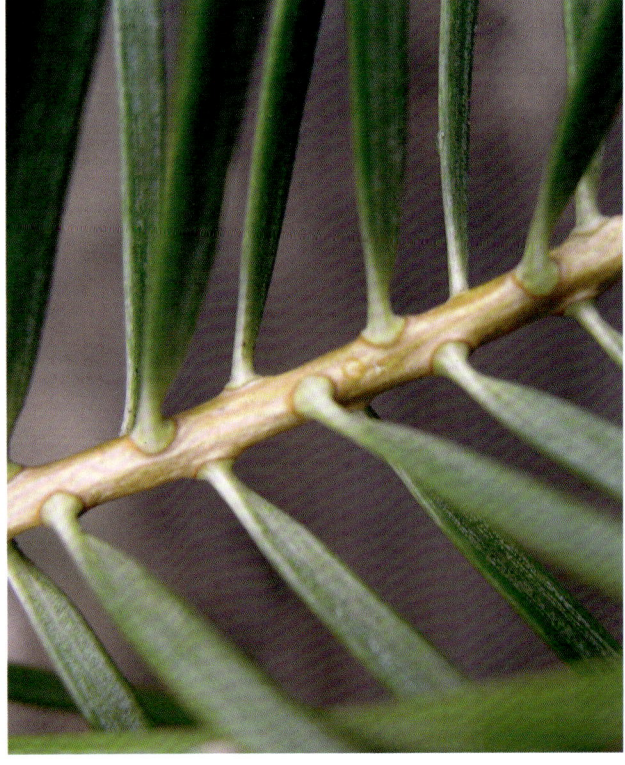

All firs have flat needles, which you can notice when you try to roll one between your fingers. Mountain alpine fir (*Abies bifolia*) has a single white line on the dorsal side of the needle and two beneath, while white fir (*A. concolor*) has two white lines only on the underside of the needle. The cones differ in color as well: mountain alpine fir cones are a dark purple-gray, while white fir cones vary from a golden green to purple.

Where, when, and how to wildcraft

Find firs growing in subalpine mountain forests or up at treeline. Gather the animal-strewn fresh resinous cones from the forest floor at the end of summer or fall. Gather the young tips of the branches in late spring or the

Fir needles are flat, and when placed between the fingertips will not roll like pine or spruce needles.

needles all year long. Pick the bright green soft tips off various branches, tasting each tree to find the flavors you like best. White fir has a lemony scent and flavor, while mountain alpine fir has more of a strong balsam aroma. Gather resins and fallen branches and twigs for their medicinal aromatics.

Medicinal uses

The mentholated aromatics of fir species can be useful as a replacement for other trees exotic to our region such as eucalyptus or camphor. Fir infusions are lovely with cream and a dollop of honey, and helpful when cold season strikes. Blend the warming aromatics into herbal steams to help release stuck phlegm in the lungs or open up the sinuses. Try combining usnea with the fir twigs or needles for even more lung and sinus rejuvenation. The fresh needles and twigs also can be brewed in a large quantity and added to baths for a sore muscle soak. The infused oils can be used for cough rubs, massage oils, or in salves to heal injuries.

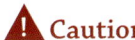 **Caution**

Fir is not for internal use in pregnancy without consulting a physician.

Future harvest

Taking needles and tips should not damage the tree. Spread out your harvest of young tips between many trees, lightly pruning the forest as you move through.

HERBAL PREPARATIONS

Tea
Hot infusion
3 tablespoons fresh needles and twigs
1 cup water
Drink 1 cup 3 times a day.

Tincture
1 part fresh needles, twigs, or resin
2 parts menstruum (75% alcohol, 25% distilled water)
Take 20–40 drops 3 times a day.

Oil
Infuse with fresh needles, twigs, or resin.

fireweed

Chamerion species
willowherb
PARTS USED leaves, flowerbuds, flowers

Find a stand of blossoming fireweed and lie down beneath it.
The sight of the fuchsia flowers against the blue sky is nourishment for the soul.

How to identify

Fireweed is a staple wildflower of the west, growing erect with four-petaled fuchsia flowers blossoming from the bottom up to the tip of the raceme. Young spring shoots of fireweed poke through old leaves, next to the first yarrow and dandelion leaves. The young stalks have a reddish coloring that disperses into the green leaves. Both stems and leaves are smooth and hairless. The leaves are long and lanceolate; some have slightly toothed margins and look similar to willow leaves. Each leaf has a pronounced white midvein, and they spiral alternately up the thick stem.

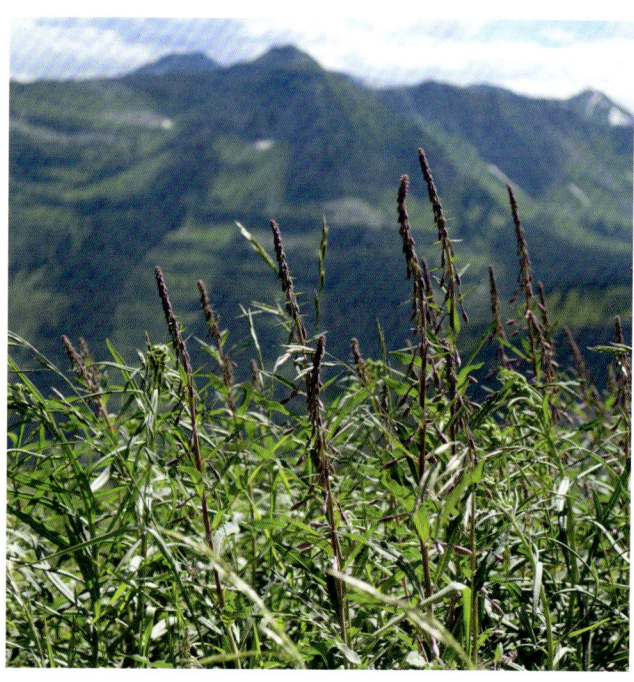

You needn't wait for the flowers to blossom when gathering fireweed; the leaves and flowerbuds also make good medicine.

Where, when, and how to wildcraft

Obviously, old burn sites are a common place to find fireweed thriving. It likes the cool, moist mountain air and is usually found at the edges of woods, in pasturelands, near waterways, high on rocky slopes, or along roadsides. Gather the flowering and budding tops of the plant in summer. Pick tall flowering plants that are not yet withered. Cut the stem above where the leaves begin to look old, or above where the plant has gone to seed, taking the vibrant leaves, flowers, and flowerbuds. Dry the herb by bundling it and hanging it. Once dry, garble the leaves, flowers, and flowerbuds from the thick central stalk which can be composted.

Medicinal uses

Fireweed is known for its anti-inflammatory properties when used internally and externally as teas, tinctures, or washes. It has an affinity for reducing swelling in the pelvic regions, making it ideal for prostate or bladder infections. A tea or tincture can be used internally for afflictions like colitis, ulcers, candida imbalance, and irritable bowel syndrome, soothing the inflammations while supporting the body's ability to fight infections.

For infants, soak a cloth in a bowl of fireweed tea and wash those red crevices that accompany diaper rash or yeast infections, or that often occur in between the neck rolls.

Leaves and flowers can be infused into oils for use in fungus-fighting salves. They also make a really lovely addition to smoking blends, giving body to the smoke and offering the beautiful magenta of the flowers to the mix.

Future harvest

Clipping the shoots back in early spring helps to stimulate growth, so no need to worry about overharvesting the shoots. Be mindful of the other early growth around you in the spring by walking with care.

Fireweed blossoms from the bottom up, and they say that once the last flower opens, the first snow is days away.

HERBAL PREPARATIONS

Tea
Hot infusion
2 tablespoons fresh or dried leaves, flowers, and flowerbuds
1 cup water
Drink as needed.

Tincture
1 part freshly cut leaves, flowers, and flowerbuds
3 parts menstruum (75% alcohol, 25% distilled water)
or
1 part dried leaves, flowers, and flowerbuds
5 parts menstruum (60% alcohol, 40% distilled water)
Take 20–40 drops 3–5 times a day.

Oil
Infuse with freshly wilted or dried leaves, flowers, or flowerbuds.

Erythronium grandiflorum

PARTS USED leaves

Chase glacier lilies up the mountains in spring. When one spot is done blooming, another stand will be blossoming higher up the mountainside.

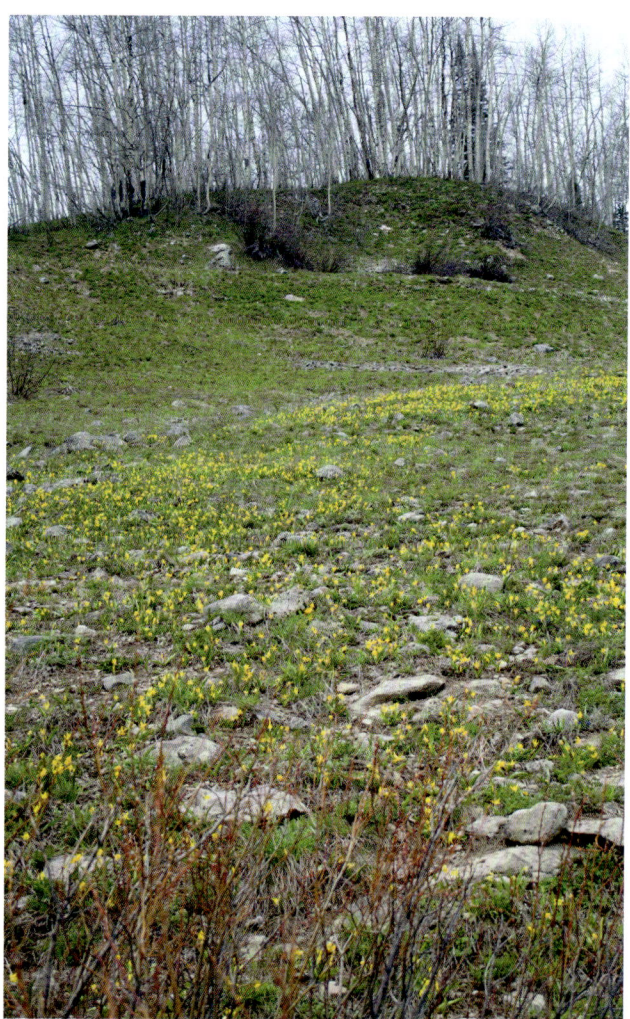

A field of glacier lily sprouts up right after spring snowmelt in the mountains.

How to identify

Glacier lilies are one of the first flowers to spring up after the long winter's snow cover finally melts, their yellow six-tepaled blossoms nodding to the ground below. The stem can vary in length, supporting one or two bent-over flowers. A single pair of narrowly oblong or elliptic leaves arises from the bulb (technically a corm). Leaves are glossy, smooth, and vibrantly green. The higher in elevation the plant grows, the more dwarf it becomes.

Where, when, and how to wildcraft

Walk through a high mountain meadow in late spring, and with any luck, glacier lilies will be there to delight you. Find them growing in the partial shade of forests, in sunny high alpine meadows, and in avalanche slide paths. The leaves can be harvested from spring into summer, even after the flower has bloomed and turned to seed. Pluck just one leaf per

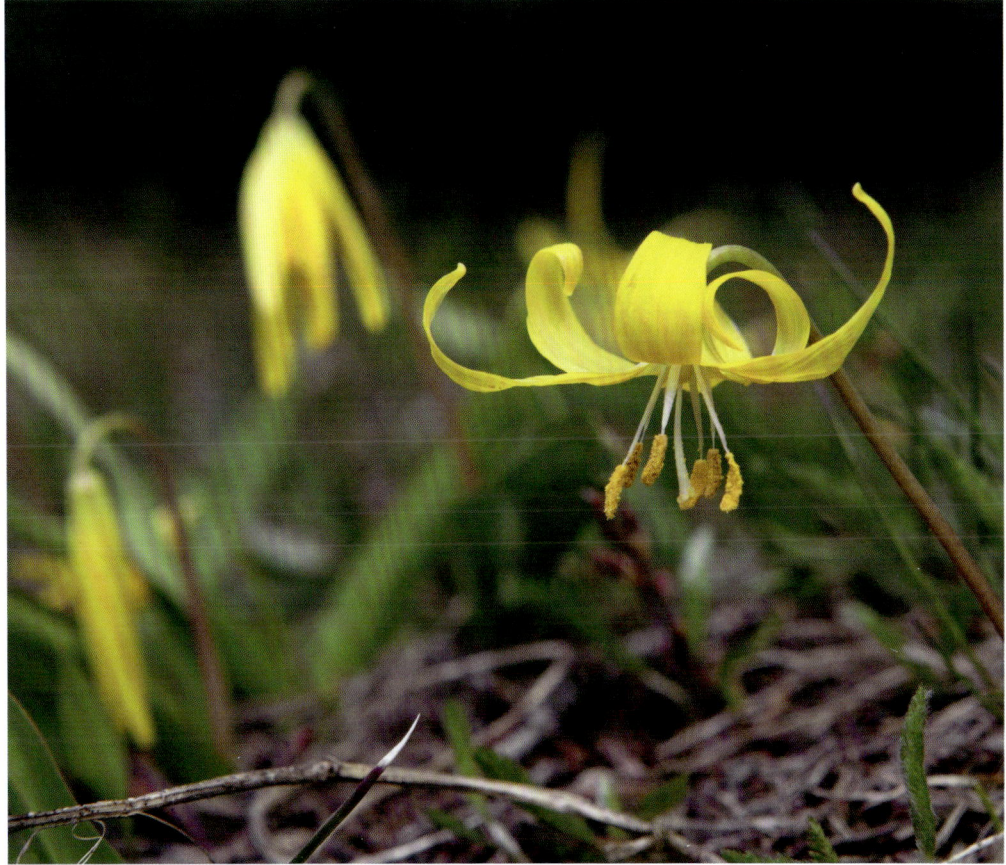

Gather one leaf per plant, and while doing so, take a nibble of the glacier lily flowers for an edible treat.

plant. Let them wilt overnight before using; this will help release some of the moisture the leaves harbor.

Medicinal uses

Glacier lily has edible flowers and roots, but not much is ever said about them medicinally. I have found that the fresh green leaves extract well in oil. I use this for skin irritations and in combination with other herbs for an antifungal salve. I include osha, beebalm, sagebrush, fireweed, and Oregon grape in what has been a superb blend for athlete's foot, nail fungus, and raw itchy skin.

Future harvest

Walk with care in the land in which it is growing, as spots preferred by glacier lily can be susceptible to erosion. One plant can take up to seven years to reach full maturity, so be gentle, take only one leaf per plant, and never pull it up from the ground. Being endemic to the higher elevations of the Rockies, this is a species best harvested strictly for its aerial parts.

HERBAL PREPARATIONS

Oil
Infuse with fresh leaves.

globemallow

Sphaeralcea species
yerba la negrita, desert hollyhock,
desert globemallow, scarlet globemallow
PARTS USED roots, leaves, flowers, seedpods

Globemallow is a much-needed demulcent herb in the dead of winter. Opening a jar filled with last spring's bright orange flowers and soft green leaves cheers my soul.

How to identify

Globemallows are native perennials with glittering scarlet-orange flowers that grow on panicles or racemes. Flowers have five petals that create a bowl-like shape with stamens that are joined as a column in the center. The foliage of the plant is soft and pubescent. Leaves of *Sphaeralcea* species can be hardly lobed or deeply lobed, and grow alternately along the stem.

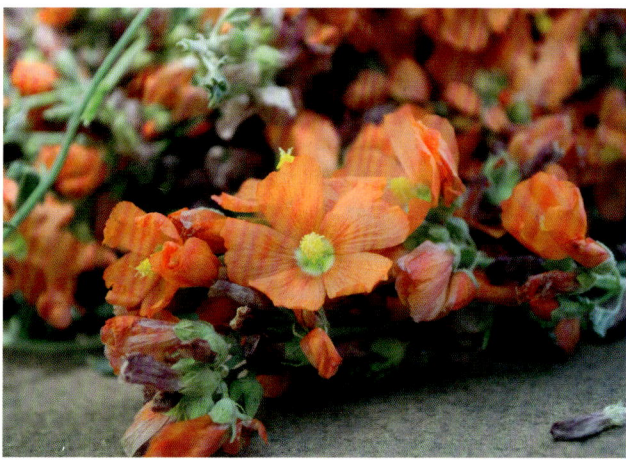

The almost iridescently orange flowers of globemallow can be confidently gathered from early spring through early fall.

Where, when, and how to wildcraft

Globemallows ornament the dry desert floor of the mountain west, blooming as early as April or May in the desert low country and still providing a bounty into early fall. Seedpods can be gathered soon after or while the flowers blossom. Clip the flowering stalks full of leaves or just harvest the blossoming flowers. Dry leaves, flowers, seedpods, and stems indoors and out of sunlight, then garble the leaves, flowers, and seedpods off the main stem after drying. Harvest roots gently and only from a few plants in each area. Chop roots before drying.

Medicinal uses

The dried powder or a moistened poultice of the roots or seedpods of globemallow can be applied to weepy wounds, sores, blisters, or infections of the skin. This mucilaginous herb acts as a drawing poultice, providing a protective layer and wicking away moisture.

Blend it with other demulcent herbs for teas to aid those dry conditions that many westerners exhibit: dry and cracked inner nostrils or nosebleeds, dry throat, chapped lips, or a chronic feeling of dehydration. Flowers, leaves, and seedpods can be used as a tea or wash for dry, itchy, inflamed eyes.

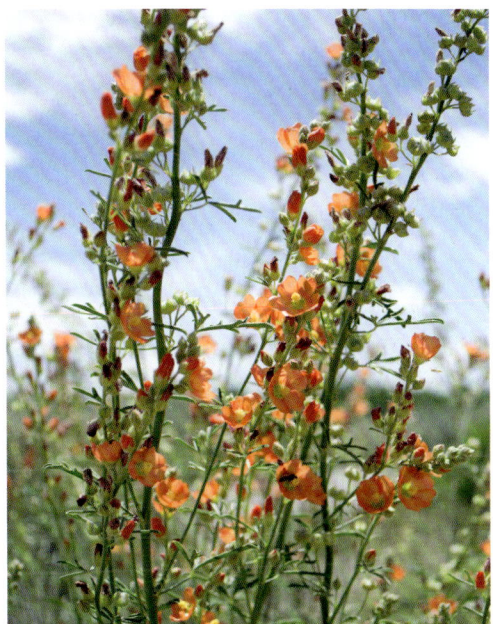

The tall species of globemallow offer a lot of foliage from one plant.

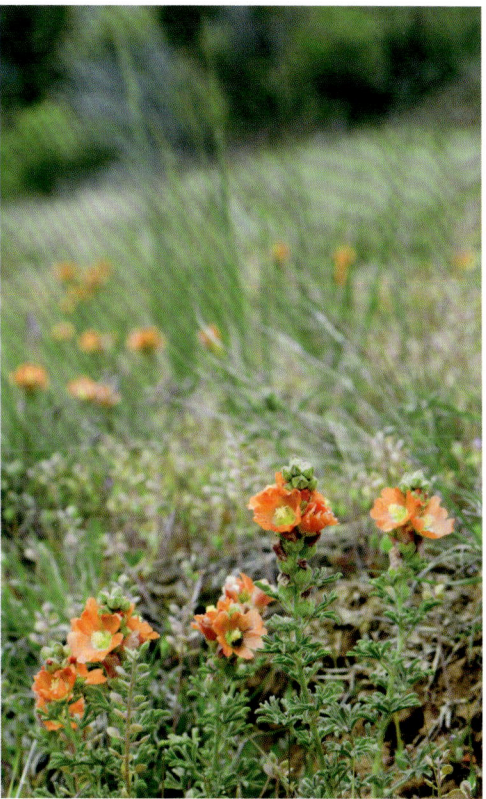

The little globemallows offer the same exact medicine, just less of it per plant.

Cold water infusions help to extract the mucilage in all its glory, as heat can damage the quality of the constituents. Make an oil extraction from dried globemallow flowers and leaves. It can be part of a skin-healing salve. These plants are similar to mallow (*Malva neglecta*) and can be used the same way, though globemallows are not as demulcent and carry more of a floral taste in tea form.

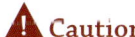 Caution

Consult with a physician if you are taking medications absorbed through the gastrointestinal tract, as globemallow can slow or extend the absorption rate, due to its mucilaginous nature.

Future harvest

This is not a plant that needs to be ripped from the ground. The aerial portions alone are enough to harvest. If digging the root, do so consciously, and never clear an area of it. Harvest roots only in an area with a hundred plants or more, and even then be sure to gather only a few.

HERBAL PREPARATIONS

Tea
Cold infusion
½–1 ounce fresh or dried leaves, flowers, seedpods, or root
1 quart water
Drink all day long.

Oil
Infuse with freshly wilted or dried leaves or flowers.

goldenrod

Solidago species

PARTS USED leaves, flowers, flowerbuds

Late summer sets in as goldenrod blossoms are ready for harvest.
Gather them quickly as they bloom from buds to flowers.

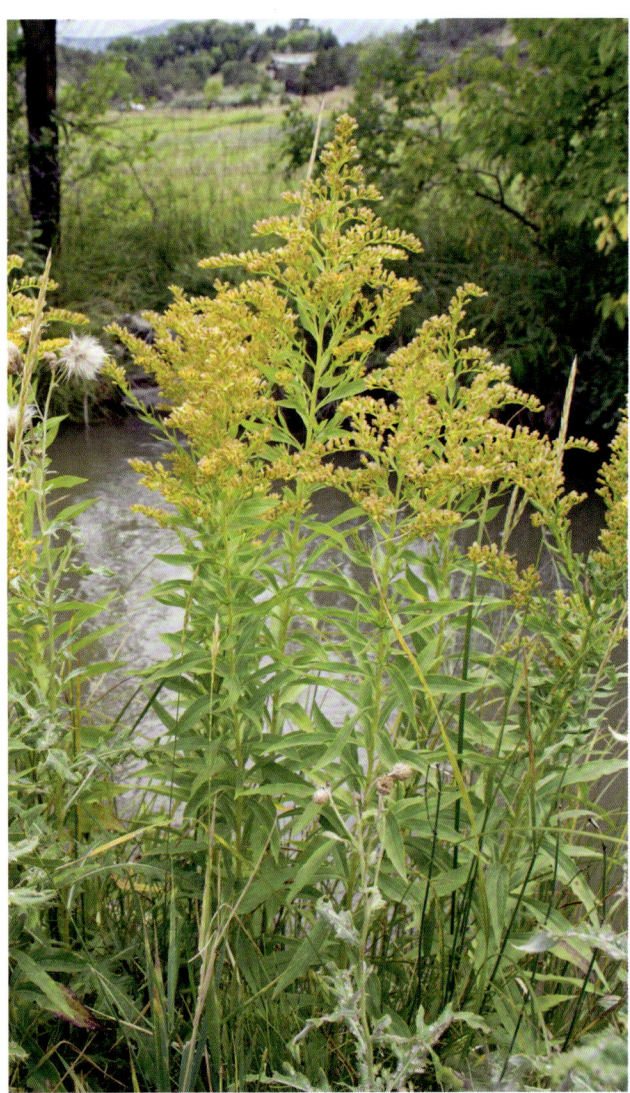

Stands of goldenrod can be found lining irrigation ditches.

How to identify

When in full bloom, goldenrod flowers light up the fence lines with their crescent-shaped heads of clustered yellow flowers. Plants range in height from just shy of a foot to more than 7 feet tall, and they form large stands—where there is one, there are usually many. The stalk is unbranched, and in some species it can be hairy, along with the leaves. Long, lanceolate leaves grow alternately up the stalk. Some leaves have smooth edges, while others are jagged. Many people blame hay fever on goldenrod, but it is a completely innocent bystander, as it is not wind-pollinated.

Where, when, and how to wildcraft

Goldenrod inhabits disturbed soils in partial to full sun, and can be located in fields, along riverbanks, and high up mountain roads. Several species occur throughout the mountain west; all are usually fully bloomed by August in most elevations, so

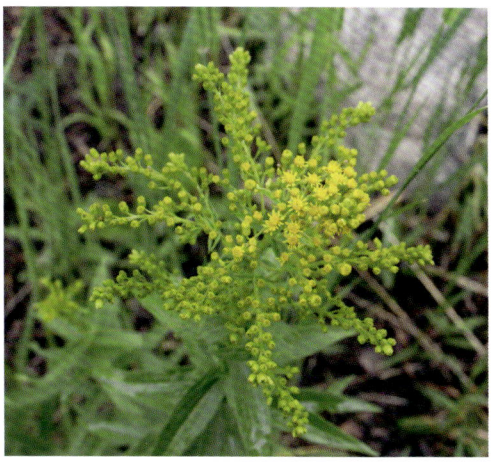

Gather the flowers of goldenrod right as they begin to bloom; this lets them dry without completely fluffing out.

prime harvesting season begins in July and can last late into September.

To gather goldenrod I simply cut the budding or flowering tops at their peak showing. I use them fresh in tinctures, oils, or honey. The leaves can be gathered and dried for teas. Flowers will go to seed and fluff out as they dry, making them unsuitable for tea. Gather when the flowers are still tight in buds, just as some are starting to bloom.

Medicinal uses

Fresh leaves and flowers are good for teas, but they can also be dried and stored for the future. Goldenrod is a useful astringent when allergies strike. The cooling bitterness of goldenrod can be particularly beneficial in fevers accompanied by body aches, nauseous stomach, or diarrhea.

Goldenrod can be used similarly to arnica when infused in oil, providing stimulation and circulation to the area of application. The oil works well on overworked joints that hurt, especially when combined with *Maianthemum* species or alder. Goldenrod as tincture, tea, infused oil, or liniment is also helpful when you feel exhausted, especially in combination with a tired lower back and achy feet.

⚠ Caution

This plant is in the Asteraceae, which can be problematic for people who have an allergy or sensitivity to sesquiterpenes.

Future harvest

By taking only the flowerheads and leaves, the plant is not put into much jeopardy. Be mindful of the smaller, native species and harvest more abundantly from the taller ones.

HERBAL PREPARATIONS

Tea
Hot infusion
2 tablespoons fresh or dried leaves
1 cup water
Drink 3–4 times a day.

Tincture
1 part freshly chopped leaves and flowers
2 parts menstruum (75% alcohol, 25% distilled water)
or
1 part dried leaves and flowerbuds
5 parts menstruum (60% alcohol, 40% distilled water)
Take 10–20 drops 3 times a day.

Oil
Infuse with freshly chopped or dried leaves and flowers.

grindelia

Grindelia species
gumweed, tarweed
PARTS USED leaves, flowers, flowerbuds

Another plant I can never get enough of, even with the basketloads I take home each summer. I find new uses for grindelia every year—this time it's a love affair with infused honey.

How to identify

Grindelia is a small bushy-looking yellow-flowered aster. Its stems are highly branched and full of alternate leaves. Leaves are lanceolate, toothed, and mostly lack a petiole. The yellow disc and ray flowers protrude out of the resinous, sticky, green involucre of bracts. Notice the scaliness and recurved tips of the cupped bract. Flowers vary between species, some (such as *Grindelia nuda* var. *aphanactis*) lacking ray flowers.

Where, when, and how to wildcraft

Throughout the mountain west, find grindelia growing abundantly and robustly in abandoned lots, along roadsides, and in alleyways. Grindelia is ready for wildcrafting in late summer when the sticky yellow buds are beginning to blossom. Bring clippers or scissors to snip the resinous flowering tops and buds, or clip a small bouquet of the stalks with leaves attached.

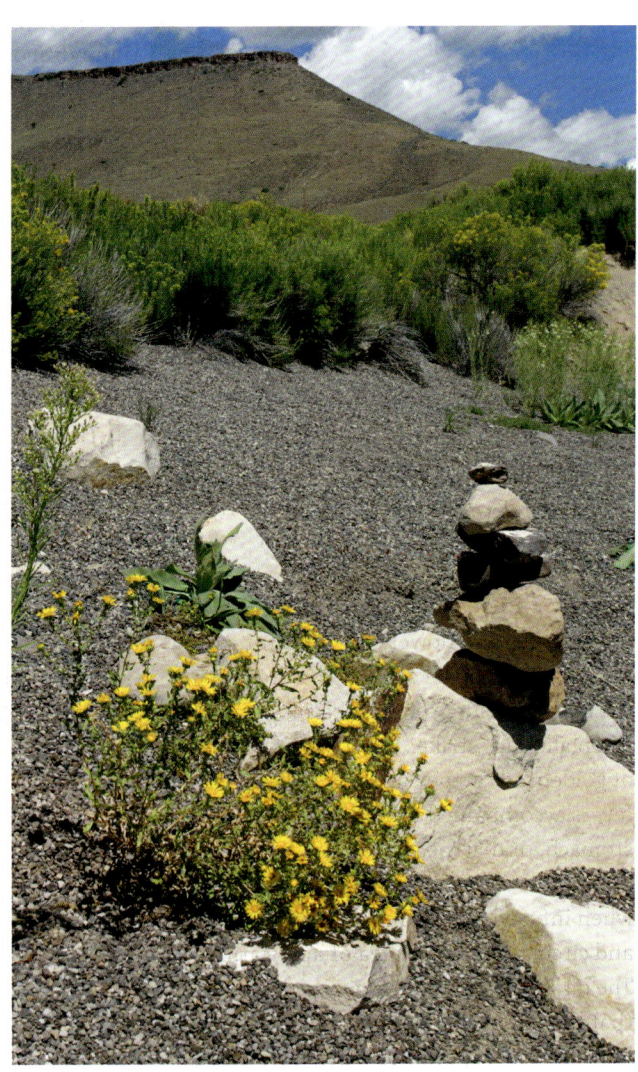

Grindelia squarrosa loves reclaiming disturbed soil.

It's a good idea to have a bottle of rubbing alcohol on hand for squirting on your fingertips, postharvest, to help work off the sticky resins.

Medicinal uses

Grindelia is a key ingredient for many cough syrups, which can be made from the fresh flowering tops in an extraction of alcohol. Use in combination with a mixture of syrups like cherry flower, twig, or berry; plantain; horehound; and hyssop. The tinctured grindelia works well with the respiratory tract as an expectorant, providing a moistening relief to the tissue and helping to loosen mucus when the cough is stuck and dry.

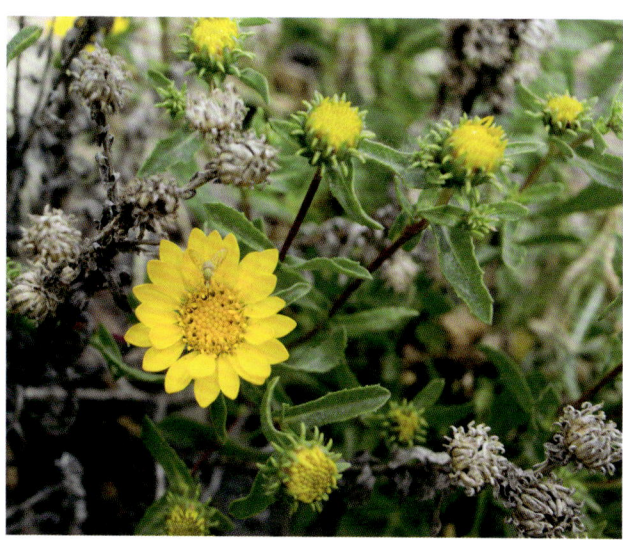

The sticky, resinous flowerbuds of gumweed will leave your fingers tacky and beautifully aromatic.

An infused honey of fresh or dried grindelia is marvelous. It can be used in cough syrups, added to teas, combined in tinctures to create elixirs, or blended with facial care products. Be pleasantly surprised by how strongly the aromatics are preserved in taste and smell.

Grindelia-infused witch hazel provides a perfect toner for sun-damaged, aged, or combination skin associated with chronically inflamed conditions such as acne, eczema, or psoriasis. Try it blended with rose hydrosol for a toning spritz.

Oils infused with grindelia can be used for salves, creams, and serums. It has a healing quality comparable to calendula and can be used as its wild replacement. It acts as a superlative healer to the mucosal and epidermal tissues.

Grindelia makes a quite bitter tea that—though it can be healing when taken internally—is best used as a wash for wounds, or combine the dried herb with others for a healing sitz bath. Try using grindelia in facial steams for purifying and toning the face.

Caution

Grindelia has some potential to be irritating to the kidneys due to its high resin content. Those with a sensitivity to plants in the Asteraceae should avoid it.

Future harvest

Gathering the flowering tops should pose no threat to this rather weedy friend.

Tea
Hot infusion
1 tablespoon chopped leaves, flowers, and flowerbuds
1 cup water
Drink 3 times a day or as needed for coughs.

Tincture
1 part fresh leaves, flowers, and flowerbuds
2 parts menstruum (90% alcohol, 10% distilled water)
or
1 part dried leaves, flowers, and flowerbuds
5 parts menstruum (80% alcohol, 20% distilled water)
Take 20–40 drops as needed.

Oil
Infuse with fresh or dried leaves, flowers, and flowerbuds.

hawthorn

Crataegus species

PARTS USED twigs, flowers, fruit, thorns

Whenever there is a situation affecting the heart, whether emotional or physical, hawthorn is the first herb I turn to.

How to identify

Approximately six species of *Crataegus* inhabit the mountain west. A deciduous tree or shrub, hawthorn produces either red or black berries with large, hard seeds. Some berries are large enough that they resemble crabapples, but you'll know they're not by the large, 1- to 2-inch thorns found on most branches of hawthorn. Leaves are ovate, with either subtle jagged edges or definably larger serrations around the tip and occasionally lobed margins. Small white flowers bloom in clusters; each has five petals, resembling a miniature apple blossom.

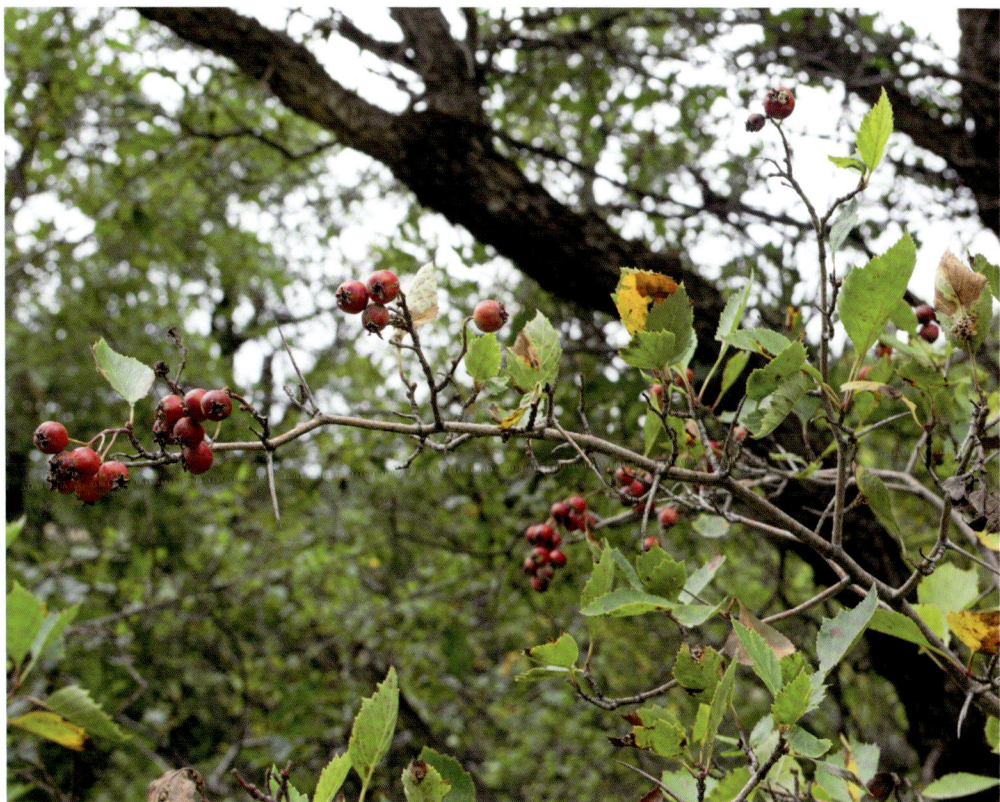

The sharp thorns of hawthorn can be more than an inch long.

Where, when, and how to wildcraft

Hawthorns are found near riverbanks, on the forested hills of the mountains, and in thickets through canyons. Rarely is a single tree found growing alone, which makes it easy to collect an abundance of berries. The berries begin to ripen in late August or September, depending on your location and elevation. Gather the berries when they are deep red or black, being sure to mind the long thorns that arm most branches. If you find most berries are too high to reach, spread a blanket or sheet around the base of the tree and shake the ripe berries down.

Flowering twigs can be collected in spring. Clip the ends of flowering branches when the trees are displaying their delicate white blooms.

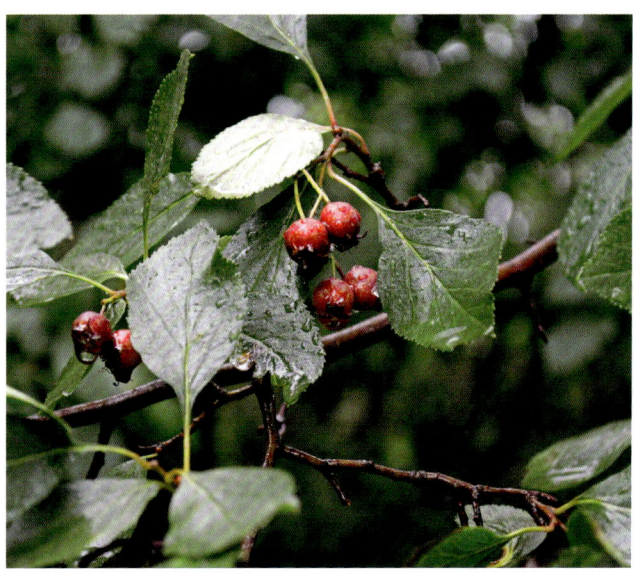

Crataegus species brighten the mountain west with their berries each fall—if it looks like a small crabapple but grows on a thorny tree, it is probably hawthorn.

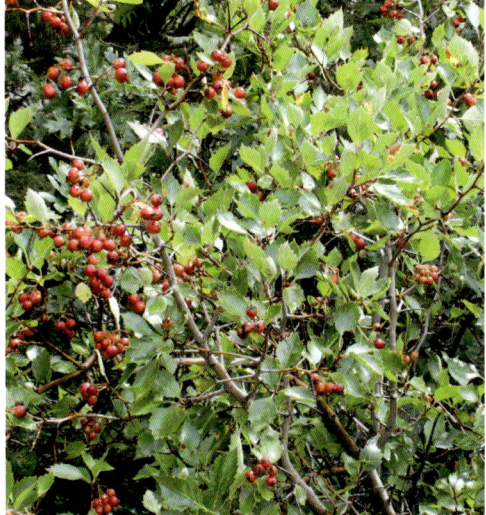

A blight that causes browned leaves and flowers affect hawthorns. Be sure to collect only from healthy specimens, like this one.

Medicinal uses

The berries, twigs, thorns, and flowers of hawthorn have a strong affinity for the heart, helping to heal emotional wounds and strengthening the physical organ. The berries have been proven to act as a trophorestorative, improving the heart's circulation and its ability to uptake oxygen. Hawthorn helps to dilate blood vessels.

Hawthorn berries can be a useful remedy for individuals who are anxious or feel the weight of the world too keenly. It is an herb I turn to when major trauma happens in someone's life, such as death, heartbreak, or shock, and for sufferers of post-traumatic stress disorder.

The cooling energetics and slightly moistening actions of hawthorn make it a favorable additive to summer teas, iced or hot. It blends well with mallow, rose, pineapple weed, and wedge of lemon. The tart, pectin-rich berries can aid in digestion or be used in bitter formulations.

Extractions of hawthorn can include any combination of berries, thorns, flowers, or twigs. Extract the berries in alcohol, vinegar, or honey or simmer them into a syrup. Make hawthorn honey starting in the spring with the fresh flowers, along with a few twigs, and then add the fresh berries in the fall.

An infused oil can be used in protective balms or anointing oils. Powdered hawthorn berries are a luscious ingredient to add into skincare products like masks, scrubs, and serums. The powder is pectin-rich and full of flavonoids, which benefit the skin. Try combining the powder with raw honey, jojoba oil, or glycerin; other powdered herbs like mallow or aloe; or powdered clays for a mud mask.

Caution
This herb will not help serious heart conditions.

Future harvest
Always leave berries behind for the animals.

HERBAL PREPARATIONS

Tea
Hot infusion
1–3 teaspoons flowers or thorns
1 cup water
Decoction
1 ounce fresh or dried berries, twigs, or
  thorns
1 quart water
Drink 1–2 cups 3 times a day.

Tincture
1 part fresh berries, twigs, thorns, or flowers
2 parts menstruum (75% alcohol, 25%
  distilled water)
or
1 part dried berries, twigs, thorns, or flowers
5 parts menstruum (60% alcohol, 40%
  distilled water)
Take 30–60 drops 3–5 times a day.

Oil
Infuse with fresh or dried flowers, twigs, thorns, or berries.

horehound

Marrubium vulgare

PARTS USED leaves, stems, flowers

Horehound has a long-standing use in cough drops for its superb ability as an expectorant. Helps dampen a throat tickle, too!

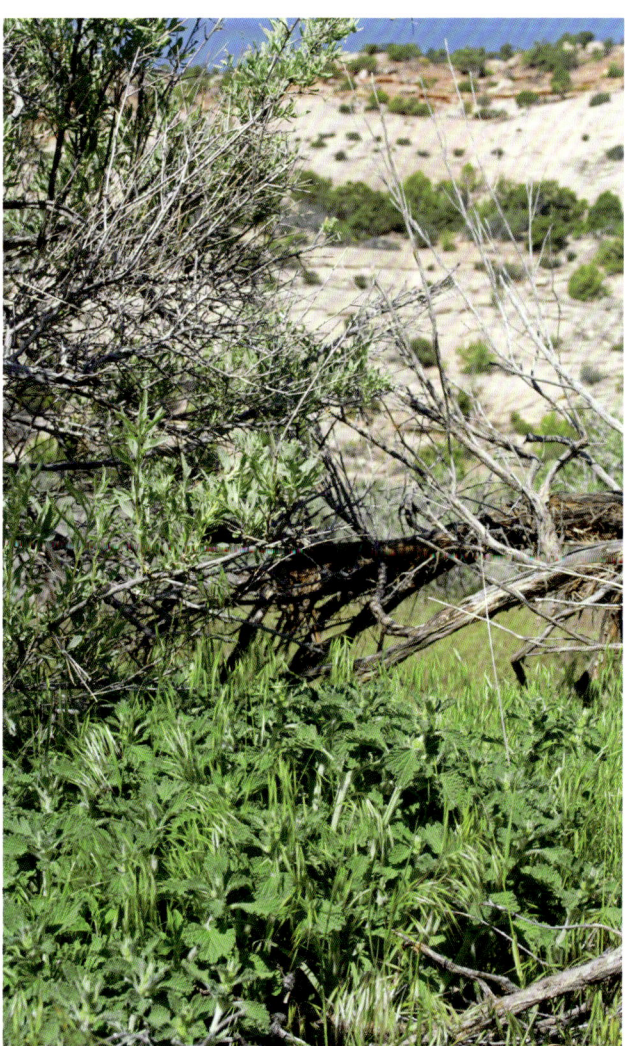

A weedy friend of the mountain west, horehound grows abundantly in the lowlands, deserts, and canyons.

How to identify

This greenish gray plant has a stem covered in woolly white hairs that make it glisten silver in the sunlight. As a member of the mint family, it has the characteristics of a square stem and opposite leaves. The soft, fuzzy leaves are toothed, rounded, and crumply-looking because of the deeply impressed veins. Undersides of the leaves are lighter in color. Find the flowers growing in rounded, ball-like clusters that surround the stem. They are small, white flowers, with sharp bracts that make it a poky and clingy burr once dried.

Where, when, and how to wildcraft

Find horehound in abandoned places of the west. It will take over disturbed spaces in urban or agricultural areas. It likes dry soil and lower elevations such as the Front Range of the Rockies and the desert west.

Harvest from spring until midsummer. Simply clip or pinch the top few inches of

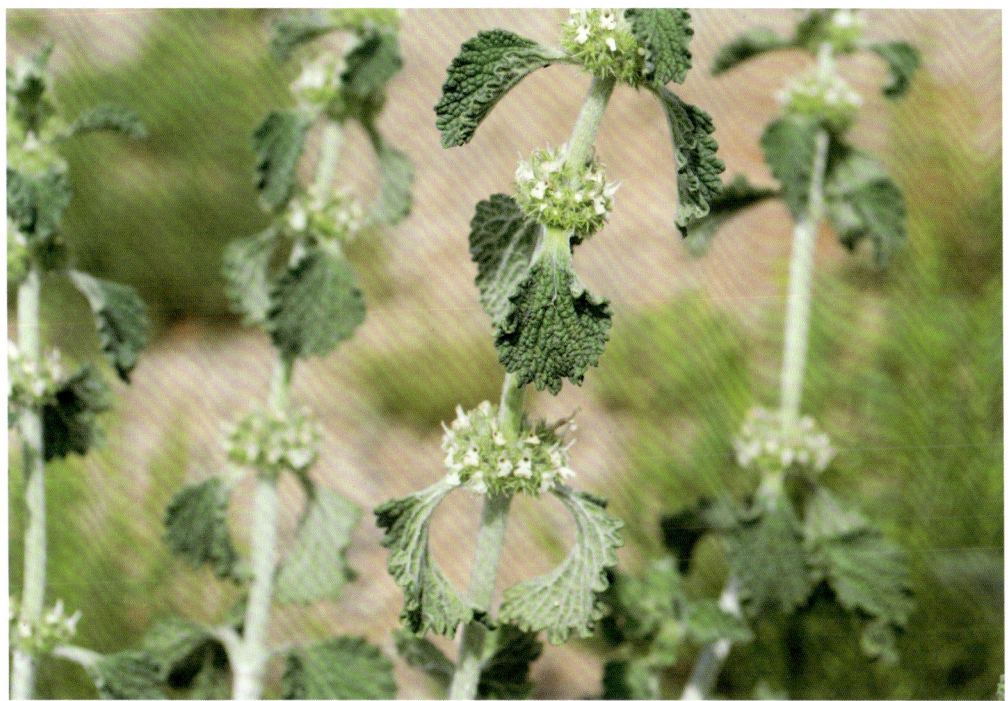
The silverish hue of horehound comes from all the little hairs that grow all over the stems and leaves.

the plant, which will harbor a lot of foliage. Spread on mesh or wire racks for drying.

Medicinal uses

Horehound can be a superb herb to use when bronchial infections are creeping into the lungs. It helps to expectorate and thin the mucus to make it easier to cough up and out. An infused honey or syrup is great to have on hand for a raspy voice or irritating cough. It has a long history of being widely and commercially used in cough drops. Adding honey or other moistening herbs, such as Siberian elm or globemallow, can be an excellent balance to the bitter and drying properties of horehound.

Future harvest

This grows as a prolific weed in parts of the west. Always respect its habitat but feel free to take plenty.

HERBAL PREPARATIONS

Tea
Hot or cold infusion
1–2 tablespoons fresh or dried leaves, flowers, and stems
1 cup water
Drink 3 times a day.

Tincture
1 part fresh leaves, flowers, and stems
2 parts menstruum (75% alcohol, 25% distilled water)
or
1 part dried leaves, flowers, and stems
5 parts menstruum (60% alcohol, 40% distilled water)
Take 15–25 drops 3 times a day.

Oil
Infuse with fresh or dried leaves.

Equisetum species

PARTS USED aerial portions

Horsetail, being high in minerals like silica and calcium, is a must-have in assisting the healing of connective tissue or bone injuries.

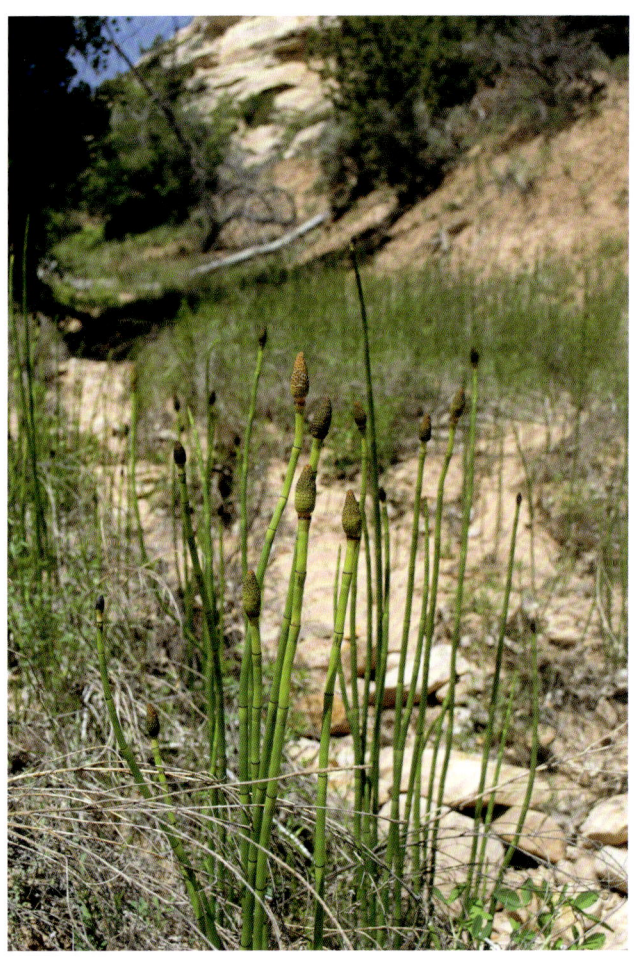

Sometimes you will stumble upon horsetail that appears to be growing in the dry, desert landscape. However, if you pay attention to your surroundings, you will notice that the dry path you are hiking is no doubt transformed into a flowing waterway when the rains come.

How to identify

If you have ever walked along the bank of a river or stream, you surely have noticed horsetail. It is a plant that has a look all its own. It is almost prehistoric, or out-of-this-world-looking when compared to the flora growing around it. Some species are single, slender stalks that are jointed together, others have jointed stems that branch out at every joint along a central stalk. *Equisetum arvense* and *E. palustre* have the look of a horse's tail with their long, strand-like branches. *Equisetum laevigatum*, *E. variegatum*, and *E. hyemale* have the slender single stalks that are jointed together. Each of these stalks can be pulled off and separated from the plant.

Where, when, and how to wildcraft

Find horsetail along waterways, where it thrives on the shorelines. Harvest from spring until late summer. As the seasons progress, the higher you climb in elevation the younger the horsetail becomes. Harvest by picking or trimming the stems a few inches from the ground. Species that have whorled branches should be picked while the branches reach for the sky.

Medicinal uses

The joints can be picked apart, the tender pieces that fit into each other are tender enough to nibble and suck on, creating an herbal juice in your mouth with little taste. This is a great source of silica and is best taken by eating or drinking in tea infusions. Silica helps the body absorb calcium properly. Horsetail happens to be high in both silica and calcium, making it a superb herb to use in mineral-building tea blends. Use when there is a degeneration of bones or injury resulting in cartilage damage, fractures, or breaks. It can help strengthen connective tissues. Horsetail can be extracted in vinegar, but it is best used in tea form through either an infusion or a decoction.

Horsetail can also be combined with other herbs such as stinging nettle, wild rose, and globemallow for a hair rinse. Make a hot infusion of the herbs, creating a tea that you can drink while taking a bath and use as a final rinse before leaving the tub.

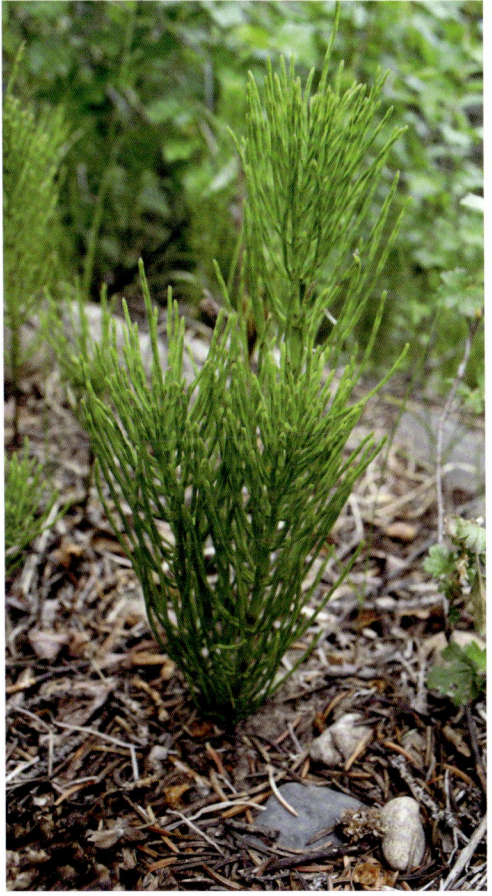

Young *Equisetum arvense* ready for a light picking in the spring.

Hair Rinses

A hair rinse is a creation of dried herbs that through various means nourishes the scalp and hair. Some herbs to use include horsetail, alfalfa, and stinging nettle; they provide hair-vitalizing minerals such as silica and calcium. Others such as globemallow, mallow, and Siberian elm bark help to hydrate dry locks.

To begin, blend your herbs together and store in a glass jar. Add 1–3 tablespoons per cup of hot water and steep for 15 minutes. Strain well, sip a bit if you'd like and then pour over your head after or during a shower. Wring your hair out without rinsing for maximum benefits.

Not only is it beneficial to pour a hair rinse over your head after a shower, but it is a tea blend I drink as well. Nourish your insides and exterior beauty simultaneously.

For many applications, horsetail should be dried and ground to powder. Add the powder to tooth-brushing blends. Infuse it in oil and add it to salves. It is beneficial in an oil or glycerin base for healing stubborn wounds and burns. Also it promotes elasticity in the skin and can help heal sun-damaged skin.

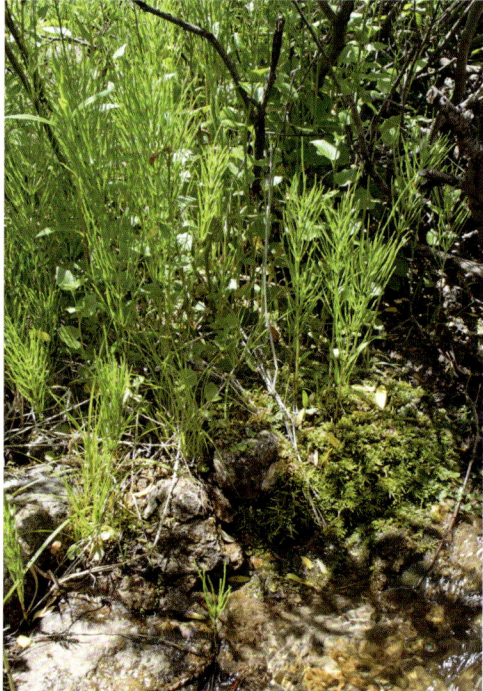

A creekside thick with horsetail; if gathering, make sure to leave enough of the plant behind for it to maintain a healthy life.

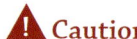 **Caution**

Gather horsetail only from areas where the watershed is clean. Horsetail can absorb heavy metals and chemicals from the soil, as well as unwanted nitrates.

Large amounts of horsetail can be potentially irritating to the kidneys or urinary tract due to the high mineral content.

Future harvest

Be careful not to rip the plant from the ground; you want to be sure the stand remains healthy and continues to flourish.

HERBAL PREPARATIONS

Tea
Hot infusion
2 tablespoons fresh or dried aerial portions
1 cup water
Drink 3 times a day.

Vinegar
1 part fresh aerial portions
4 parts vinegar
Take 1 tablespoon 1–3 times a day.

Oil
Infuse with fresh or dried aerial portions of horsetail.

hyssop

Agastache species
horsemint
PARTS USED leaves, flowers

Hyssop leaves release a light licorice-like flavor when crushed and chewed.

How to identify

The most common hyssop in the Rocky Mountains is nettle-leaf giant hyssop, *Agastache urticifolia*, which has leaves that look like stinging nettle without the stingers. Leaves are wider at the base, ovate, and toothed all the way to the tip. When you come across a stand of hyssop, you may think it is mint or possibly catnip on steroids. Giant hyssops can grow upward to 3 feet or more. When you smell a crushed leaf, you will notice it isn't mint-like, but mustier like catnip with a hint of licorice. The eastern slope of the Rockies has a species, *A. foeniculum*, which also has stinging-nettle-shaped leaves, and super-strong licorice-fennel-like aromatics and taste. For identification, this can be differentiated from *A. urticifolia* by its size—it tends to get to only about 3 feet or less in height.

Flowers become whiter as they are exposed to the hot sun, whereas the newly bloomed spikes are light pink or lavender. The flowering spike never seems to bloom entirely at once. Upon closer inspection you will notice the trumpet shape of the flowers and the extra long stamens and stigmas peeking out.

Where, when, and how to wildcraft

Find hyssop's tall blossoms waving in the wind from late spring at lower elevations

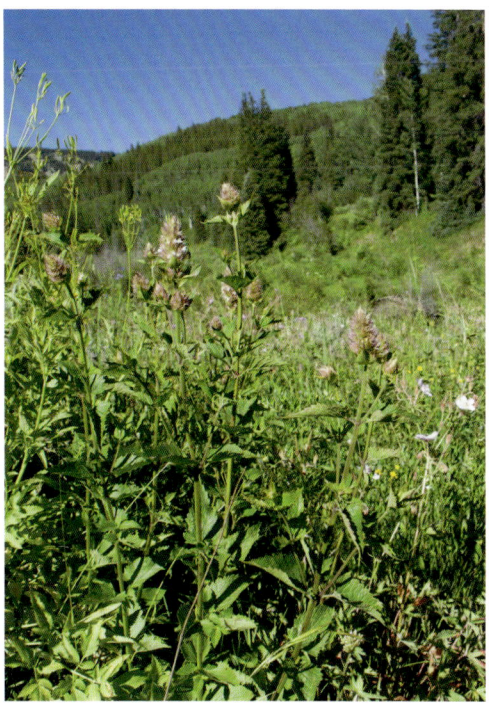

Mountain hillsides are often full of fragrant hyssop.

through summer higher up in the mountains. Look for it in lush mountain meadows and in the partial shade of woodlands. Harvest the aromatic budding flowers when they are in full bloom on a sunny dry day. Leaves start to lose their flavor from the heat of summer; they are best gathered early in that season.

Pinch or cut off some of the flowering stalk and some leaves. Take only a little from each plant in a large stand.

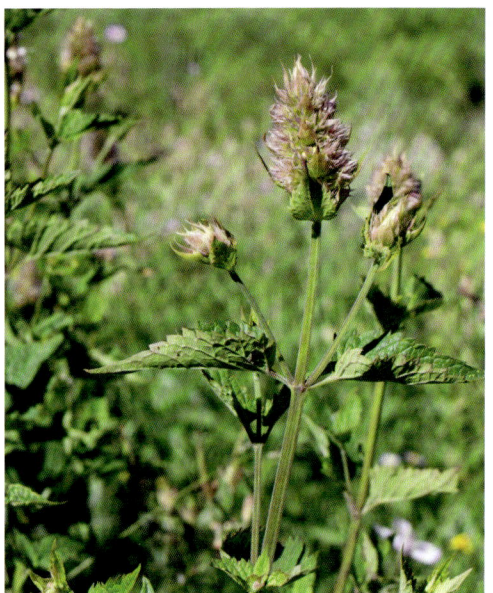

The alternate leaves give hyssop a resemblance to stinging nettle before the flowers bloom.

Medicinal uses

The aromatic leaves and flowers of hyssop, while fresh or dried, make lovely tea or honey. The flavor is licorice-like with a slight mustiness. It works well against coughs, providing some soothing relief to the chest. Hyssop can be used in fever formulas, as it can help bring about sweating and has a calming effect. The aromatic properties can be useful in dispelling gas or settling an upset stomach.

Future harvest

The reason you never see only one hyssop plant is because it spreads through underground roots called rhizomes. Since the plant is not spreading strictly by seed, it is okay to gather flowerheads, but be respectful of the pollinating insects and leave plenty of flowers behind.

HERBAL PREPARATIONS

Tea
Hot infusion
2 tablespoons fresh or dried leaves and
  flowers
1 cup water
Drink 3 times a day or as needed.

Tincture
1 part fresh leaves and flowers
2 parts menstruum (75% alcohol, 25%
  distilled water)
or
1 part dried leaves and flowers
2 parts menstruum (60% alcohol, 40%
  distilled water)
Take 20–40 drops 3 times a day.

Oil
Infuse with fresh or dried leaves and flowers.

juniper

Juniperus species
PARTS USED twigs, leaves, fruit

The blue cones or "berries" of juniper have a pungently warm and bitter action, making them useful in formulas for creating better digestive flow.

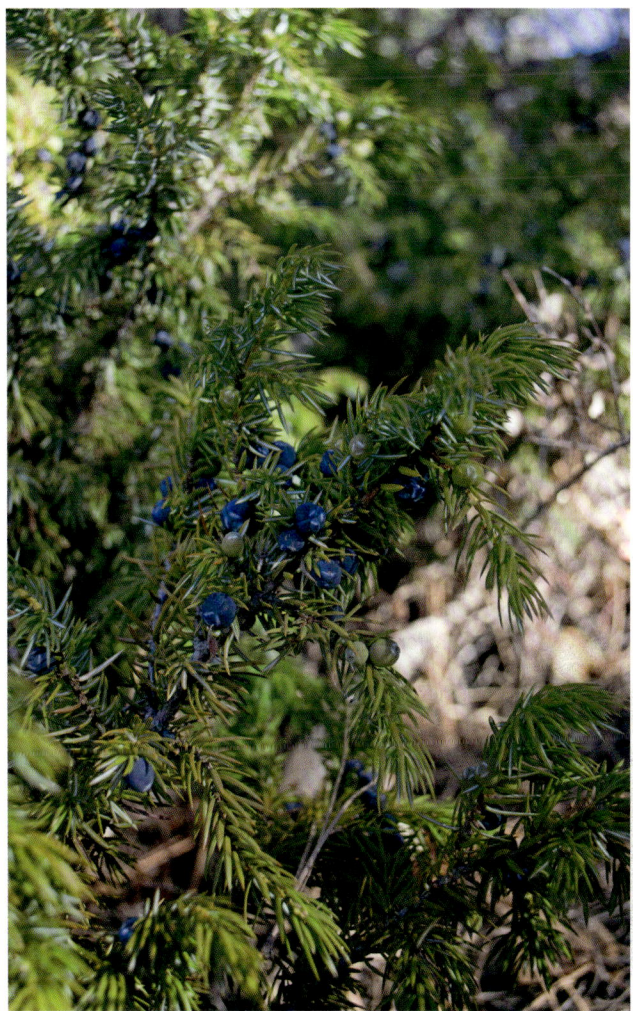

The bright royal blue berries of juniper are best gathered toward the end of fall, when the cool nights have made them sweeter and more flavorful.

How to identify

Juniper grows either as a ground-dwelling shrub or as a trunked tree. Branches have scaly evergreen leaves that are rough or needle-like. The berries are in fact soft, flesh-covered cones. All species of juniper have green immature berries that ripen to a chalky deep royal blue. Common species of the mountain west are Utah juniper (*Juniperus osteosperma*), common juniper (*J. communis*), and Rocky Mountain juniper (*J. scopulorum*).

Where, when, and how to wildcraft

Juniper can be found all over the mountain west and southwestern Canada. Find it growing in landscaped yards or clinging to canyon walls. Juniper likes a dry climate, growing alongside piñon pine or sagebrush. Branch tips and leaves can be collected all year, but gather the berries when they reach a royal blue color in late fall through to early spring. I gather juniper berries by raking my fingers through the leaves, releasing the berries into a basket I hold below. Clip the branch tips and take some leaves when gathering the berries.

Medicinal uses

Juniper is one of the first herbs I turn to for bladder infections, as long as the person does not have a kidney infection or weakness going on at the same time. As an antimicrobial herb, the crushed berries combine well with uva-ursi, mallow, and dandelion leaf for a tea to drink. A lovely bitters can be made from the berries as well. Juniper combines well with other conifers, especially piñon or fir. Try using an already-infused juniper honey to blend with the tincture for a delicious bitters elixir.

Topically, it can also be used in antifungal formulas. Oil infused with juniper berries or leaves combines well in salves or creams that soothe dryness and protect the skin from the elements of sun, wind, and cold. A spritz of hydrosol helps to rejuvenate the skin and soothes sunburn.

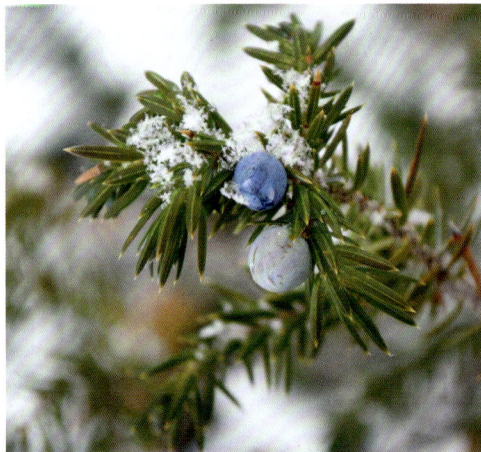

Juniper berries, twigs, and needles can be gathered throughout the winter.

Use the fresh twigs and leaves to inhale in a pot of herbs when a cold or sinus infection has you plugged up. Add in usnea or stored-away mallow for their properties of hydrating dry tissue.

Juniper branches can be bundled along with artemisias or other aromatic plants of the west for a smudge stick. Burn to clear bad energies from a space.

Caution

Pregnant women or people with known kidney disease should not consume juniper berries or foods that include them. Juniper is not recommended for long-term use.

Future harvest

Junipers provide a lot of food for animals during the winter months. Be mindful of where you are foraging and harvest only where berries are plentiful.

HERBAL PREPARATIONS

Tea
Hot infusion
1 teaspoon fresh or dried berries
1 cup water
Drink 3 times a day at onset of bladder infection, for 1–2 days only.

Tincture
1 part fresh berries
4 parts menstruum (75% alcohol, 25% distilled water)
Take 10–20 drops 3 times a day for no more than 3 days.

Oil
Infuse with fresh or dried twigs, leaves, or berries.

---

linden

Tilia species
American basswood
PARTS USED flowers

Linden helps to calm and nourish the heart and nervous system. Do try by taking a deep inhale when blossoms are fresh.

How to identify

Linden trees are tall, full-looking trees, often with low branches and short trunks, growing to heights between 30 and 100 feet. The densely branched trunk is straight; often, more than one trunk comes from one spot. The bark varies by species. It is gray or brown in color and can be furrowed, fissured, or may have flat ridges. The leaves are heart-shaped with unequal bases and are serrated around the margins. They may be smooth on top with soft hair on the underside. Flowers are a pale yellow with five petals and hang in clusters on a stem from a leaf-like bract. Bracts are long, narrow, and pale in color compared to the vibrant green leaves. The flower stem attaches to the center vein of the bract. Nuts are round and hard, containing a pair of seeds.

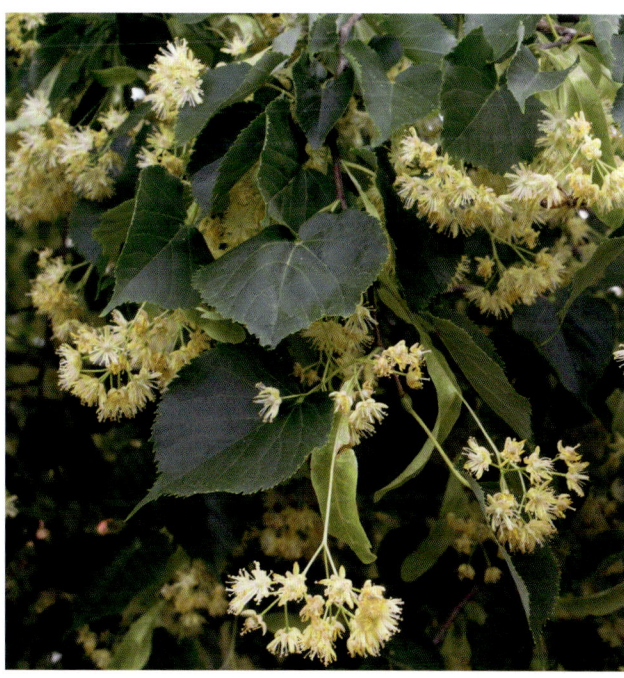

Find linden trees planted throughout towns and cities of the west.

Where, when, and how to wildcraft

The scent of linden trees reaches you long before you turn the corner and realize the entire street is lined with this beauty. Flowers begin blooming in late spring and continue into midsummer. The blooms of a particular tree, however, can be gone quickly—be ready to harvest as soon as you begin to enjoy their sweet aromatics in the air. Harvest in summer from a tree that is loaded with highly aromatic flowers. It is very easy to pick a lot of flowers quickly from a large, old tree. Gather nuts in late summer, and crack them open with your teeth to get to the small seeds inside.

Medicinal uses

When the heart needs more flow of vital forces, or love, linden can be a perfect addition. The flowers have a calming and sedative effect that can be brought on by just smelling the fragrance of the flowering tree. Linden can be beneficial for the overagitated or restless adult or child, bringing relief to panic attacks, nervous tension, and anxiety.

With slightly demulcent properties, linden is another lovely herb to use when blending teas in the dry states of the west. It has uplifting and relaxing actions, along with cooling energetics. Linden-infused honey is a delicious addition to teas, syrups, or elixirs when there is a fever, cough, or stuck mucus in the lungs or nose.

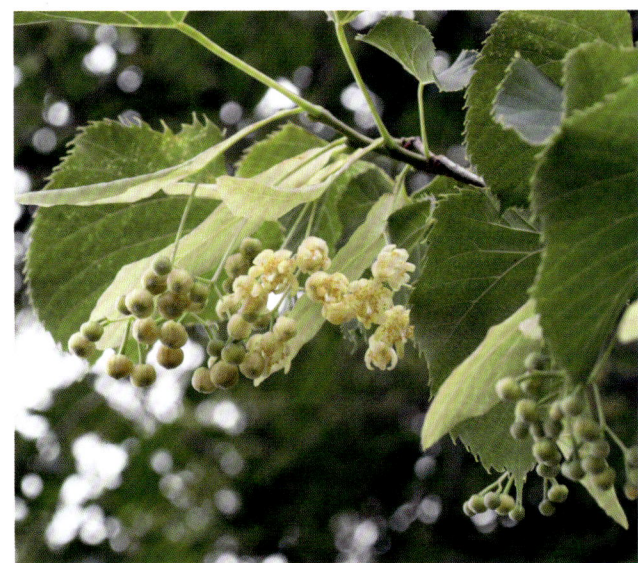

The sweet fragrance of linden flowers fills the air in the spring and early summer in lower-lying towns of the mountainous west.

Caution

Consult with a physician if you are taking medications absorbed through the gastrointestinal tract, as linden can either slow or extend the absorption rate, due to its mucilaginous nature.

Future harvest

Linden trees are generally not found growing wild in the mountain west. Be leery of gathering near heavily trafficked roads, landscaped buildings, and municipal areas. Find a happy tree in the yard of someone who does not use chemicals on their lawn, and ask permission to gather there. Linden flowers provide a lot of nectar for bees, so be careful of these buzzing friends and try not to take too much from them.

HERBAL PREPARATIONS

Tea
Hot or cold infusion
2 tablespoons fresh or dried flowers
1 cup water
Drink as needed.

Tincture
1 part fresh flowers
2 parts menstruum (75% alcohol, 25% distilled water)
or
1 part dried flowers
5 parts menstruum (60% alcohol, 40% distilled water)
Take 20–40 drops as needed.

Oil
Infuse with fresh or dried flowers.

mallow

Malva neglecta
cheeseweed, common mallow
PARTS USED roots, leaves, flowers, seedpods

Mallow is one of the great demulcent weeds of the west, completely
underutilized and hugely abundant. Check your yard for this lovely medicine!

How to identify
Mallow has palmate leaves with a texture of soft velvet from the tiny hairs that can be found on most of the plant. The rounded edges of the leaf are scalloped, making the leaf look ridged. Leaves stem from long petioles arising from a taproot. The plant forms basal leaves at first, and then leaves grow alternately up the flowering stalk. Flowers are white to soft pink and usually have darker pink or purple stripes radiating from the flower's center to the heart-shaped tips of the petals. Seedpods are disc-shaped and look like a cheese wheel.

Where, when, and how to wildcraft
This introduced weed grows all over the west, primarily below 8000 feet. Mallow is a drought-resistant plant that does well in rocky or dry, disturbed soils. It is mostly found near places that have been frequented by people and is not so common in the

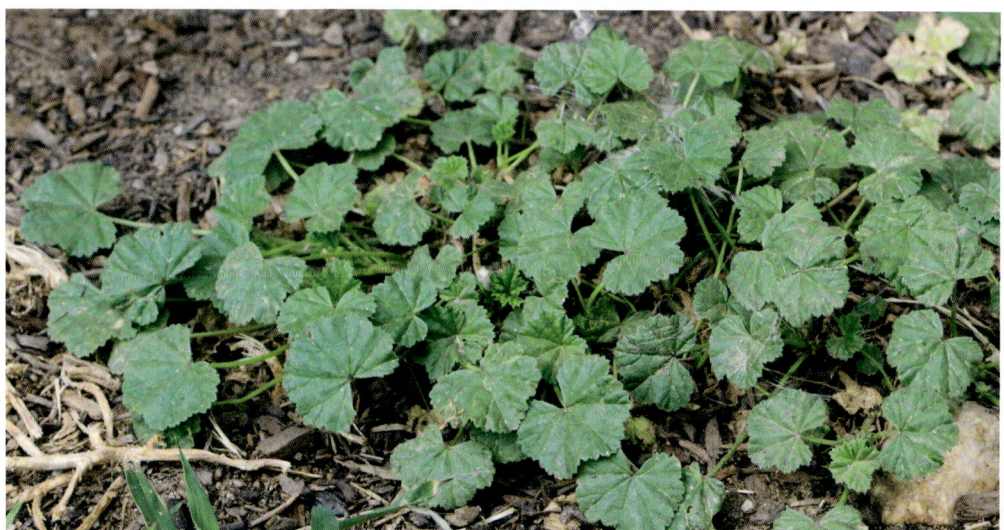

An abundance of mallow graces the mountain west, harboring in alleyways, across open fields, and at the edges of parks. Mallow is a plant to gather all through the summer for its leaves, roots, flowers, and seedpods.

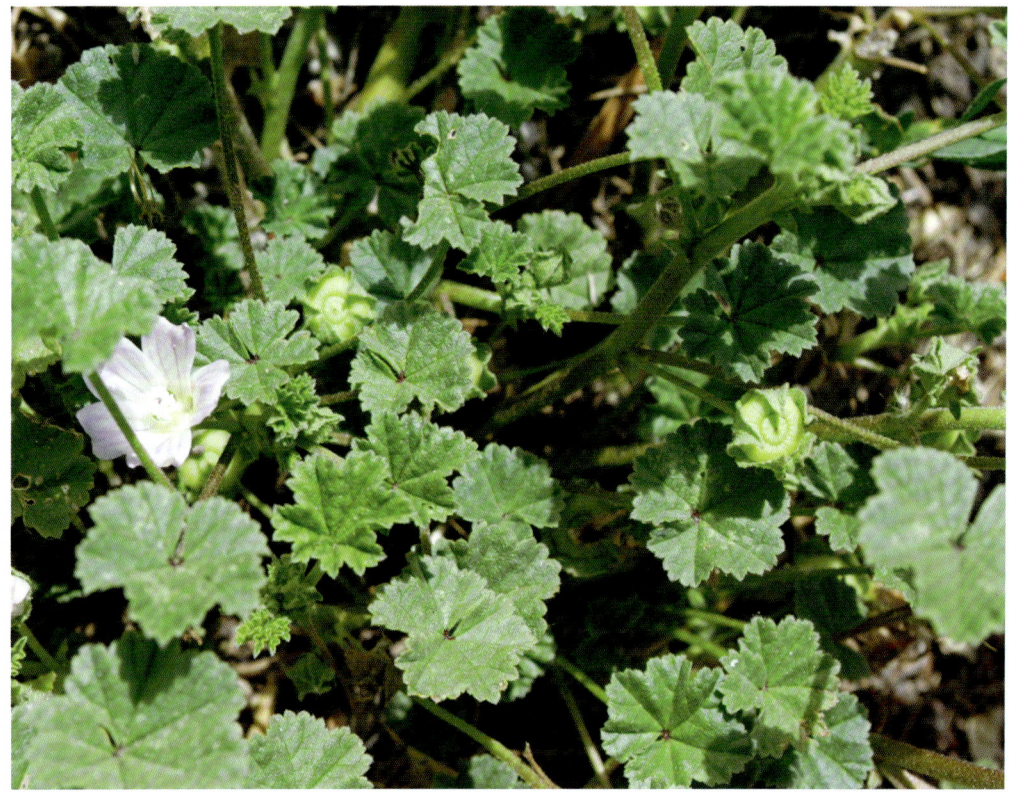

Pick the greenest leaves, the blossomed flowers, and the seedpods to make a cold infusion that will provide extra hydration for you on the driest days.

wilderness. Gather the basal leaves and roots in spring, the flowers in summer, and then toward the summer's end, the seedpods. The whole fresh plant can be uprooted from spring through summer and is entirely medicinal. The cheese-wheel-looking seedpods are a favorite foraged treat and can easily be gathered by plucking.

Mallow leaves and stems are full of minerals, which show the efficiency of the root system for pulling them out of the soil. This also means you should not harvest near contaminated soils or old mines.

Make bundles of fresh herb for a simple way to dry and crumble the leaves. Simply clip the plant about 4 inches down along the main stalk. Always look for stems abundant in foliage. Tie the clipped ends tightly together and hang the herb bundle upside down, in a dry spot that is out of direct sunlight. In about a week the leaves will be dry enough to crush off the stems and store in a clean jar.

Medicinal uses

Mallow may look like a common weed, but in fact it should be treasured as one of the west's best herbs for the constitutionally dry individual. It is a demulcent herb that brings much needed moisture to the internal systems of the body. Signs of dryness where mallow is beneficial can be nosebleeds, itchy skin, dry lips, sore throat, dry unproductive cough, or constipation. A cold infusion that is left to steep for at least 25 minutes can bring major relief when drunk regularly or daily.

Teas can also be used for inflammations or infections of the urinary tract, gastrointestinal tract, or lungs. Dry itchy eyes can be relieved with a rinse of a thoroughly strained tea of mallow leaf or root.

The leaves, fresh or dried, can form a poultice for bringing down topical inflammation or relieving pain. This can be useful with bug bites or stings, or weeping or infected wounds. The fresh leaves can be juiced for the ultimate green goodness. Used internally or externally, this slightly gooey liquid is superb for infections of any mucous membranes or sunburns. Freeze it in ice-cube trays for later use.

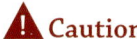 Caution

Consult with a physician if you are taking medications absorbed through the gastrointestinal tract, as mallow can either slow or extend the absorption rate, due to its mucilaginous nature.

Future harvest

Mallow is a nonnative, hardy-growing plant. You need not worry about harvesting the whole plant; however, as it grows annually, gathering all the seedpods for consumption can limit next year's growth. If you would like to propagate mallow, let the plant self-seed, replant seeds, or use cuttings.

HERBAL PREPARATIONS

Tea
Cold infusion
1 ounce fresh or dried leaves, root, flowers, or seedpods
1 quart water
Decoction
3–4 tablespoons fresh or dried root
1 quart water
Drink the quart throughout the day or as needed.

Oil
Infuse with fresh leaves, flowers, or root.

Mormon tea

Ephedra species
jointfir
PARTS USED stems

The unique appearance of Mormon tea makes it an easy herb to spot while moving through the desert landscape.

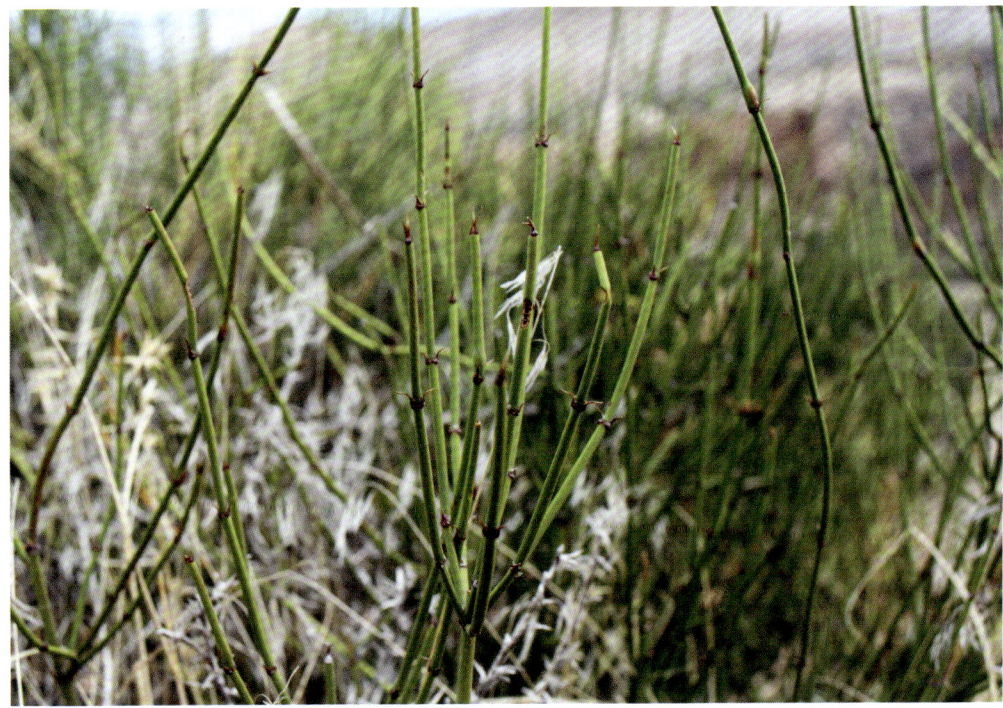

Mormon tea is a plant lacking all the obvious, usual parts, such as noticeable leaves and flowers.

How to identify

A unique desert-residing shrub, Mormon tea can be distinguished by its jointed green stems that appear leafless and without flowers. This prehistoric-looking plant does in fact have leaves; however, they are small and scale-like, fused closely around the stem. It is the junctions of these leaves that make Mormon tea stems appear jointed. *Ephedra* is a gymnosperm, meaning it produces spores that look more like a cone than a flower. The male and female cones of Mormon tea make this plant more similar to a pine or juniper tree than a flowering plant.

Where, when, and how to wildcraft

Mormon tea can be harvested anytime throughout the year in the desert lowlands of western Colorado, Utah, and Nevada. Even with snow covering the ground, Mormon tea should still be visible with its green antenna stems branching toward the sky. Clip sections of the jointed stems from many different shrubs, trying not to impact one area or a single plant too much.

Medicinal uses

Mormon tea stems can be chewed while you hike through the desert, giving a pleasant taste and maybe even a touch of energy.

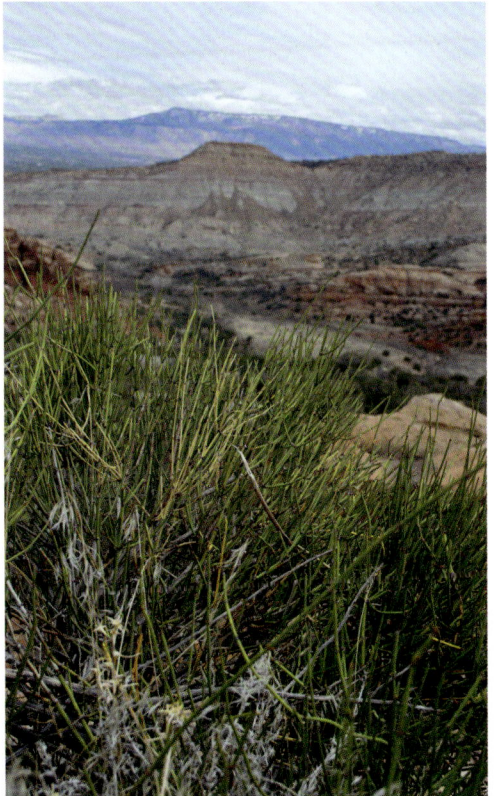

This alien-looking plant, Mormon tea, is a desert native and has a long-standing use as medicine by Native Americans and Mormon settlers.

Chewing the stems can also help if you are suffering from allergies, relieving clogged sinuses and a runny nose.

Drinking the tea or taking tincture of Mormon tea has provided relief from the symptoms of allergies or a cold. Its high calcium content is a good addition in nourishing tea brews. This herb has diuretic, astringent, and anti-inflammatory properties, which make it useful in urinary tract infections.

Caution

Make sure you are gathering only the wild varieties of *Ephedra* species. *Ephedra sinica*, often used in ornamental plantings, is far more potent and a rather different medicine. It is very stimulating and should be used only with professional guidance.

Future harvest

Mormon tea should be harvested with care. Trim only a few inches from each plant, spreading your harvest out throughout many stands.

HERBAL PREPARATIONS

Tea
Hot infusion
1 tablespoon fresh or dried stems
1 cup water
Drink as needed.

Tincture
1 part fresh stems
2 parts menstruum (75% alcohol, 25% distilled water)
Take 10–20 drops 3 times a day.

Oil
Infuse with fresh or dried stems.

motherwort

Leonurus cardiaca
lion's tail, lion's heart
PARTS USED leaves, stems, flowers

Motherwort helps to soothe the anxious and worried mindset occasioned by parenthood and life in general.

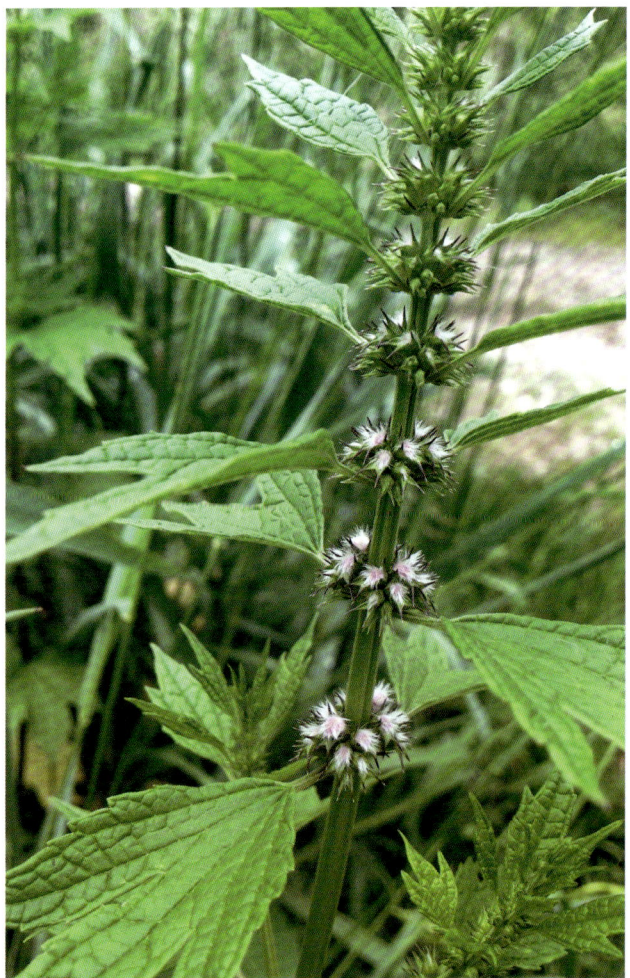

Chewing on the bitter leaves of motherwort brings an immediate calm to the entire body.

How to identify

Motherwort is part of the mint family, and in North America it is a weedy perennial. The more mature lower leaves tend to be palmately lobed, while the younger leaves that grow closer to the top are trilobed. Leaves have impressed venation and grow opposite along the square stem. Flowers are pinky purple and two-lipped with flower parts in fives. The calyx becomes very spiky when dried and will tend to stick to clothes or shoes.

Where, when, and how to wildcraft

Motherwort likes to grow in disturbed areas at lower elevations. Find it on the borders of trails or woodlands. Harvest when the leaves are vibrant, from spring until late fall. Leaves can be dried, but preparations such as oil infusions or tinctures made with fresh leaves are much stronger. The whole plant can be cut fresh and tinctured.

Medicinal uses

Motherwort is a very bitter, drying and cooling, nervine herb that acts upon the nervous system, bringing relief to anxiety and dampening stress responses. It is well suited for nervous sweaty palms, anxious new parents, highly strung individuals, or the frazzled burnt-out student. A few drops of tincture or sips of tea instantly bring a calm to the body. It combines well with skullcap, wild rose, and valerian flowers for a calming tea or tincture formula.

Motherwort can be used for relieving menstrual symptoms, such as cramping and bloating. For women going through perimenopause it can be a cooling herb which relaxes the nerves and helps during hot flashes. The leaves and flowers can be infused into oils for uterine belly rubs or cramp-relieving salves. This herb has a profound effect on circulation.

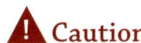 Caution

Not for use in pregnancy, and caution is advised in perimenopausal women, as motherwort has been shown to increase menstrual flow.

Future harvest

Motherwort grows as a wild weed, and a mint family plant at that. Harvest as much as you'd like.

Nervine

Herbs that are relaxing, calming, or nourishing to the nervous system are nervines. They can be sedative (hops), muscle-relaxing (pedicularis), sleep-enhancing (valerian), or calming to the nerves (skullcap). Some nervine herbs, such as wild mint or beebalm, can also stimulate the nervous system, promoting circulation.

HERBAL PREPARATIONS

Tea
Hot infusion
1–3 tablespoons fresh or dried leaves, stems, and flowers
1 cup water
Drink as needed.

Tincture
1 part fresh leaves, stems, and flowers
2 parts menstruum (75% alcohol, 25% distilled water)
or
1 part dried leaves, stems, and flowers
5 parts menstruum (60% alcohol, 40% distilled water)
Take 10–20 drops 3 times a day or as needed.

Oil
Infuse with fresh or dried leaves, stems, and flowers.

Sorbus scopulina
rowanberry, fireberry
PARTS USED fruit

*The tart, astringent medicine of mountain ash berries lends itself well
to vinegar extractions and sipping tonics for supporting the immune system.*

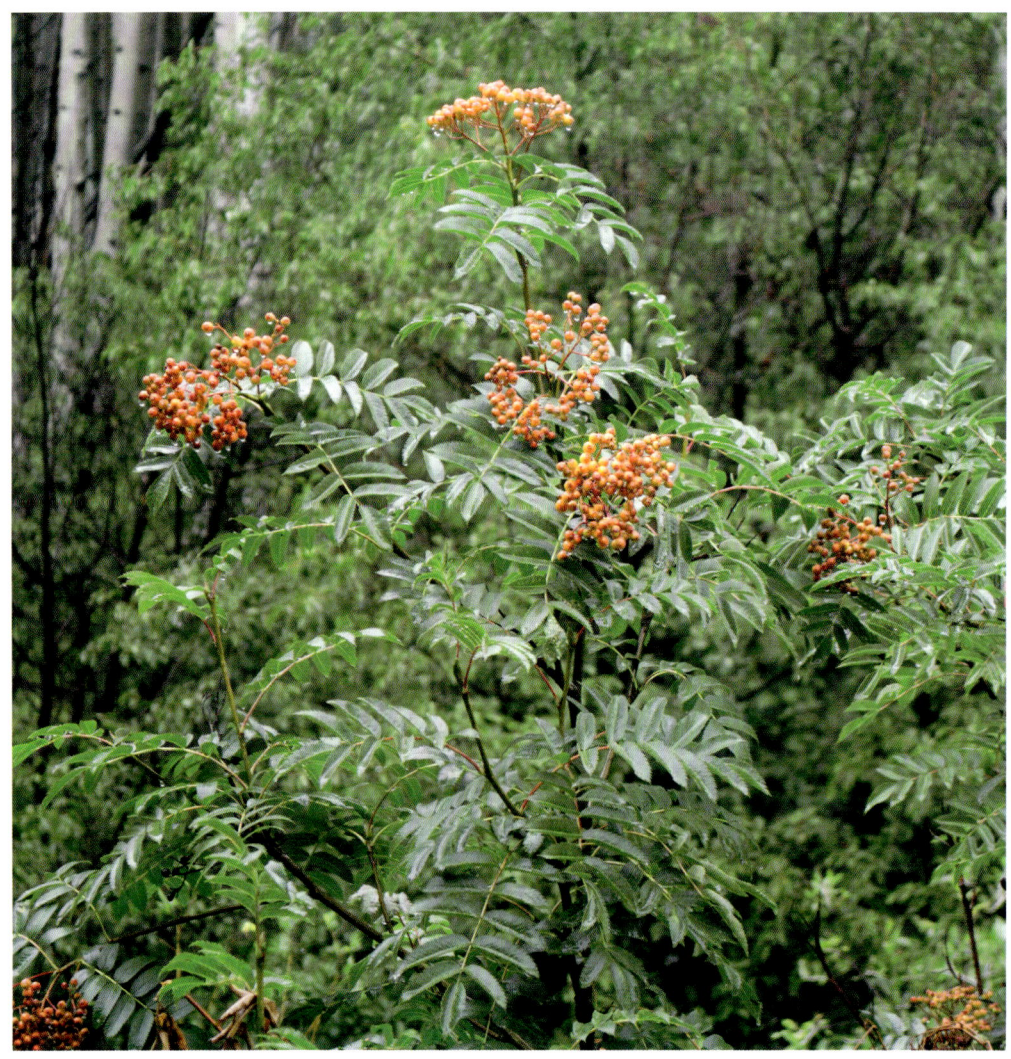

Mountain ash is a common shrubby tree at higher elevations in the mountain states.

How to identify

Mountain ash is a shrub-like deciduous tree, capable of reaching moderate heights of up to 20 feet. Leaves are made up of nine to 12 pinnately compound, lanceolate leaflets with serrated margins. The entire leaf grows alternately along the branches. The tree resembles an elder (*Sambucus*) with its clusters of white flowers and compound leaves; however, mountain ash has more leaflets than elders, and if you rub the leaves of mountain ash, they do not give off the distinct unpleasant odor that elder leaflets do. Being a member of the rose family, the berries look like miniature apples, growing in clusters, turning from fiery orange to red when ripe.

Where, when, and how to wildcraft

Find these trees at the openings of conifer forests in the foothills and mountain valleys. Berries are best gathered after the first few frosts; cold snaps set the sugars in the fruit, which softens the berries and renders them less sour. Watch your step, though, as the trees often grow on rocky slopes. European mountain ash (*Sorbus aucuparia*), a common ornamental, can be used similarly.

Mountain ash berries grow in clusters, making them easy to gather quickly. Snip the clusters into a basket and pick the berries off the stems at home. When processing your harvest, discard any hard or discolored berries, along with the stems. The berries go quickly, so time your harvest right; wait until after at least one frost before you gather.

Medicinal uses

Mountain ash berries are bitter and somewhat acrid, providing a circulatory action. This makes the berries useful for bitters formulas, helping the flow of digestion. Tincture of the astringent fruit can be helpful for sore throats. Berries are also high in flavonoids and are immunostimulating, making them useful for recovering from illness. An infused honey of fresh mountain ash berries can be made in the fall for use in teas or elixirs.

Caution

Mountain ash leaves, seeds, and bark contain a small amount of cyanogenic glycosides, which can convert into a potentially toxic substance in the human body. Although mountain ash is regarded as completely safe to use, large quantities of seeds eaten at one time could be toxic.

Future harvest

Gathering the berries should have no implications, but as always, leave some behind to support wildlife.

HERBAL PREPARATIONS

Tincture
1 part fresh berries
2 parts menstruum (75% alcohol, 25% distilled water)
Take 10–20 drops 3 times a day.

Vinegar
1 part fresh berries
4 parts vinegar
Take 1 tablespoon 1–3 times a day.

---

mullein

Verbascum thapsus

PARTS USED roots, leaves, flowers

Flowers for the ears, leaves for the lungs, and roots for the spine make mullein mighty fine.

How to identify

The mighty mullein is a biennial plant, having thick, long, fuzzy basal leaves in its first year. The leaves are pale green and covered in hairs that make them soft to touch. The following year it will send up a giant stalk that will be studded with little yellow flowers. Flowers will start blooming in summer, one by one, the whole stalk never flowering all at once. While some flowers bloom on the tall dense stalks, many will be in bud and others will have gone to seed. Stalks are usually singular, but sometimes a plant sends up several tall spires.

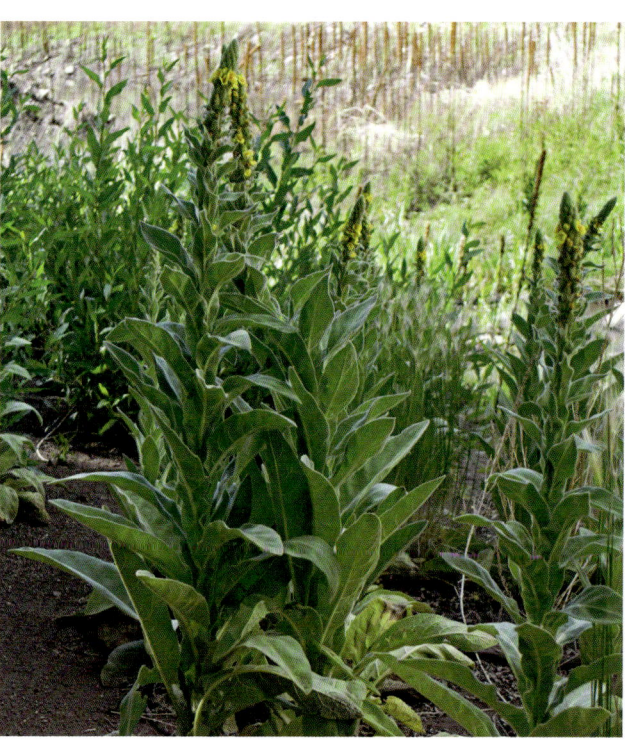

Find mullein growing out of control in disturbed areas.

Where, when, and how to wildcraft

Find mullein taking hold along roadways, helping to clear exhaust from the air. The pollutants from the road are something we do not want to take home, so harvest your mullein far from where cars travel.

Gather the roots of first-year mullein in the spring or fall. Dig up the young rosettes for both the roots and leaves. Roots can be chopped up fresh and then dried. Gather the flowers by plucking them one by one out of the stalk. Flowers can also be dried and stored for later infusions.

Medicinal uses

Mullein has many uses that are valuable to each of us at some point in our lives. Take for instance that first earache of a child—the

Ear Oil

Ear oils should be in every new mother's medicine kit. Many children will have at least one earache or infection during childhood. This can accompany teething, come on with viruses, or be associated with other issues relating to cranial bone structure or fluid retention. Combine the following ingredients, fresh or dried, in a glass jar:

- Mullein flowers act as an analgesic, are antiviral, and bring circulation to the ear.
- A clove of garlic brings its warming and extra pathogen-fighting ability. Chop and dry, or roast garlic clove at 250°F for at least 10 minutes first.
- Cottonwood buds reduce the inflammation and relieve the pain, while also carrying antimicrobial properties.
- Beebalm can be another powerful addition to bring warm circulation to the area and act as an antifungal or antimicrobial agent.

Pour your oil of choice, such as olive oil, over the herbs, so that they are covered in 3 times the amount of oil. Place jar in double boiler, and let the mixture heat for at least 2–4 hours. Strain your oil extremely well, using a coffee filter or tea bag.

If you used fresh herbs, reheat your oil to separate any leftover water. After warming for at least an hour, pour off the top oil, leaving any residual cloudy oil behind—this is the trapped water that gets stuck at the bottom of the jar.

Let your oil cool before using in the ears. Test warm oil on the inside of your wrist for temperature first before administering. Place 3 drops into the ear canal, and cover with a cotton ball. Keep head tilted so that the oil can move its way in. Apply this as needed for earache pain relief.

Caution: Use ear oil only if you are certain there is no perforation to the ear. If you choose to warm your oil, be very careful it isn't too hot. Do not use cottonwood buds if you are allergic to aspirin.

flowers infused into oil make such a lovely pain-relieving remedy. Use it along with dry or roasted garlic (never raw garlic, which kept in oil raises the possibility of botulism); fresh twigs and buds of aspen, willow, or cottonwood; and fresh or dried leaves of beebalm. The pain-relieving properties of the mullein flowers help to soothe the inflamed middle ear.

Mullein root provides support to the structure of the body as an internal or external remedy. Extract it with alcohol for use as a tincture or liniment. An oil infusion can be made for use in salves or massage oils.

Mullein offers a sense of alignment when you are feeling out of sorts at the structural level. Use it during or after bodywork sessions to help maintain the benefits of the treatment. It can encourage lubrication to spinal vertebrae, fascia, and joints, improving health of cartilage, which could possibly be from it giving increase in synovial fluid. It is good for structural alignment, spinal injuries, bruises, nerve injuries, and swollen joints that are weak and painful. Mullein root and Saint John's wort flowers, along with an antispasmodic like hops or nonnative lobelia, can dull nerve pain such as sciatica, relieve or unkink a stiff neck or muscle spasms, and can assist in bringing you back to a more balanced state.

The leaves are famous for soothing coughs, helping to moisten up the lungs and loosen stuck mucus. They are also popular in smoking blends; I find it to be quite harsh in larger quantities.

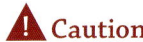 Caution

The seeds of mullein are toxic and should not be consumed. The dried hairs of the leaves can be irritating, both internally and externally. Because of this, it is important to make sure to strain your tea of mullein leaves through a fine strainer, such as a coffee filter or tea bag.

Future harvest

Mullein is one of the hardiest, tallest, and loveliest perceived noxious weeds around. It's often targeted for spraying with herbicides, so be careful where you gather; keep away from deformed or yellowing plants.

If you want to create a neighborhood of mullein in your own yard—which I will warn, city officials have been known to discourage—simply take home dried tops of the stalk and shake the seeds over your yard.

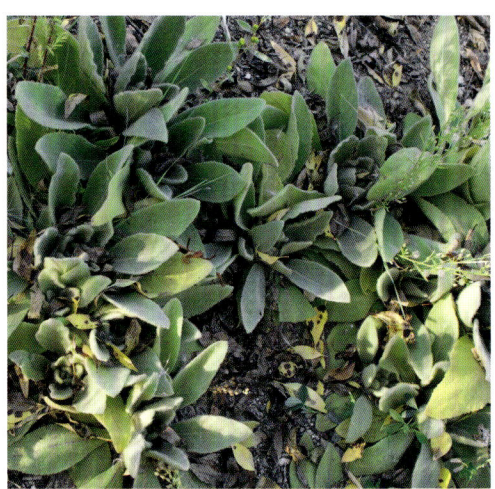

The best time to harvest the roots of mullein is in the plant's first year of growth, when it shows only the rosette of leaves.

HERBAL PREPARATIONS

Tea
Hot infusion
2 tablespoons fresh or dried leaves
   or flowers
1 cup water
Decoction
1 ounce fresh or dried root
1 quart water
Drink 1 cup 3 times a day.

Tincture
1 part fresh root, leaves, or flowers
2-3 parts menstruum (75% alcohol, 25% distilled water)
or
1 part dried root, leaves, or flowers
5 parts menstruum (60% alcohol, 40% distilled water)
Take 20-40 drops 3 times a day.

Oil
Infuse with fresh or dried root, leaves, or flowers.

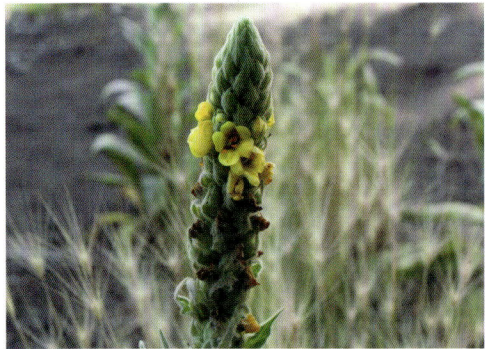

Flowers of *Verbascum thapsus* need a gentle but sturdy pinch to be plucked off the stalk.

northern bedstraw

Galium boreale

PARTS USED leaves, stems, flowers

A simply useful herb, full of nutrients, northern bedstraw can be found in many places throughout the Rocky Mountains.

How to identify

Northern bedstraw has small skinny leaves, growing in whorls of four at each node along the stalk. Leaves are toothless but have fine hairs along their edges. Stems are smooth and square, becoming branched only toward the top, where flower clusters form. Flowers are white with four white petals and pointed tips.

Where, when, and how to wildcraft

Northern bedstraw can be found on mountain slopes, throughout conifer and aspen forests, or in moist meadows with partial shade. The young tips of the plant are best before the plant buds, blooms, and goes to seed; gather them then. Collect flowers and leaves when they are present. Simply clip off the part of the plant you are interested in.

Medicinal uses

Since northern bedstraw is such a prevalent plant of the

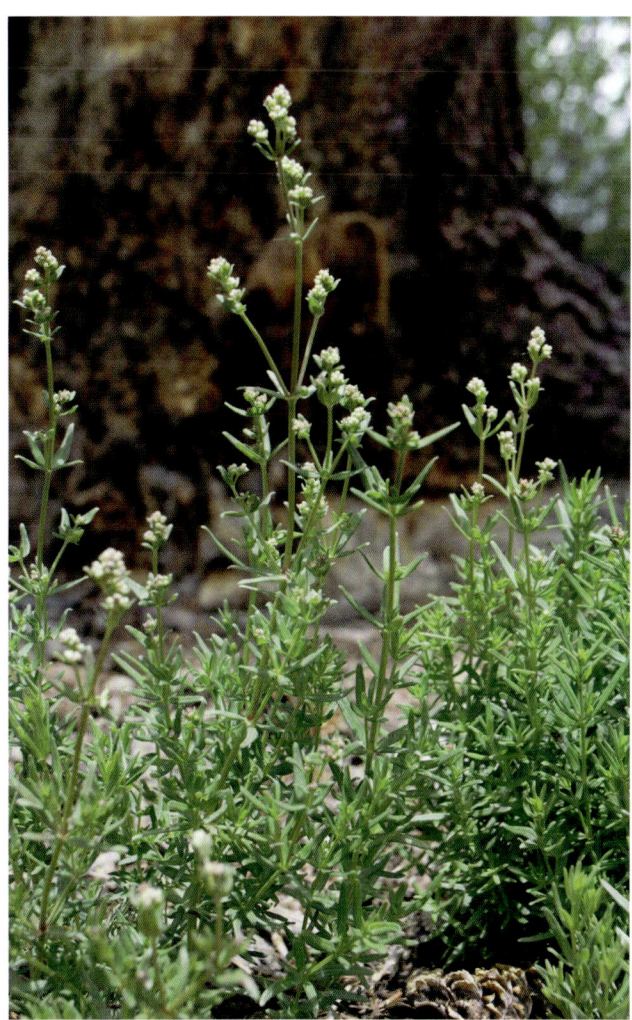

Find little patches of northern bedstraw around the base of conifer trees or spread throughout meadows.

west, it is easy to harvest bundles as needed. The fresh plant is best to use for making tea, adding to soup stocks, infusing into vinegars, or juicing for its large vitamin and nutrient content.

Sip an infusion of fresh or dried northern bedstraw to help relieve bloating, for internal ulcers of the mouth or stomach, and to relieve swollen glands. It is a cooling and drying herb that can also be applied fresh as a poultice to skin irritations. The fresh or dried plant can be infused into oils for use as a skin regenerator. It can relieve skin issues such as psoriasis, eczema, boils, cysts, or wounds.

Future harvest

Northern bedstraw is a hardy perennial that grows in colonies through a horizontal root system and also spreads by seed. Your wildcrafting will have minimal impact on it, particularly if you harvest only the stalks.

HERBAL PREPARATIONS

Tea
1 tablespoon fresh or dried leaves, stems, and flowers
1 cup water
Drink as needed.

Vinegar
1 part fresh leaves, stems, and flowers
4 parts vinegar
Take 1 tablespoon 1–3 times a day.

Oil
Infuse with fresh or dried leaves, stems, and flowers.

Quercus species

PARTS USED bark, twigs

Oaks come in all shapes and sizes, and the bark and twigs
of every species can be utilized as medicine for easing pain.

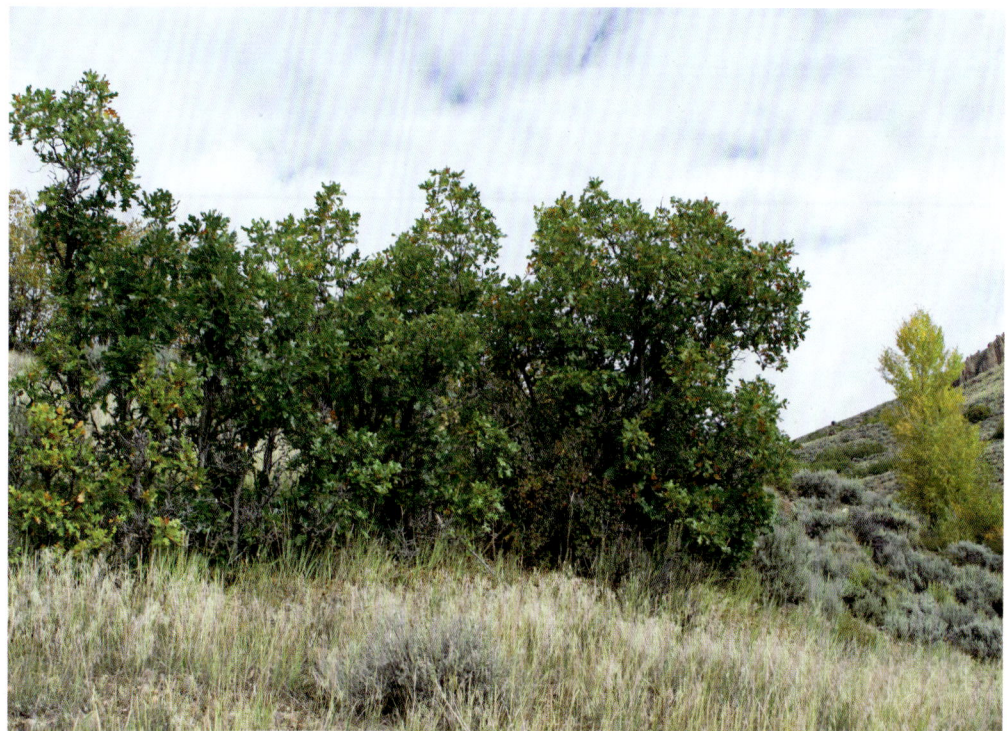

Stands of scrub oak fill pockets of the mountain west, growing among the juniper, serviceberry, and sagebrush.

How to identify

Many oaks tower above all the other trees in the neighborhood. These tall oaks have large, deeply furrowed trunks that rise to many branches. The leaves are lobed, thick, and shiny. The fruits are acorns, which vary in size and shape depending on habitat and species.

Our oaks of the wild west are much smaller and scragglier than the larger landscape specimens. Scrub oak (*Quercus gambelii*) is our most widespread native shrubby tree in the lower western Rocky Mountain states. It averages heights of 10–30 feet, growing much taller if it has an adequate water source. Leaves have the common trait of family members in the Fagaceae, with anywhere from seven to 11 deep lobes; they are a deep green and so shiny they look waxy.

The scraggly scrub oak forests are nearly impassable, and the hillsides they cover are lit up each autumn with their red fall color. The acorns are under an inch in size with a scaly cap that covers about a third of the nut. Acorns start out green and turn brown with age and ripeness.

Where, when, and how to wildcraft

Scrub oaks grow on dry hillsides in the southwestern portion of our region, in large stands among sagebrush, serviceberry, and prickly pear. Gather the bark or twigs in spring or fall when the sap is running rich in the tree. Twigs can be chopped into small pieces for drying or using fresh. The fresh bark can be peeled from the branches and used dried or fresh.

Medicinal uses

All species of *Quercus* can be used in the same ways. I use oak bark in my formulations for teas that ease sore throats, swollen glands, or diarrhea. The anti-inflammatory and astringent properties of this cooling bark are also fitting for sitz baths, wound soaks, or jock itch. Oak bark or twigs can be infused into oils for pain-relieving rubs or salves. The powdered herb can be used for first-aid application to open wounds, burns, or sores. It helps to stop the bleeding, lessen the pain, and astringe the wound.

Caution

The tannins in oak can be irritating to the stomach when drunk in large and frequent amounts.

Future harvest

Trimming a few branches from each tree or collecting windfallen branches will have no effect on the vitality of oak trees. Always make sure to gather bark with the tree's life in mind. Peel from pruned or fallen branches. Never peel or girdle the trunk of a living tree.

Oregon grape

Mahonia repens
grape root
PARTS USED roots, leaves

*The evergreen leaves of Oregon grape would flag
this amazing medicine all year round, if not for the snow.*

How to identify

Oregon grape is a bit of a misleading name for a plant that grows so low to the ground with no vines attached. The compound leaves are evergreen and reminiscent of holly leaves; they are deep green, waxy-feeling, and thick with jagged edges that can be sharp to the touch. The small flowers are bright yellow and carried in a dense raceme. Berries start out green but turn a deep purplish blue when fully ripe. When the inner root bark is scratched, it will show bright yellow.

Where, when, and how to wildcraft

You will find Oregon grape growing in pine forests, rocky slopes, and sagebrush lowlands. Gather the roots and leaves in spring and fall.

Roots are thin and long and shallow in the ground. Be gentle when tugging up this root—it grows more like a runner, and other plants around can easily be disturbed. Carefully dig around the base of a mature plant until you

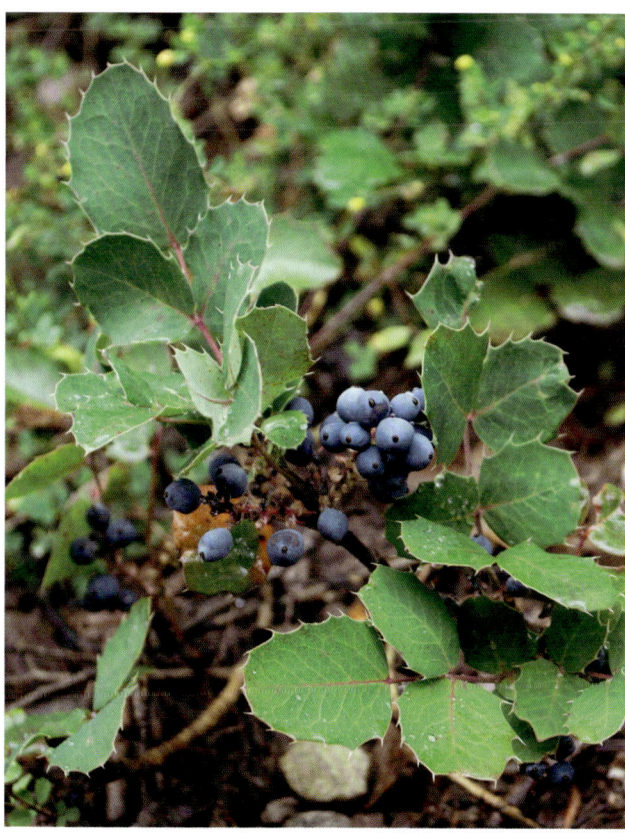

Find the tart, bright blue berries of Oregon grape in late summer and fall. They could be a nice addition to a bitters formulation involving the root.

come upon one of its rhizomatous runners. Cut off a section of the root, taking this as your medicine, and leaving at least 6 inches

Mountain Bitters: Sore Throat Elixir

This elixir can be used as a daily bitter tonic to take before or after meals. Cottonwood buds, Oregon grape root, wild hops, and alder in a tinctured bitters formula can be very stimulating to the appetite, while supporting more bile secretion, which helps with digestion.

Additionally, this same bitters formula can also work well for sore throats and coughs. It has a drying and warming action that may be helpful when a fever is present accompanied by a sore throat. This sounds counterintuitive, but since cottonwood acts as a diaphoretic and increases the body's temperature slightly to help it fight infection, it will cause you to sweat, which in turn will cool you down. Oregon grape and cottonwood have drying properties that may decrease the mucus drip that is irritating the throat. All the herbs have an anti-inflammatory nature and can help soothe those painfully red mucous membranes.

I have found that the addition of wild hops to the mixture helps to relieve coughs. By increasing the body's ability to expectorate what is agitating the respiratory tract, the coughing fits or spasms are calmed.

To prepare this elixir, either mix equal parts of the individual herb tinctures together, or combine equal parts of all the dried herbs together with the fresh cottonwood buds in winter to make a tincture. Fill a jar tightly with herbs and cover them with a menstruum of at least 80% alcohol. Take 5–10 drops before each meal or as needed to aid digestion or fight a fever, sore throat, or cough.

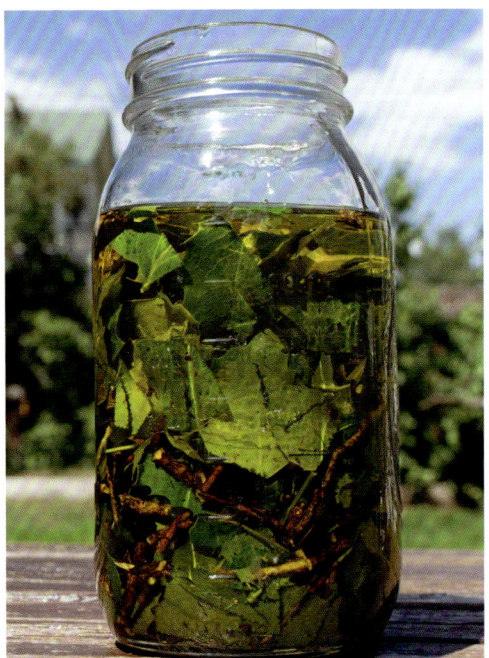

Fresh leaves and roots of *Mahonia repens* infusing in oil.

of root on each plant. In this way you can harvest from a stand without taking too much life force. Or if you are not using the leaves for medicine, replant the root crown. Clip off a section of the root as harvest, leaving a few inches attached to the leaves and root crown for replanting.

After digging up the root, process while fresh, as the dried roots become incredibly solid. Chop up into small pieces, dry, and store. The leaves are easily dried on a screen, but do be careful of their poky edges. The berries can be collected in late summer when plump and deep blue in color.

Medicinal uses

Oregon grape root is thought to clean up invasive microbes in the digestive and respiratory tracts. It is especially useful when illness presents a stagnant, damp heat, like that of a sore throat or stomach ulcers.

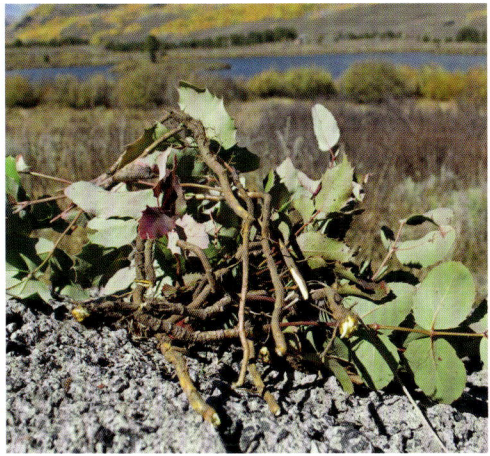

Fresh roots show the yellow constituent, berberine, which will make your tincture a golden color.

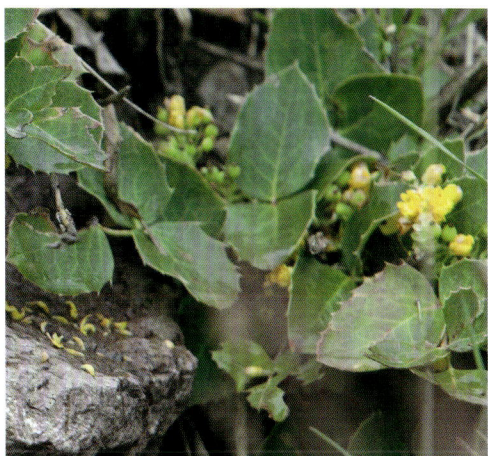

Oregon grape in flower during the early summer months.

Having such a bitter taste is also beneficial for secreting more bile from the liver and gallbladder, offering another layer of assistance with digestion, and aiding in the breakdown of fats for better absorption. An oil of the fresh leaves and roots makes a great addition to antimicrobial and skin-healing salves, working well with itchy spots related to skin conditions such as eczema.

⚠ Caution

Do be mindful that bitters can cause an increase in stomach acid, which may worsen or exacerbate conditions such as gastroesophageal reflux disease (GERD), ulcers, or acid reflux. Oregon grape can also speed up the metabolism of certain medications in the liver; check with a healthcare practitioner if you are on a prescription.

Future harvest

Gather Oregon grape roots only when a large amount is growing throughout a vast area. Look for dense stands covering an area where you can count more than a hundred plants.

HERBAL PREPARATIONS

Tea
Decoction
1 ounce fresh or dried root
1 quart water
Drink 1 cup 3 times a day.

Tincture
1 part chopped fresh root and leaves
2 parts menstruum (75% alcohol, 25% distilled water)
or
1 part chopped dried root and leaves
5 parts menstruum (60% alcohol, 40% distilled water)
Take 10–20 drops 3 times a day.

Oil
Infuse with fresh or dried root and leaves.

osha

Ligusticum porteri
bear root, Porter's lovage, chuchupate
PARTS USED roots, leaves, flowers, seeds

A revered plant that needs to be respected, guarded, and tended. Check your patches every year, and make sure you see more plants returning, not fewer.

How to identify

Certain identification is mandatory for osha, as poison hemlock (*Conium maculatum*) can be mistaken for it quite easily. There are a few guidelines to consider when out to harvest osha. Most of the time, but not always, poison hemlock grows under 7000 feet and osha is found growing over 7000 feet. This can vary by latitude, though, as I have seen poison hemlock growing at 9000 feet in New Mexico.

The leaves of osha are dissected, fern-like, with many highly lobed leaflets. Its many small, white flowers grow in the typical umbel formation of the Apiaceae. Plants grow in rhizomatous clumps, with many rootlets coming off the main plant. The crown of the root has many hair-like strings that are leftover pieces of fiber from the previous years of stalk growth. The stalks are hollow and die back to the ground each year. A plant takes seven years to reach maturity and has many years of life after that.

Where, when, and how to wildcraft

Osha is an herb specific to damp mountain climates, high places that receive a good amount of rain or snow. Once you are able to accurately identify osha, and you happen to be in a place where it grows abundantly, take only a small piece of root from a very

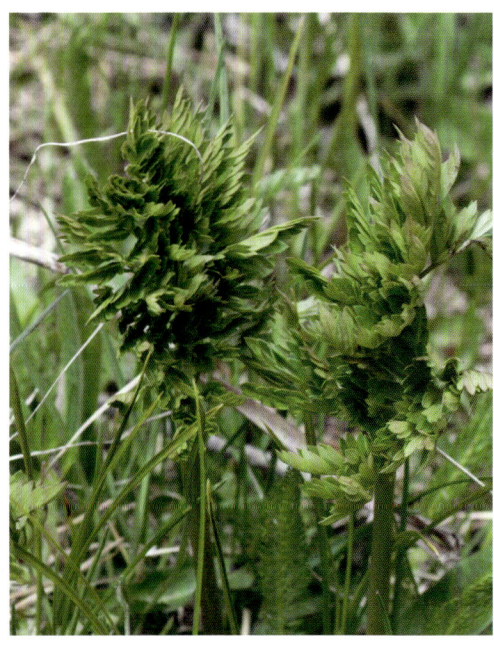

The fragrant young leaves of osha in spring will guide you to the right spot for harvesting.

few plants, leaving the rest of the stand alone. Move on to another stand, and harvest from it, respectfully; and so on. Harvest the leaves from spring until fall; use fresh in medicine-making or dry for smoking blends and teas. Loosen roots with a sturdy stick, bone, or piece of antler, as metal digging tools can injure the plant. Using a sharp knife, cut the root away from the plant. Don't try to pull or rip it out of the ground.

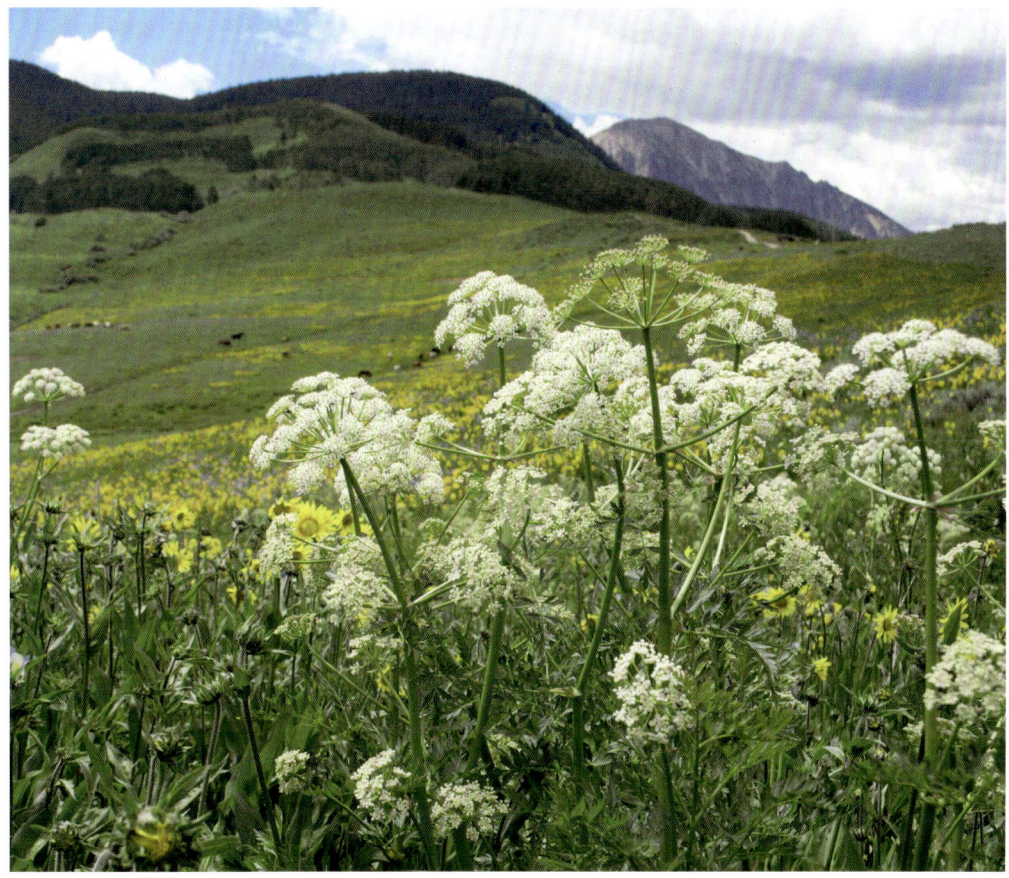

Ligusticum porteri blooming among Colorado wildflowers in the peak of summer.

Medicinal uses

The osha plant is sacred and should be venerated as such. Small amounts go a long way. For this special medicine of the mountains, try to reuse the root for more than one application. Osha root is said to be dug up by bears in the spring and is their ritualistic awakening tonic to clear out the hibernated winter's bowels. It is a spicy, aromatic, and oily root with downward-flowing actions.

Osha root has many uses, from soothing the aggravation of sinus and lung infections, to calming digestive tract woes and clearing fungus of the toes. Osha is a drying, warming, aromatic, and circulating herb. It is the first medicine I reach for when I feel like I am catching a respiratory illness. Simply chewing a small piece of root and sticking it in your lip like a tobacco chew can be a curative for coughs, sore throats, and upset stomachs; hold it there overnight or throughout the day.

Tincture, elixir, infused raw honey, and root chews are convenient ways to quickly administer a helpful dose of osha. These are especially handy for another nifty trick of osha—it has the ability to help balance people when they are having altitude sickness.

Infused honey or maple syrup is one of my favorite methods of administering osha. The honey mixed into warm water or tea can

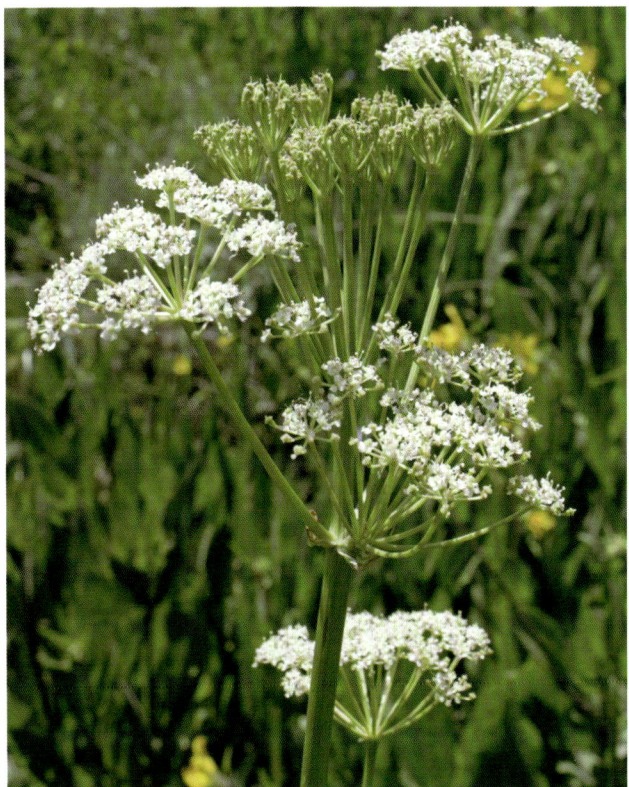

Seeds of osha beginning to form. Seed identification is very important when harvesting from the Apiaceae.

infections. Osha tea can also help to quell a nauseous stomach and reduce vomiting.

The root can be used for those who are trying to quit tobacco-containing products. It helps to heal the lungs and work out the crud for smokers, and is useful when combined with spikenard and usnea. Leaves can be used for smoking blends. They add a sharpness and body to blends that have flowers such as fireweed, pedicularis, rose, or pearly everlasting. For those who use chewing tobacco, the root can be a spicy and flavorful replacement in the lip as a dip.

Use the leaves for teas and oils. They can also be added to root tinctures and honeys. Osha root can be infused into oil for antifungal blends or antimicrobial salves or skin applications. The root can be lit and used for a cleansing smudge stick

be taken for colds and flu viruses. Combine it with other herbs for fighting respiratory illness: plantain, mallow, or grindelia to accompany a dry cough; yerba mansa, beebalm, balsamroot, and usnea for fighting bronchial against illness and bad energies. Leaves can also be bundled fresh along with artemisias and juniper for a smudging stick.

Remember to find ways to reuse the osha roots you have. After using a piece of osha

Elixirs

Elixirs can be made in various ways. For a simple elixir, extract an herb in alcohol first, then after straining the herb out, add honey for a sweetened taste (an infused honey could be used instead of plain raw honey). Herbs infused into honey can also be strained out of the honey and covered with brandy to make an elixir. Try formulating herbal blends; for example, grindelia extracted into alcohol and chokecherries infused into honey can be combined for a flavorful medicinal cough syrup.

root in a quart of hot or simmering water—even a jar of cold water extracts this root well—simply pull the root out after you have infused it for at least 20 minutes, let it dry, and reuse it when another bout of the cold has you wanting osha tea.

I infuse dried or fresh roots into honey at a 1:4 ratio. I place my jar of osha honey into a water bath—a pot or crockpot with water—at its lowest temperature, leaving it to infuse in the warmth for at least a day. I then take the chopped roots out of the honey and turn them into candied osha pieces by drying or dehydrating them. Or I fill a new jar with the honeyed roots and cover them with brandy, making an elixir. Sometimes I add other herbs to the elixir, like redroot or alder, which bring lymphatic support while fighting illness.

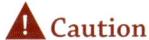 Caution

Osha can help to bring on a delayed menstrual cycle. Internal medicines made from fresh osha root should not be used in pregnancy in large doses or at all in delicate pregnancies.

Future harvest

Osha is fast becoming a popular herb in the alternative healing market. It is also a threatened plant, and its existence depends on me and you. This is not a plant to go making money off of just because you found a pristine mountainside loaded with it. These roots hold a lot of medicine; a little goes a long way. Absolute respect is needed, both for the plant and the land it grows in. Take only a small rootlet from each plant and harvest only when you are in an area where it grows abundantly. Look for large fields of more mature plants located off the beaten track. Be sure that the stand you harvest from is not also being harvested by someone else.

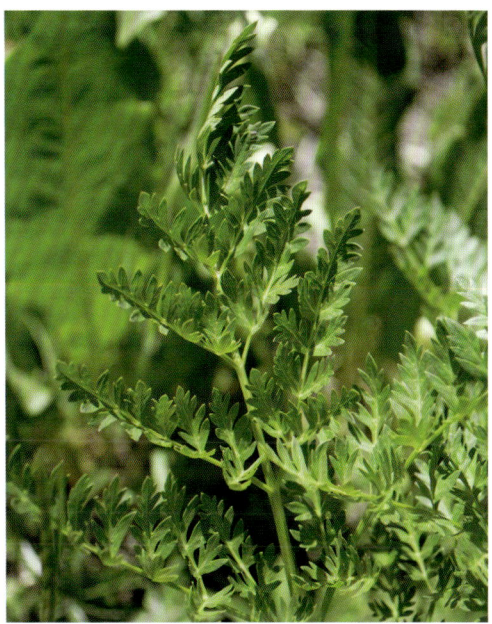

Become familiar with the leaves and smell of osha, so as not to be misled by poison hemlock.

HERBAL PREPARATIONS

Tea
Hot or cold infusion
1 tablespoon fresh or dried root, flowers, seeds, or leaves
1 cup water
Drink 1 cup 3 times a day.

Tincture
1 part fresh root or leaves
2 parts menstruum (85% alcohol, 15% distilled water)
or
1 part dried root or leaves
5 parts menstruum (70% alcohol, 30% distilled water)
Take 10–20 drops 3 times a day.

Oil
Infuse with fresh or dried root or leaves.

Prunus persica

PARTS USED twigs, leaves, flowers, fruit, pits

Peach season is highly anticipated all summer long. As people wait
for the fruit to ripen, I go out and harvest the leaves for blending into teas.

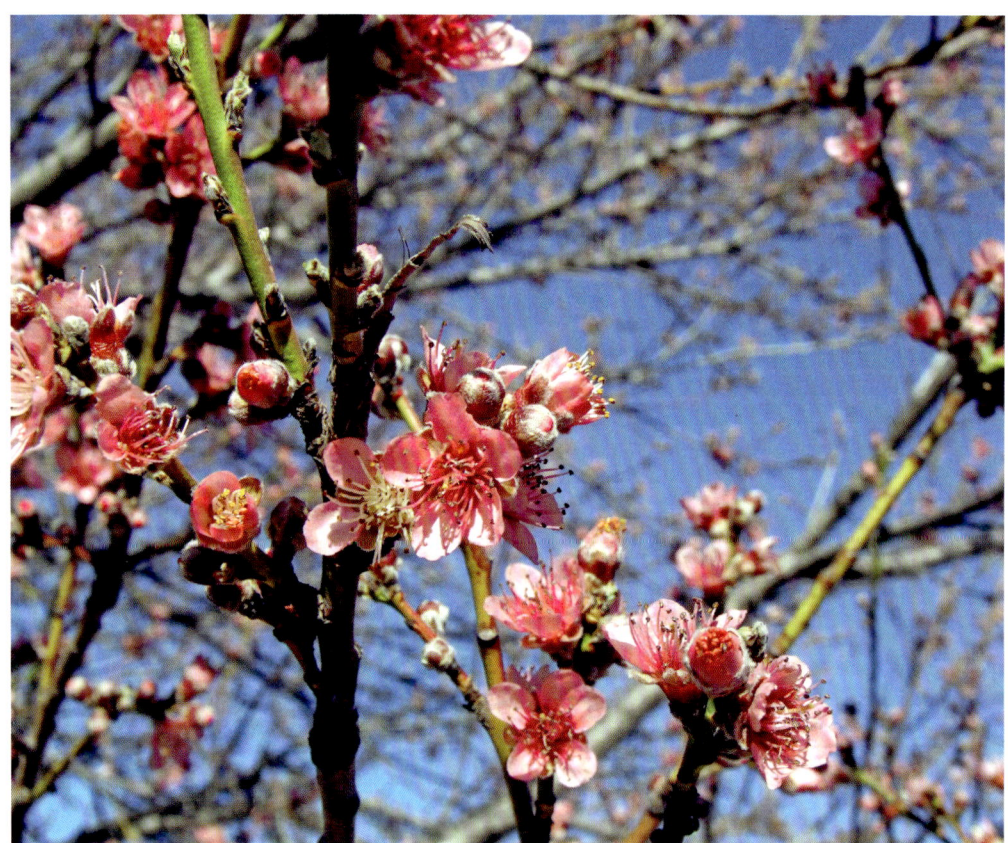

A feral peach tree loaded with spring blossoms.

How to identify

A tree of the rose family, peach has beautiful light pink blossoms of five petals with many stamens. The trees can be hard to differentiate from other species by blossom alone, but when the long, curved, simple leaves sprout from the branches, it becomes easier to identify. The branches create a broad canopy for the fruit to ripen under. When peaches are ripe, they are orange, yellow, and red with a fuzz covering the soft, fleshy skin. A type of stone fruit, each peach has a hard, ridged pit at the center.

Where, when, and how to wildcraft

Feral peach trees can be found in the rich-soiled farming communities of the lower slopes. If you can't find a wild-growing specimen, many farmers will let you go into the you-pick orchards during the spring and summer to let you gather peach leaves, or if you are lucky, blossoms. Gather the leaves after the tree has blossomed in the spring or summer, or collect the blooms and twigs in spring. The leaves and blossoms can be dried for tea blending, and the fruit can be harvested in late summer and used for its cooling medicine. There is medicine in the core of the fruit as well, so keep your pits and add those into a jar for tincturing.

Medicinal uses

Peach leaves, flowers, twigs, fruit, and pits are all very cooling and bitter, ideal in the overheated days of summer. The gentle, nourishing relief that peach leaf brings to the body makes it a useful remedy for those experiencing grief, sadness, or loss. It is a calming nervine that helps to release the tied-up tensions of the body brought on by disease or intense incidents such as death or divorce. A tincture can be made of the leaves and flowers in the spring, or try infusing honey with the blossoms to create a peach elixir.

The fruit and pit can also be incorporated into flavoring formulas to carry that sugary peachy sweetness. The moistening component comes out more with use of the fleshy parts, making the fruit useful for coughs and inflamed gastrointestinal tracts. The leaf can be crushed and used as a poultice for insect bites.

Future harvest

When taking leaves from branches, do not strip only one branch. Move throughout the tree to harvest, or better yet, spread your picking out through an entire orchard.

HERBAL PREPARATIONS

Tea

Hot or cold infusion
2 tablespoons fresh or dried leaves or
  flowers
1 cup water
Drink 1–2 cups 3 times a day.

Tincture

1 part fresh leaves, flowers, twigs, fruits, or
  pits
2 parts menstruum (75% alcohol, 25%
  distilled water)
or
1 part dried leaves and twigs
5 parts menstruum (60% alcohol, 40%
  distilled water)
Take 20 drops 3 times a day.

pearly everlasting

Anaphalis margaritacea

PARTS USED leaves, flowers

Smoking blends are increasingly popular alternatives to tobacco or cannabis—a new option without the head buzz. Pearly everlasting flowers increase the chances of its being a cough-free experience.

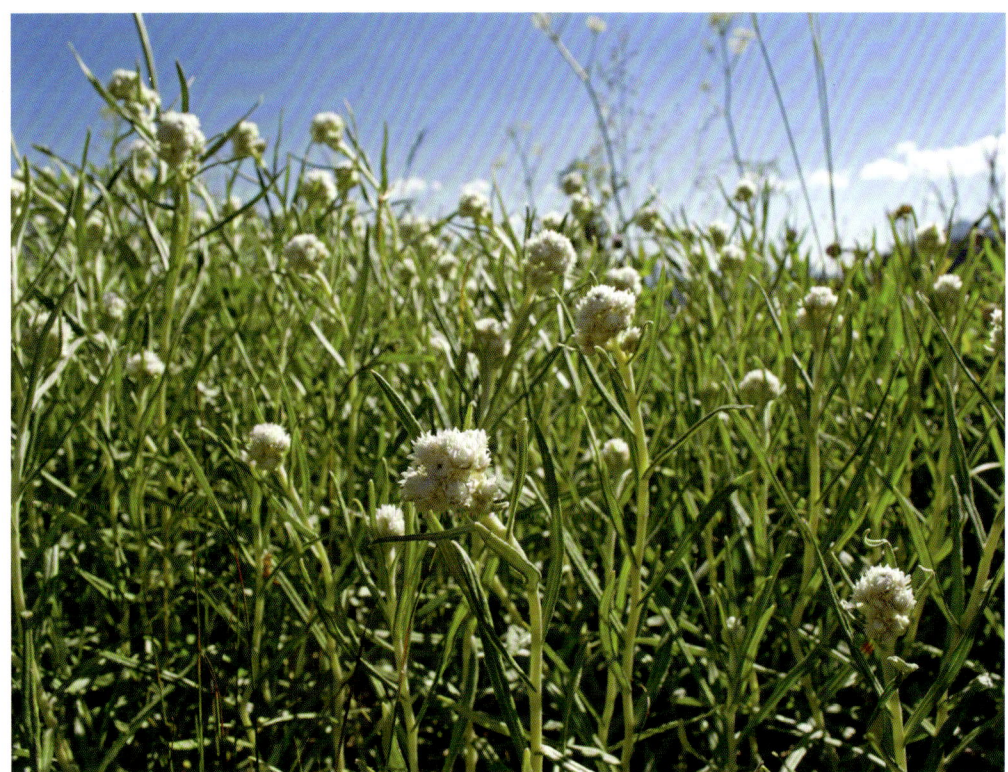

When the flowers of *Anaphalis margaritacea* feel almost dry to the touch, it's prime time for picking.

How to identify

In late summer, the long-lasting pearly white blossoms of *Anaphalis margaritacea* can be seen dotting the mountainsides. A touch to the flower blossoms makes your senses go soft—they are silky and will remain pristine until late fall. Growing in rhizomatous clumps, pearly everlasting is hardly ever seen alone and will mostly be found in abundant stands. The leaves are thin, lance-shaped, and grow alternately along the stalk. Fine woolly hairs coat the stalk and undersides of the leaves, giving pearly everlasting a silvery green color.

Where, when, and how to wildcraft

Silky white patches of pearly everlasting can be found blooming through the mountains in late summer as the first few cold nights begin to set in. This is the ideal time to harvest. Gather the flowers by pinching just under each cluster. Leaves can be gathered as well.

Medicinal uses

The flowers of pearly everlasting look fresh when dried. They are beautiful when preserved in herbal flower arrangements. Try hanging a bouquet of blooming yarrow, wild beebalm, pearly everlasting, wild hyssop, and a few sprigs of farm-fresh lavender. Once dried, the bouquet makes a gorgeous gift that provides a soft floral fragrance and helps keep a home clear of unwanted energies.

The stalks, leaves, and flowers can be combined with artemisias and juniper branches and braided with sweet grass for a smudge bundle that burns well and smells delightful. Pearly everlasting flowers and leaves have been traditionally used in smoking blends by Native Americans. As an inhaled smoke, pearly everlasting has been used to assist with coughing fits and clearing the lungs.

As a tea or tincture the leaves and flowers can relieve coughs or asthma, through shrinking and soothing the inflamed mucous membranes. Infused oils of the plant are useful in healing salves for burns.

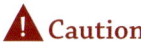 Caution

This is a member of the Asteraceae, which can cause allergic reactions in sensitive individuals.

Future harvest

Pearly everlasting is a bountiful plant in the mountain states. Collection from one stand will provide plenty for drying, usually without looking like you made a dent in the stand.

HERBAL PREPARATIONS

Tea
Hot infusion
2 tablespoons fresh or dried leaves and
    flowers
1 cup water
Drink 3 times a day.

Tincture
1 part fresh or dried leaves and flowers
5 parts menstruum (60% alcohol, 40%
    distilled water)
Take 10–20 drops 3 times a day.

Oil
Infuse with fresh or dried leaves and flowers.

Pedicularis species
lousewort, betony, elephant's head
PARTS USED leaves, flowers

The body-relaxing effects of pedicularis can be enjoyed in herbal smoking blends.

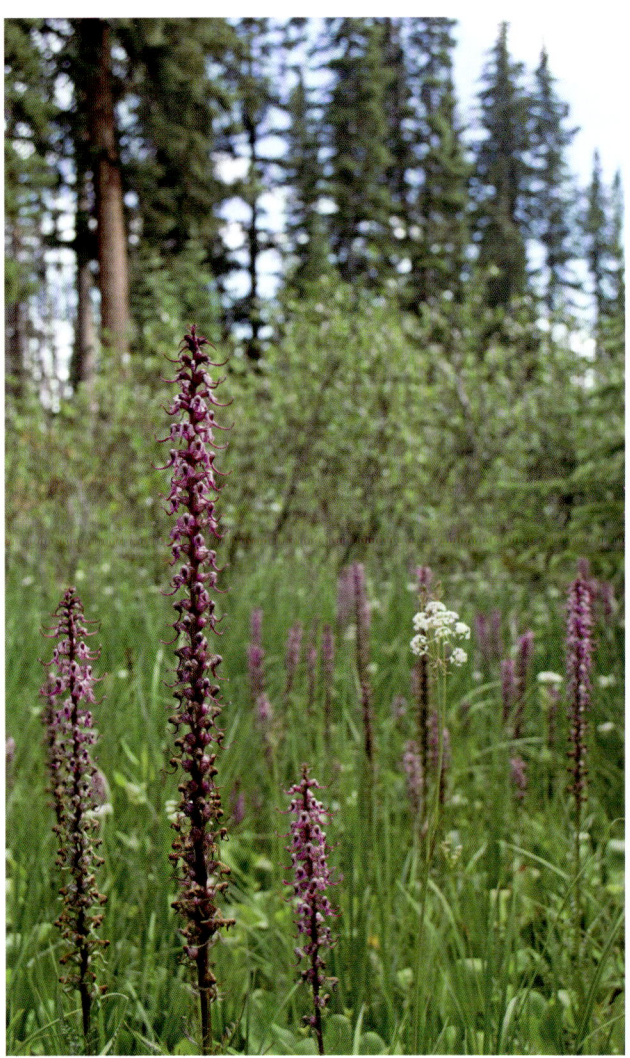

Pedicularis groenlandica is exquisite in its beauty. Please harvest only where there is an absolute abundance.

How to identify

Pedicularis species vary widely throughout the mountain west. The leaves of some, such as *P. procera*, *P. sudetica* subsp. *scopulorum*, and *P. groenlandica*, can look like a clumped bunch of fern fronds before the inflorescence shoots up. Leaves are elongated, have serrated margins, or are highly divided and feather-like.

Flowers come in a variety of colors from yellow to magenta. Each dense inflorescence has many tiny hook-shaped flowers. Some species have inflorescences which are tightly clustered, while *P. racemosa* has white flowers growing interspersed between leaves along a raceme.

Where, when, and how to wildcraft

Most species can be found in areas where there is plentiful rainfall or in riparian areas. *Pedicularis groenlandica* grows in marshes or rich riparian areas around 9000 feet. Other species can be found at high elevations throughout moist forests or wet meadows. Chew the leaf of almost any pedicularis and you'll find a watermelon aftertaste, followed by its bitter principles, giving off a gentle, sweet relaxation to the body. Some species have more of the watermelon essence than others.

Gather the leaves from spring until fall and the flowers during late summer. Delicately handle the plants, clipping just the flowerheads or taking only a few leaves from each plant.

Medicinal uses

Pedicularis species are among the great muscle and mind-body relaxants. Plants have been described by many herbalists as creating an almost loopy sedative quality, encouraging a profound full-body relaxation response. Pedicularis offers a variety of different ways to achieve this. The dried flowers and leaves can be used in smoking blends to promote mental relaxation as well as an overall feeling of slight sedation. A tincture or teas are also useful forms for internal dosage.

Smoking Blends

Most herbs you can drink as a tea are also smokable. The aromatics come through in an obviously burnt, but pleasurable way. The actions and energetics of herbs come through the smoke and can actually have an effect similar to the tea. Take for instance the smoke of pedicularis flowers. It's an excellent body and mind relaxant, taking you slightly away from the chaos of the world. Smoking wild rose can bring an ease to the heart or fill your body with love. Pineapple weed or skullcap can be calming to nerves; osha leaves, with their expectorant and bronchial-dilating tendencies, could bring some respiratory relief.

When thinking of herbs to blend, think of how they would grind up for use in a pipe or to roll in papers. Flowers and leaves do best, with roots being more difficult for obvious reasons.

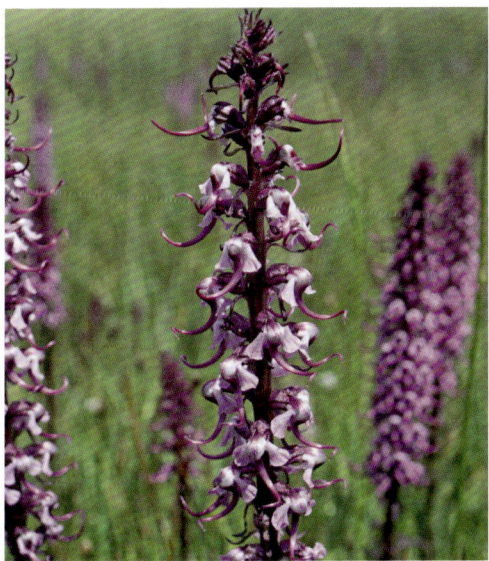

The stunning flowers dry well and hold their peculiar elephant's-head shape.

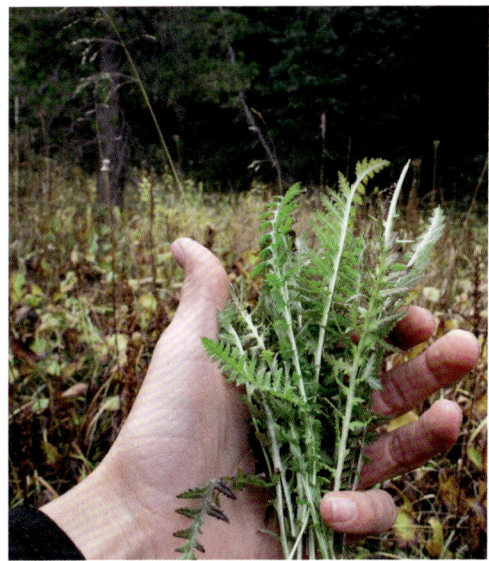

Green leaves of pedicularis can still be gathered into autumn and used for medicine.

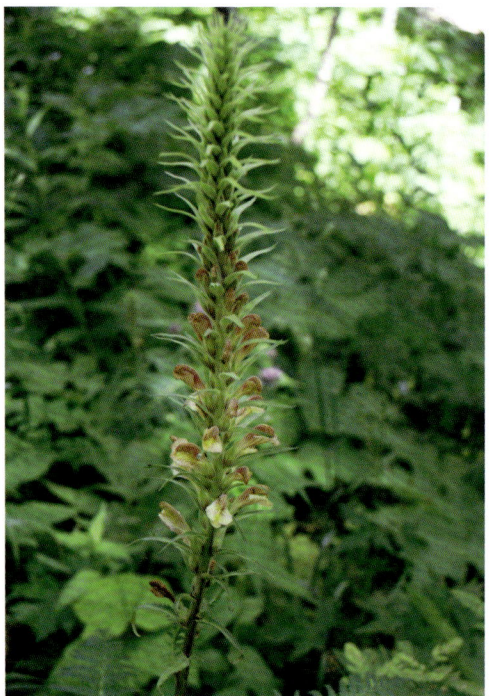

The biggest of the louseworts is *Pedicularis procera*.

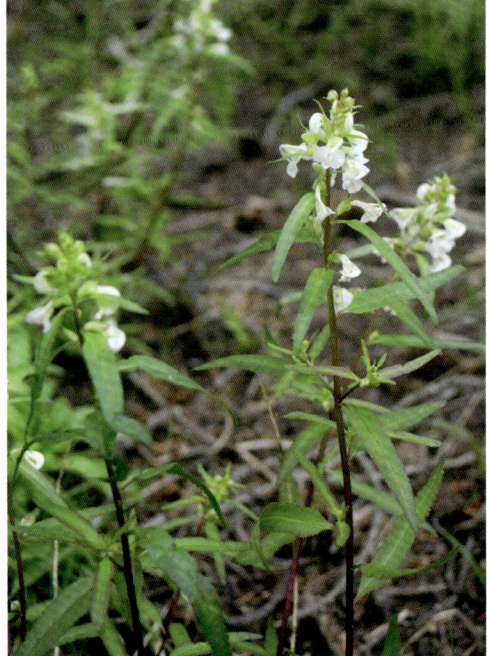

Pedicularis racemosa (curly lousewort) has white flowers that have a rounded curve to them.

An infused oil of pedicularis leaves and flowers applied topically can provide relief where there is a muscle spasm, tension, or stiffness. A liniment extraction works similarly.

⚠ Caution

Pedicularis is a hemiparasitic plant that grows from a host plant and can carry constituents of that plant. Be very cautious harvesting near plants that are toxic or have alkaloids that can be harmful if ingested. Look for another area to harvest if something like aconite or water hemlock is growing nearby.

Future harvest

Harvest with care and an eye toward leaving all but large stands untouched. Be especially conscious of the delicate wetland soils and other species growing nearby.

HERBAL PREPARATIONS

Tea
Hot infusion
2 tablespoons fresh or dried leaves and
   flowers
1 cup water
Drink 3 times a day.

Tincture
1 part fresh leaves and flowers
2 parts menstruum (75% alcohol, 25%
   distilled water)
or
1 part dried leaves and flowers
5 parts menstruum (60% alcohol, 40%
   distilled water)
Take 10–20 drops 3 times a day.

Oil
Infuse with fresh or dried leaves and flowers.

---

pine

Pinus species

PARTS USED twigs, needles, resin, pollen

*A cup of pine-needle tea is a warming medicinal tisane
on a frigid winter's eve, full of cold-fighting vitamin C.*

How to identify

Often we look at a conifer and automatically call it a pine, when in fact it may be a tree from an entirely different genus, such as fir (*Abies*), spruce (*Picea*), or Douglas fir (*Pseudotsuga*). The needles of many *Pinus*

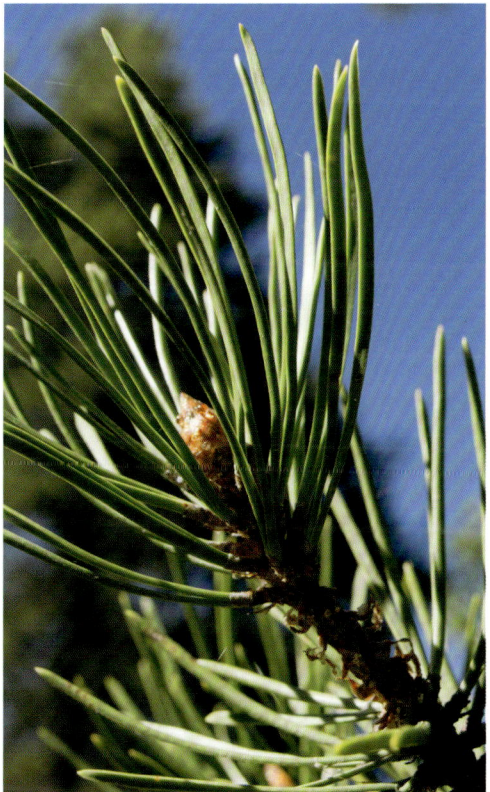

Lodgepole pines have two needles per fascicle and grow alternately on the twig.

species are much longer than those of other conifers, making the tree branches look tufted. Pine needles come in bundled sets of two as in lodgepole pine (*P. contorta*), three as in ponderosa pine (*P. ponderosa*), or five as in limber pine (*P. flexilis*) and whitebark pine (*P. albicaulis*).

The male cones, technically catkins, are soft, shed pollen in the spring, and lengthen before falling off the tree. Female cones are woody and scaly, with pine nuts nestled in between the scales. The nuts are either covered by a hard protective shell, or flattened, with a wing for wind dispersal of the tiny nut. Some pines, such as the lodgepole, have female cones that remain tightly closed for years, opening only in the event of a forest fire. The heat of the fire will open up these so-called fire cones, releasing seeds to help reseed forests after a burn.

Where, when, and how to wildcraft

Pines are found in abundance throughout the mountain west. Ponderosas are the most widespread, occurring at lower elevations and in drier climates, including Nevada and Utah. Lodgepoles can be found throughout at higher elevations, while whitebark pines are found primarily in the northern Rockies, intertwined with limber pines. Whitebark pines grow at elevations close to 12,000 feet in some places.

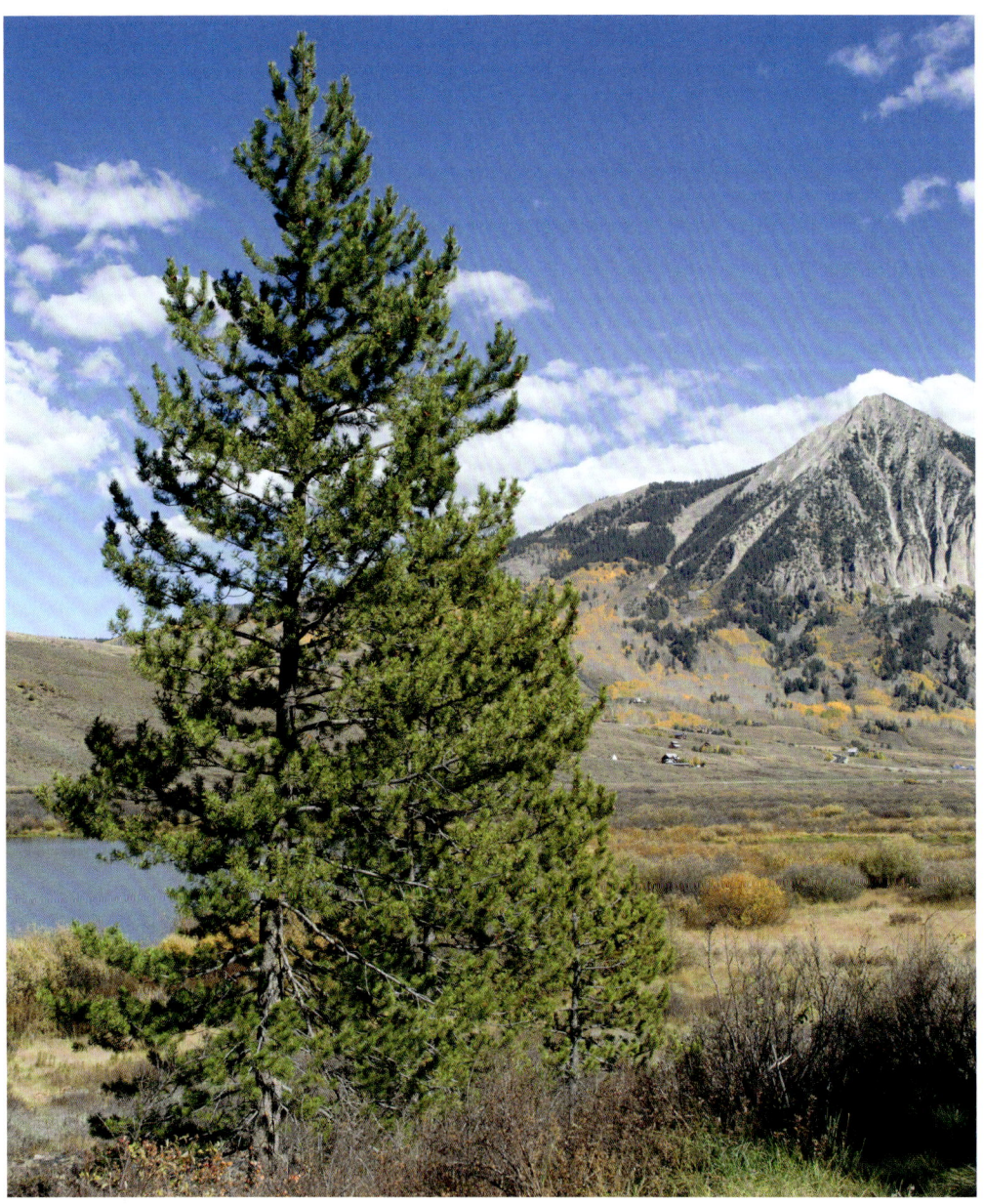

Pinus contorta is a common pine in the mountain west. It is one of my favorites to chew on while snowboarding down a mountain.

Gather male cones in spring, when they are short, in tight clusters, and full of the powdery yellow pollen; touch the cone cluster, and if powder puffs off into the air, they are ready. Resin is easily gathered in the spring or fall, when it is dripping from wounds in the trees. Gather female cones, for their nuts, in the fall. Needles can be gathered year-round.

Clusters of male cones can be clipped with pruners. A glass jar works best to gather

Processing Pine Pollen

In the spring, you will notice the male cones loaded with yellow pollen. Ponderosa and lodgepole pines are my favorites and can harbor the most pollen. First you need to know when the pollen should be there, and this happens between April and July. You may first notice the pollen on cars around the neighborhood; this is your signal to get out there before it all blows away.

Pine pollen can be collected while cones are on the tree or collected off the tree at home. In order to collect pine pollen directly from the trees, have a paper bag, plastic bag, or deep bowl on hand. Bending a branch so that its cone clusters are inside the bag or bowl, shake the branch vigorously, releasing the pollen into the collection container. It will take the shaking of many branches from numerous trees to collect a substantial amount.

To process at home, trim off the cone clusters and collect them in a plastic bag or large bowl to maintain all the pollen. Let the cones sit and dry out in a large bowl at home for a day or two. Then shake the clusters into a bowl, releasing the pollen. Store this nutritious powerhouse in the freezer for maximum freshness.

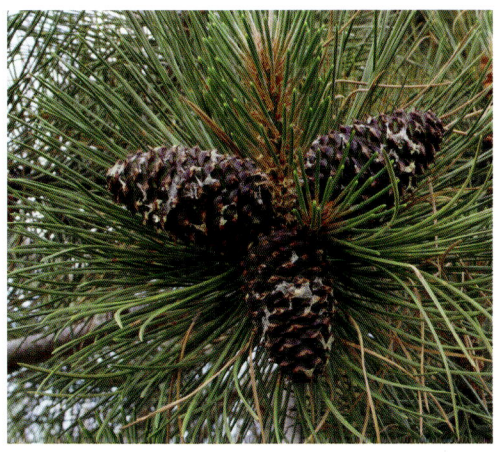

Cones of ponderosa pine are bigger and thicker than the cones of firs, Douglas firs, and spruces.

and store the sticky resin. Look for freshly trimmed branches, scarred trees, or cones that are oozing the clear resin. Needles can be gently tugged from the branches. Spread out your harvest between many trees. The younger trees, which will be easier to access, should be picked from the least, as they are trying to grow and mature.

Medicinal uses

Pinus species have needles that are high in vitamin C, which can be extracted fresh in vinegars and teas. Pine tastes lovely as an infusion or decoction, dried or fresh. It can help to expectorate coughs and can also be a mild diuretic. It can be used as a steaming herb, for inhaling—add in usnea for its demulcent, hydrating, antimicrobial assistance.

A fresh tincture or honey extraction can be made of the needles, twigs, and resin. This can be used to help move out stuck mucus in the lungs, helping to relieve coughs. The warmth of pine can encourage fevers.

The fresh needles and resins can be infused into oils for chest rubs or for an addition to massage oils. Pine helps increase circulation, providing a little warmth and help to expectorate crud from the lungs. The resin infused into oils can also be beneficial for healing chapped or dry skin. The resins of all conifers work extremely well on healing and drawing out splinters.

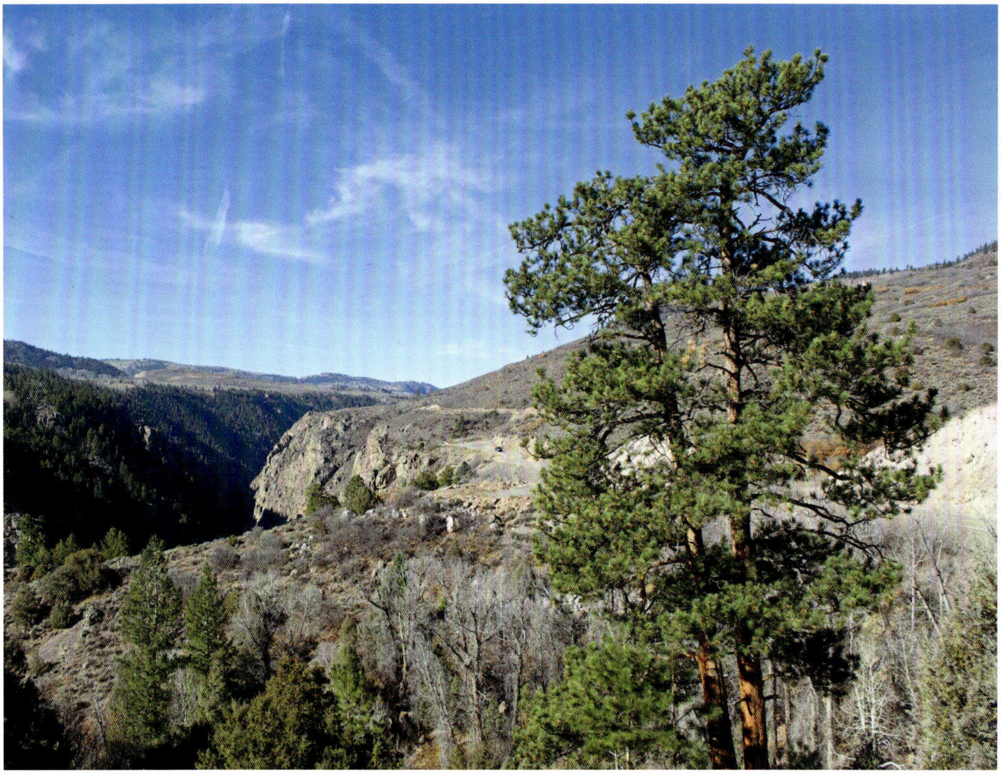

The gloriously tall ponderosa pine with its reddish puzzle-piece bark.

The pollen of pine is highly nutritious and can be extracted in alcohol or brewed as an infusion. Strain the tincture or brew through a fine strainer, such as a coffee filter or disposable tea bag.

⚠ Caution
Conifers should not be used if you are pregnant. Consult a healthcare practitioner.

Future harvest
Harvest only from trees that are not under stress from pine beetles. This invader has killed many pines in the mountain west and has also led to a lower production of cones in some species. Since pine nuts can be a substantial source of food for many bears, birds, and other critters, they are best left untouched in strained areas.

HERBAL PREPARATIONS

Tea
Hot or cold infusion
1 tablespoon fresh needles, twigs, or pollen
1 cup water
Drink 1–2 cups 3 times a day.

Tincture
1 part fresh needles, twigs, resin, or pollen
2 parts menstruum (75% alcohol, 25% distilled water)
Take 20–40 drops 3 times a day.

Oil
Infuse with fresh needles, twigs, or resin or dried resin.

pineapple weed

Matricaria discoidea
wild chamomile
PARTS USED leaves, flowers

Use pineapple weed as you would chamomile flowers,
to promote sleep or calm an upset tummy.

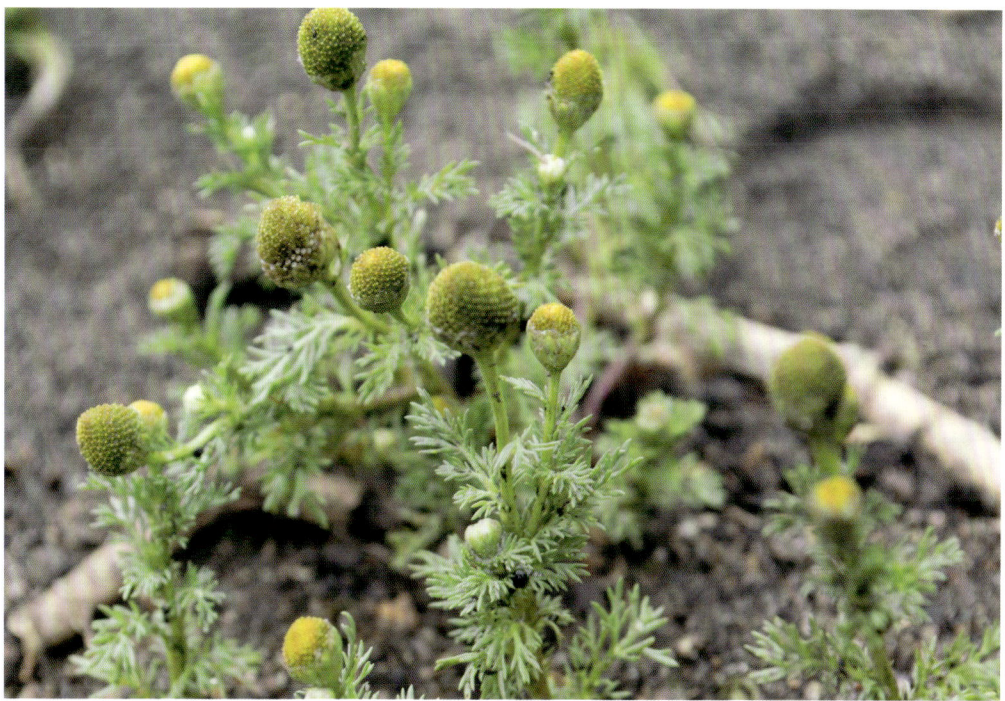

The flowers of pineapple weed may be quite small, but crush one between your fingers and inhale the sweet and not-too-subtle scent that it has to offer.

How to identify

Pineapple weed is a low-growing weed that's easy to miss even when it's right in front of you. But step on it, and it announces its presence. When crushed, the cone-shaped flowers disperse an aroma of fresh pineapple and sweet chamomile. Flowers, consisting of small tightly packed disc flowers, look like little green-yellow buttons. Pineapple weed lacks the white ray flowers of German chamomile (*Matricaria recutita*) and other species in the genus. Flat, feathery, sweet-smelling leaves are pinnately dissected and grow alternately along the flowering stalks. Many leafy flowering stalks arise from the root, making this stubby plant look full and bushy.

Where, when, and how to wildcraft

You can find pineapple weed just about anywhere throughout the mountain west, but it may not draw any attention to itself because it grows so small and close to the ground. Flowers are best harvested in the full heat of summer, as they are most aromatic at this time.

Use a small pair of scissors or your pincer fingers to gather the leaves and flowers of pineapple weed. There is no need to wash the plant matter if you harvest from a grassy spot; however, a bowl of water can be used to soak and rinse trimmings that are too sandy.

Medicinal uses

When the blues have a hold on you, a simple cup of pineapple weed tea may be all you need to release those dreary thoughts and relax. Add in some hawthorn berries, rose, and fir; this infusion is one of my favorites for healing the tender-hearted.

The teething child can benefit from the calming and pain-relieving qualities of pineapple weed, extracted in oil or glycerin and rubbed on the gums. Dip a washcloth into a tea made from the flowers, wring it out, and place the washcloth into a sealed bag for freezing. The cold, tea-soaked cloth is an excellent remedy for teething babes.

Tinctures and teas are an aid to digestion as well, because of their carminative and bitter constituents. They can also be used to get a good night's sleep, helping to calm and sedate the body.

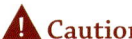 ## Caution

Pineapple weed is in the Asteraceae, and some people may have allergic reactions to this plant family. The longer you steep the tea, the more bitter it will taste.

Future harvest

Pineapple weed is abundant and happy in the west. Trimming leaves and flowers from the plant will not put a damper on its future, as it reproduces and spreads easily.

HERBAL PREPARATIONS

Tea
Hot or cold infusion
2 tablespoons fresh or dried leaves and
   flowers
1 cup water
Drink as needed.

Tincture
1 part fresh leaves and flowers
2 parts menstruum (75% alcohol, 25%
   distilled water)
or
1 part dried leaves and flowers
5 parts menstruum (60% alcohol, 40%
   distilled water)
Take 20–40 drops as needed.

Oil
Infuse with fresh or dried leaves and flowers.

Pinus species

pinyon

PARTS USED twigs, needles, resin

Resin of piñon not only smells divine but is also very regenerative and nourishing to the skin when infused in oil and used in skincare.

How to identify

Two main species of piñon grow in the mountain west: *Pinus edulis* (two-needle piñon) and *P. monophylla* (single-leaf piñon). Both are short and bushy pine trees. They do not grow in dense forests because they need space to send enormously long roots horizontally and deep into the ground to gather enough water during times of drought. *Pinus edulis* has two needles in each fascicle (the cup that holds the needles together); *P. monophylla* is unique among pine species with only one needle per fascicle. Both species have rounded resinous pinecones that are stout, measuring 1–2½ inches in length and roughly 1 inch in diameter. Inside are brown, egg-shaped seeds and their golden nut-meat, known as pine nuts.

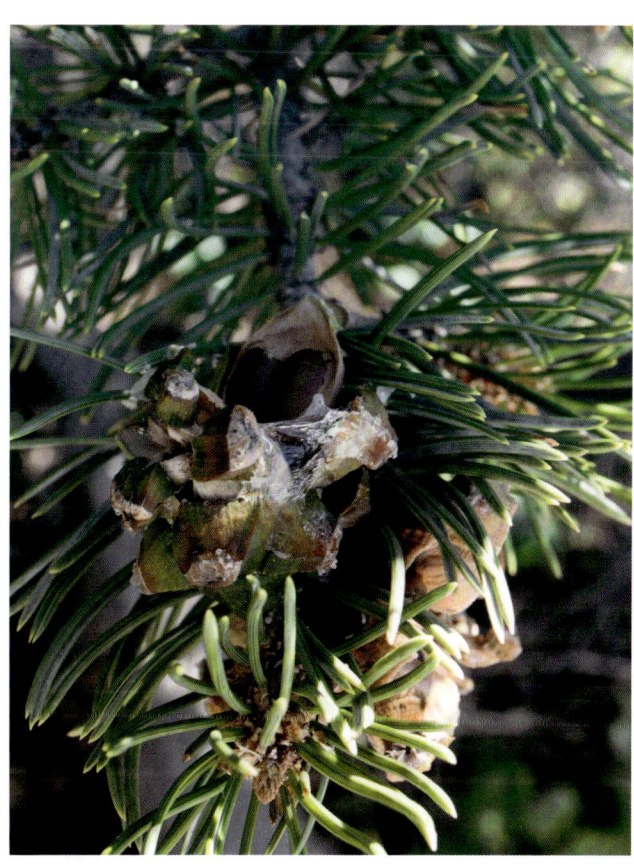

The resinous cones of *Pinus edulis* can be used for oil infusions after the nuts have been picked out and relished.

Where, when, and how to wildcraft

In the mountain west, piñon trees are primarily found in Utah, Nevada, and Colorado. Find two-needle piñon in Colorado, Utah, and parts of southern Wyoming, and single-leaf piñon in Nevada, Utah, and a small southern zone of Idaho. Piñons

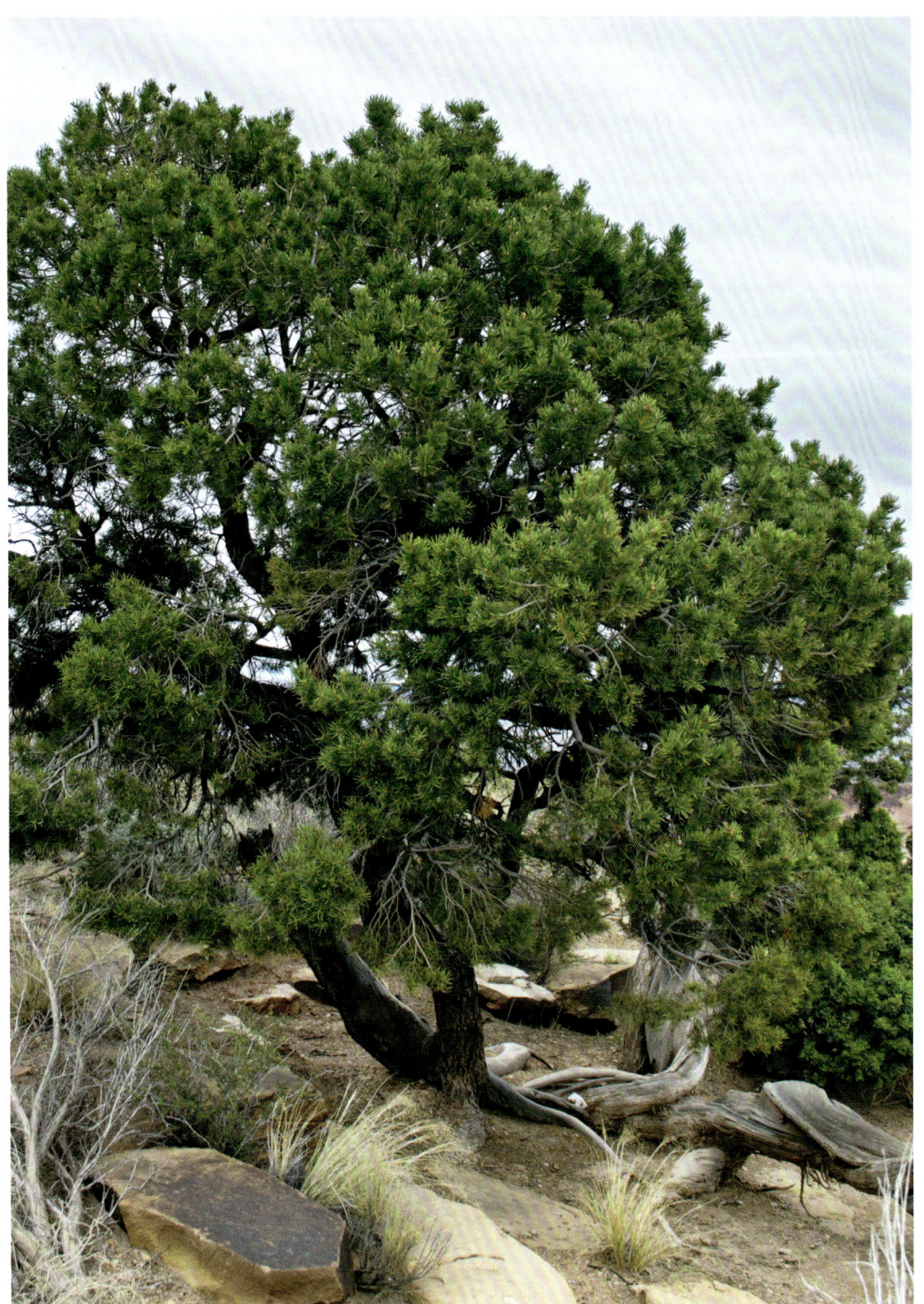

The shortened pine tree of the desert west is known as the piñon. These species are my favorites of the genus *Pinus*.

grow in the canyon lands or rocky dry soils along with junipers and ponderosa pines at 4000–9000 feet in elevation.

Gather resin in winter and needles all year long. Pull the needles gently off the branches bare-handed, but throw on some rubber gloves or disposable latex gloves if you want your hands to be functional after harvesting the cones. The delicious resin is intensely sticky.

For pine nuts, the best time is September through November. Timing matters immensely because the nuts are dispersed from the cones and quickly picked up or plucked out by birds. Gathering earlier in the season brings more abundance. One year could be a bumper crop, and the next you may not find many—or any—nuts in the cones. It is quite disappointing to crack open a pine nut seed and find it empty. It is easy to distinguish these rapscallions by the color of the shell: lightly colored shells are the fool's gold, and the darker brown shells hold the coveted meat.

Medicinal uses

Piñon is warming and highly aromatic, making it suitable for a number of applications. It helps to release stuck mucus in the chest, providing circulation and a clearing cough. Infuse oils for chest rubs or make syrups and honeys for the cold season from the needles, twigs, and resin. An infusion can be made with the needles all year long, but it is extra pleasant in the spring made with the new growth.

The distilled essential oil and leftover hydrosol of piñon is one of my most favorite scents; it can be used in a host of applications, including spritzes for the hair, face, or underarms.

Resin can be extracted in alcohol, and I love infusing large resin chunks into oils, especially coconut oil, for making superb

healing lip balms and face creams. Resin can even be used as is. I have put warmed resin on stubborn splinters that are becoming infected. The resin will help pull it out while its properties will help keep the spot clean and prevent further infection. Resin to a tree is the scab, keeping out invaders and pathogens, so be very cautious about how much you pick. Leave plenty behind to cover a tree's wound.

Caution

In an excessive amount, conifer resin can be irritating to the kidneys for some. Not for use in pregnancy.

Future harvest

Prune trees, but do not go lopping off entire branches. A lot can be gathered from many trees in an area and collecting the resin that has fallen to the sandy ground.

HERBAL PREPARATIONS

Tea
Hot infusion
2 tablespoons fresh needles and twigs
1 cup water
Drink 1–3 times per day.

Tincture
1 part fresh needles, twigs, or resin
2 parts menstruum (75% alcohol, 25% distilled water)
or
1 part dried needles, twigs, or resin
5 parts menstruum (60% alcohol, 40% distilled water)
Take 20–40 drops 3 times a day.

Oil
Infuse with fresh or dried needles, twigs, or resin.

plantain

Plantago species
psyllium

PARTS USED leaves, flowers, seeds

It's a simple pleasure to make medicine from this easy-to-identify herb,
whether it be a spit poultice, infused oil, or sun tea.

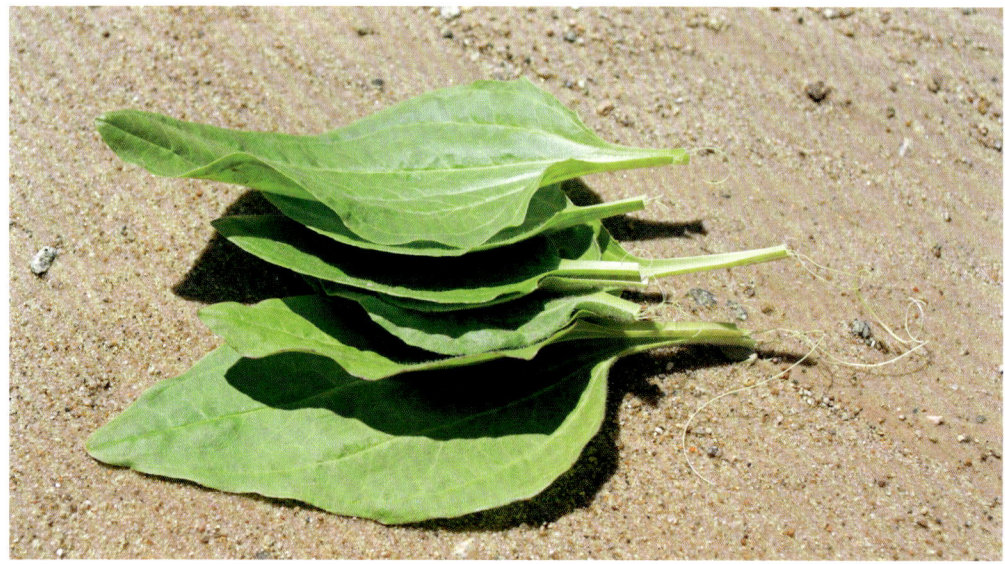

Gathering large leaves of plantain to dry and rehydrate as poultices. Notice the stringy veins of the leaves, a good sign you have identified the correct genus—*Plantago*.

How to identify

Ovate or lanceolate leaves of plantain grow in a dense basal rosette. Leaves have parallel veins that attach to thick stems. If you pull the leaves apart or break the stem, you will see that the veins are very stringy, like celery. Plantain hugs the ground, forming a mat of leaves around the leafless flowering spikes. The thin flowering spike hosts tiny white flowers that turn into brown seedpods. All plantagos can be used interchangeably.

Where, when, and how to wildcraft

Plantago seeds have been spread far and wide by the movement of people and other animals. The mucilaginous seeds easily plump up when wet and stick to fabrics, furs, feet, hooves, and wheels, which carry them long distances. Plantain can be found high up mountain trails past 10,000 feet, in the heat of the deserts, and low in the tropics. Find the best leaves in spring or early summer. Gather seeds in late summer.

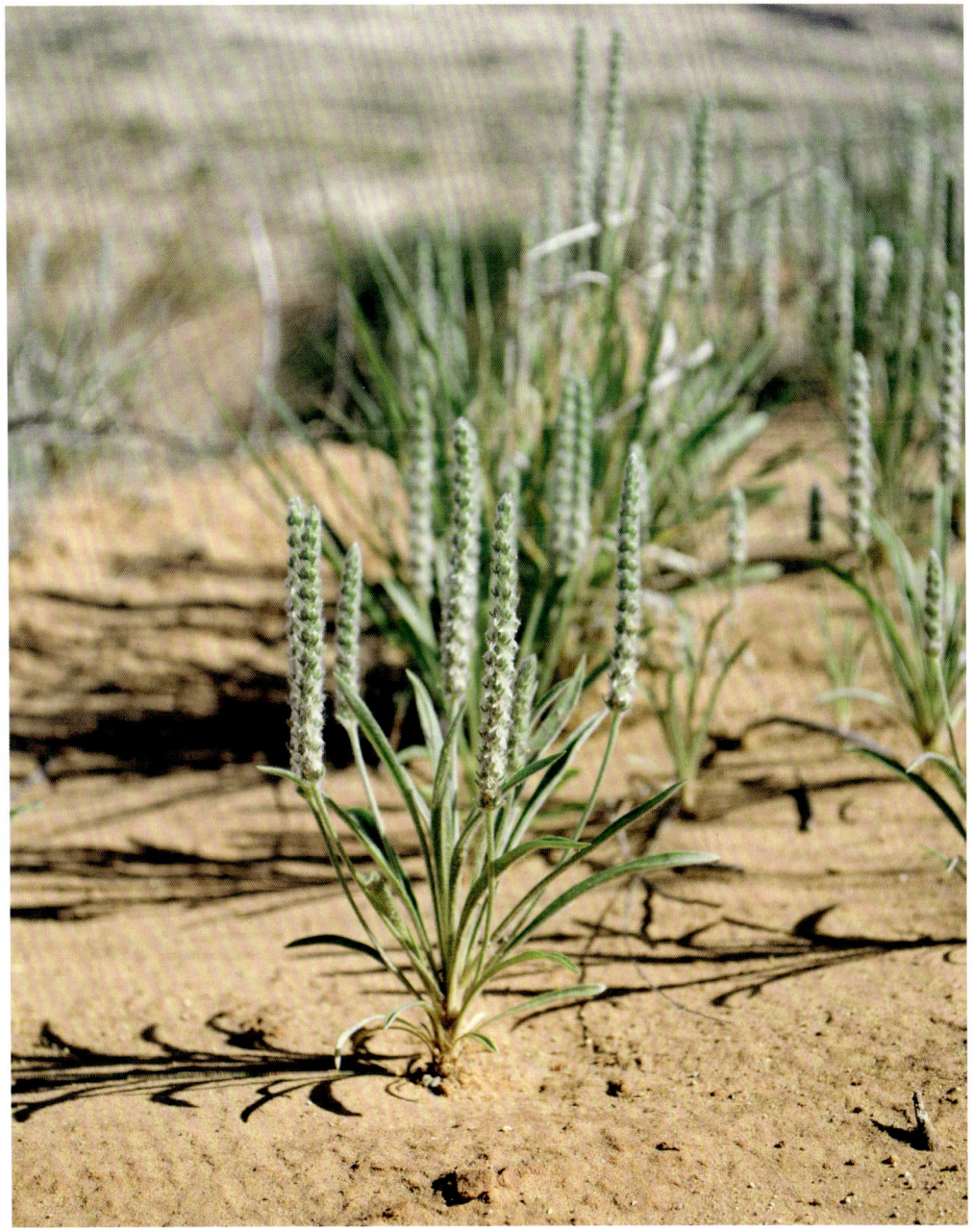

Woolly plantain (*Plantago patagonica*) in the desert of eastern Utah.

Gather the choice young leaves by plucking them at the base of the thick petiole. As plantain ages, the leaves turn tougher and more bitter. Seeds can be gathered by clipping off the seeded stalk. Take the stalk and shake the seeds off, letting them fall into a bowl. Winnow the seeds, removing all the husks, and store them in an airtight container.

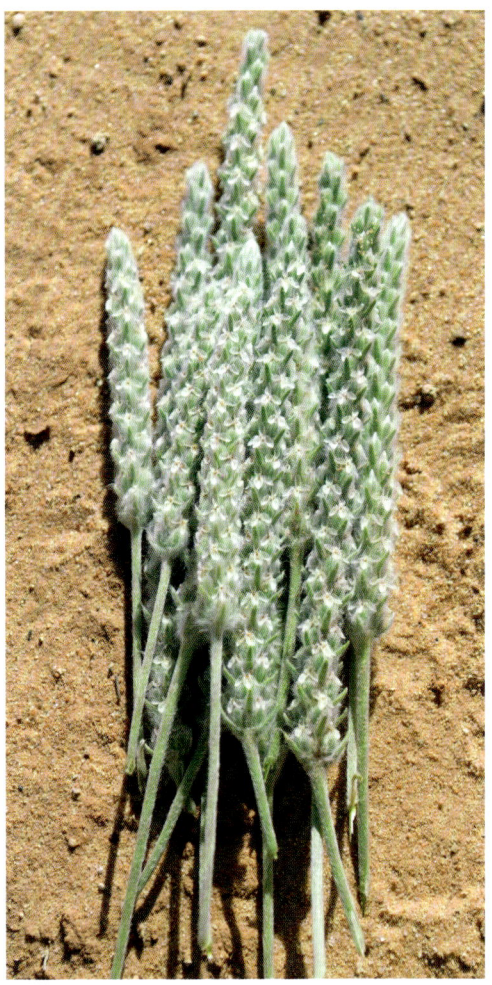

The seeding heads of woolly plantain can be used to make a demulcent tea.

Medicinal uses

Plantain is my go-to herb for any skin ailments, ragged from injury, weepy, raw, or inflamed from an infection. Make an infusion for soaking, use a poultice, or apply a salve after a wound has begun to heal. A poultice can be made by chewing up the leaves and applying them to bug or spider bites, burns, boils, blisters, or wounds, which can be especially useful while in the backcountry. Plantain can also be used in a combination with strawberry leaves, yarrow, and cottonwood bark for a postpartum sitz bath.

As a tea, plantain is very nourishing to inner tissues, such as the digestive tract and genitourinary system. The demulcent properties are rehydrating and healing. Among the demulcent herbs, fresh is always best, but dried will do just fine. Plantain tincture can be used for internal tissues that are raw and inflamed; it provides cool and moistening relief to sore throats or gastrointestinal ailments like colitis and ulcers.

Infused fresh into oil and used alongside alumroot, rose, and uva-ursi, plantain provides strong relief from bug bites or stings. This combination reduces the swelling and redness and ditches the itch.

The seeds, also called psyllium, can be used similarly to chia seeds. Make a cold infusion of them for a super-mucilaginous drink or a gel that can be applied to wounds or infections. When used in small doses, as in 1 teaspoon per cup of water, seeds can be used as a laxative and an intestinal soother. When taken in larger quantities, as in 4 tablespoons per cup of water, plantain seeds can be an antidiarrheal aid.

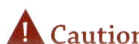 Caution

Plantain seeds promote bowel movements, so do not take in conjunction with other laxatives. Consult with a physician if you are taking medications absorbed through the gastrointestinal tract, as plantain can either slow or extend the absorption rate, due to its mucilaginous nature.

Future harvest

No worries. Plantains tend to proliferate where they grow; rarely is there a shortage of them.

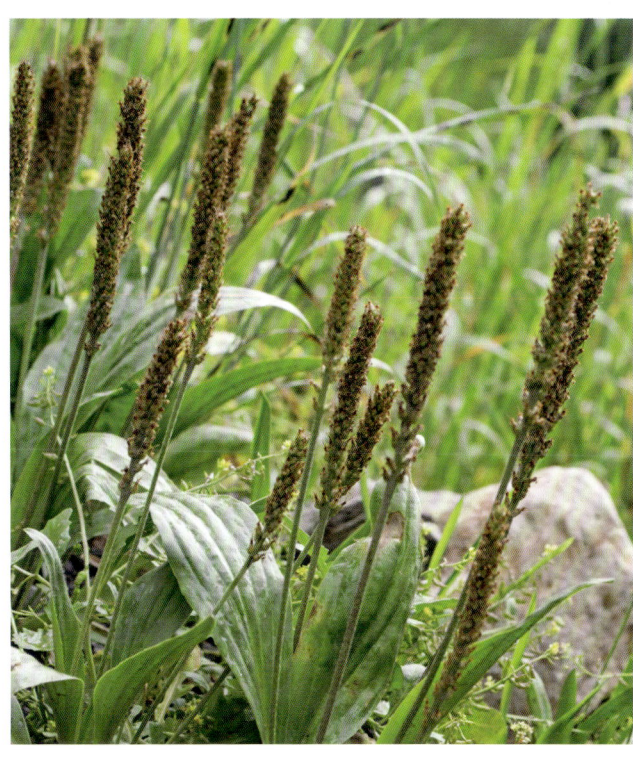

Plantago species can be found high up in the mountains. This one is dwelling over 9500 feet.

HERBAL PREPARATIONS

Tea
Hot infusion
1 ounce fresh or dried leaves
1 quart water
Cold infusion
1 tablespoon seeds
1 cup water
Drink as needed.

Tincture
1 part fresh leaves
5 parts menstruum (75% alcohol, 25% distilled water)
Take 20–40 drops 3–5 times a day.

Oil
Infuse with fresh or dried leaves.

prickly pear

Opuntia species

PARTS USED pads, flowers, fruit, flowerbuds

The slimy insides of a freshly cut pad make an excellent drawing poultice or sunburn reliever—once all spines have been removed.

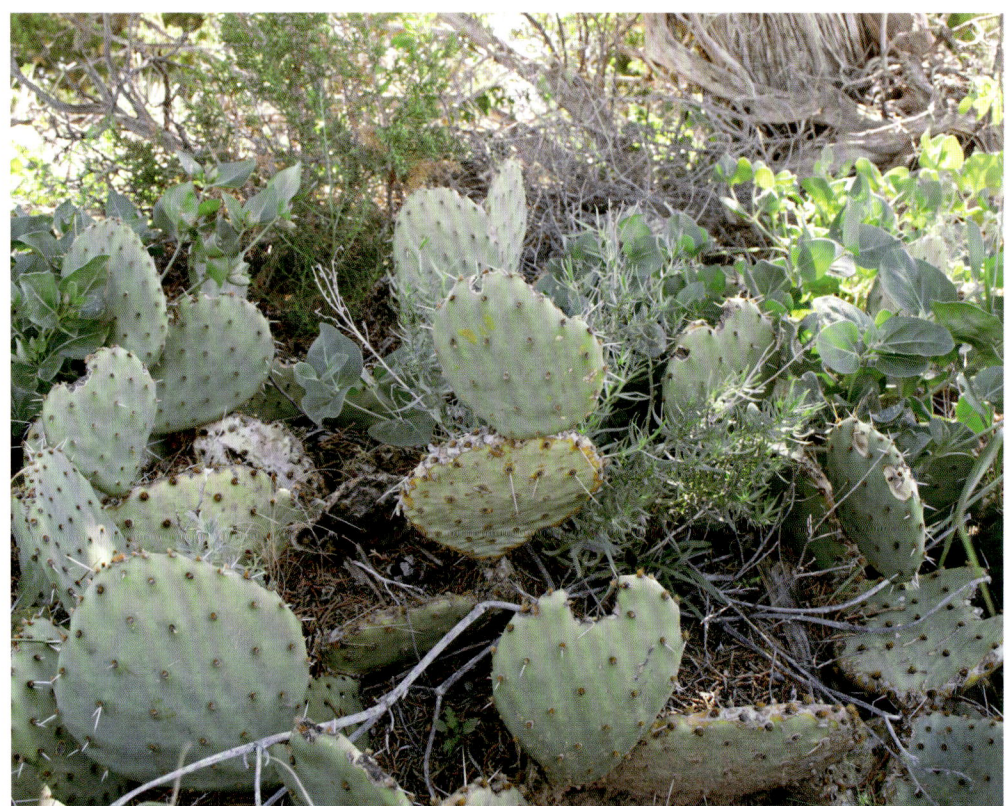

There is a lot of love inside the sharp, spiny skin of prickly pear pads. You need take only one pad from each cactus.

How to identify

Many *Opuntia* species exist throughout North America (about 200 species exist worldwide). Here in the Rockies and western deserts, they hybridize with each other making identification a little tricky sometimes. Their flat pads, known as nopales, and brightly colored fruits, called pears or tunas, are characteristic. Both the pads and fruits are covered in spines. The showy flowers vary from yellow to pink in color.

Where, when, and how to wildcraft

Find prickly pear in the desert lowlands and dry (usually south-facing) slopes of the west, in between mountain ranges, and among the sagebrush. Pads can be gathered most of the year, when there is plenty of moisture. During dry spells the pads shrivel up and are not succulent. The pears can be collected in late summer and fall.

Gather pads by clipping one free of the entire plant. The spines and glochids can then be burned off, cut out, or scrubbed away with water. Once the spines are removed, the skin can be left on or cut off before using. An easier way to harvest nopales is to leave them attached to the whole cactus while you slice into the middle of the pad, cutting the pad in half and folding it open. This way you can easily scrape out each side of the pad and get a good amount of the mucilaginous center. Once you have used this method, cut off the remaining mangled pad; otherwise, you leave the cactus vulnerable to invaders and open to infection. Cut the inner pad into thin pieces for drying. Dry in a dehydrator or oven on low heat.

Pears can be picked with a bare hand, but gloves or tongs make the experience easier and less glochid-filled. Glochids are tiny bristly spines with barbed tips, which make the pears feel very unpleasant to the touch. The cooling medicine of the pears can be used fresh for tincture or syrup, or frozen for future use. Flowers and buds can be gathered as well in the spring and early summer. Yes, they too have prickles to avoid. Flowers can be dried for blending into teas.

Medicinal uses

Make syrup from the fruits of prickly pear to create a beautiful scarlet-red remedy that can be cooling in the summer's heat. Create a cooling elixir by adding the tinctured leaves

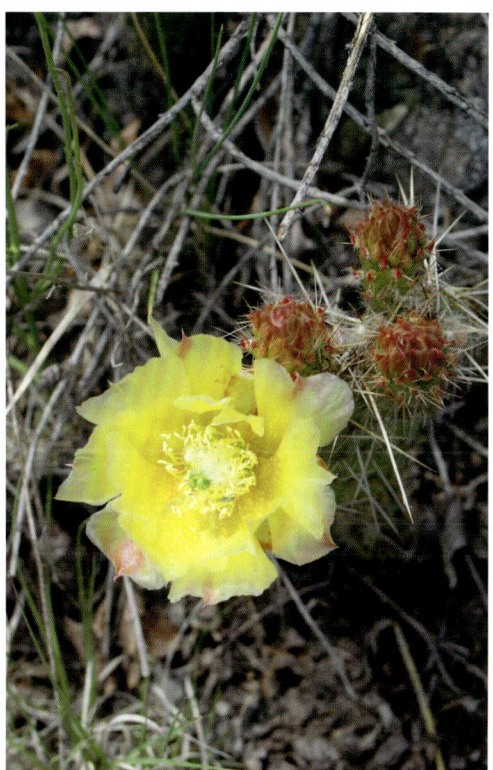

Flowers of prickly pears can be harvested ever so carefully, dried, and consumed as a demulcent tea.

of peach to the syrup (25% syrup to 75% tincture). This can bring relief from heat exhaustion.

The nopales of prickly pear can be cut open and their mucilaginous innards applied to burns or wounds while hiking in the desert. This assists in promoting healing, keeping the affected skin clean, and provides a cooling pain relief to the injury or sunburn. A pad can also be used as a hot drawing poultice to help heal inflamed and infected spider or insect bites. Slice open the cactus pad and place it in the oven or over a campfire to warm. This heated pad can also bring relief to boils.

Flowers can be dried and used for a slightly demulcent tea that can quench the thirst of the dry desert heat.

⚠ Caution

The spiny glochids (bristles) can get any- and everywhere if you are not mindful.

Future harvest

Do not take the whole cactus. They take many years to reach maturity. Leave some fruits behind for seed distribution, and if harvesting the flowers, do not take them all from one cactus. If you happen to take off a pad and are not planning on using it, place it back in the soil, and it will set roots.

HERBAL PREPARATIONS

Tea
Hot or cold infusion
1 tablespoon fresh or dried flowers, pads, or
  flowerbuds
1 cup water
Drink 1 cup 3 times a day.

Tincture
1 part fresh pears or pads
2 parts menstruum (75% alcohol, 25%
  distilled water)
Take 20–40 drops 3 times a day.

Oil
*Infuse with dried or wilted pads or fresh or
dried flowers or flowerbuds.*

purslane

Portulaca species
verdolagas
PARTS USED leaves, stems, flowers

A demulcent herb that gets plucked and chucked from most garden beds.
Don't be that person. Put purslane to its good uses, all summer long.

How to identify

Look low to the ground for a sprawling, flat-leafed, succulent green plant that has a smooth, thick, red stem, ovate leaves, and tiny yellow flowers that have five petals. The leaves rarely exceed an inch in length, and the plant itself doesn't stand more than an inch or so tall. Seeds are small and black.

Where, when, and how to wildcraft

Purslane grows all over North America in disturbed soils, preferring a warm climate. The best place to find purslane is in a garden bed, and yet it probably was not included there intentionally. City parks tend to have rogue patches sprawling through the grass lawns. Farmers are now cultivating it and adding it to salad mixes. You can find this succulent plant thriving in the heat of the summer, withstanding both droughts and scorching sun.

Trim or snap off the trailing stems of the plant a few inches

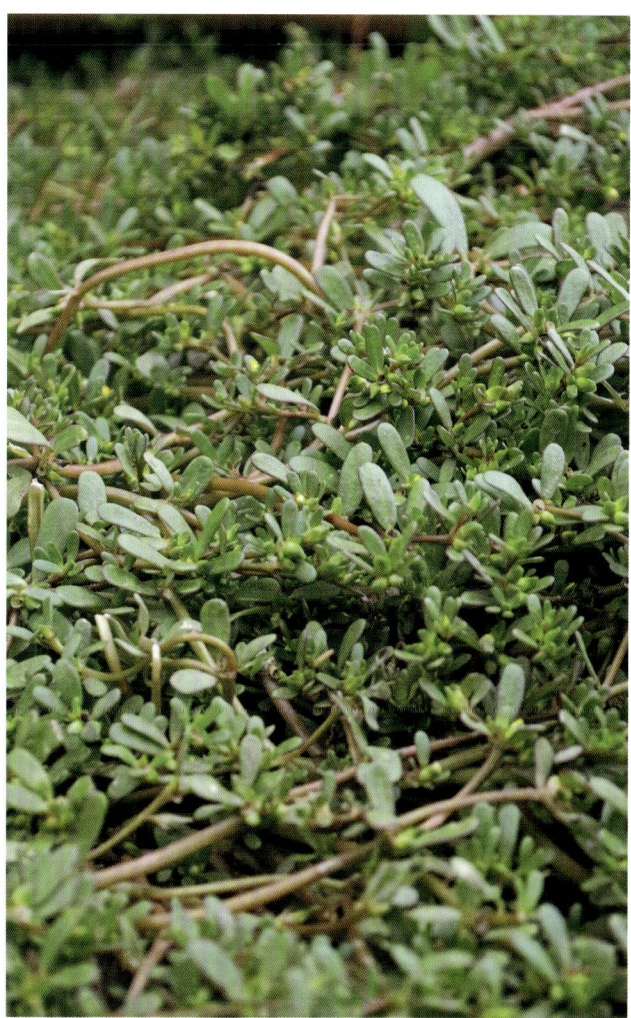

The succulent runners of purslane can be so discreet that they may be waiting for you unnoticed in your garden or front lawn.

from where they emerge from the ground. The leaves, stems, flowers, and seeds are all edible and can be dried. To make cleaning easy, soak the purslane in a water bath to loosen up any soil that is clinging to the plant.

To dry, chop up the leaves, stems, and flowers, then use a dehydrator or your oven at its lowest temperature with the door cracked open.

Medicinal uses

Purslane is loaded with vitamins and minerals but is also super-rich in omega-3 fatty acids, which makes it totally worth adding into your diet while it is fresh in the summer. It can be very healing to people who have gut troubles. Try it brewed fresh into an infusion, and sweetened with honey. Create a vinegar infusion from fresh purslane to extract its high content of minerals.

Purslane is demulcent and slick when crushed. The fresh cooling juice can provide relief to sunburns and insect bites. An oil infusion can be made for salves or serums for itchy skin or bug bites, to lessen the inflammation and the need to scratch!

Future harvest

Purslane grows pretty abundantly, and over-harvesting should not be an issue. Leave a few stems behind if you want to reseed the area.

HERBAL PREPARATIONS

Tea
Hot or cold infusion
1–2 tablespoons fresh or dried leaves, flowers, and stems
1 cup water
Drink as needed.

Vinegar
1 part fresh leaves, stems, and flowers
4 parts vinegar
Take 1 tablespoon 1–3 times a day.

Oil
Infuse with fresh or dried leaves, stems, and flowers.

raspberry

Rubus idaeus
red raspberry, wild raspberry
PARTS USED roots, leaves, stems, flowers, fruit

*An incredibly tasty, mineral-rich, apple cider vinegar tonic
can be made from a fresh extraction of the leaves and berries.*

How to identify

Wild raspberries are smaller than their cultivated relative but more mouthwatering. Depending on the elevation and climate, raspberry bushes can be quite large, maxing out at about 8 feet, or be very dwarfed on high mountain cliffs, reaching only a foot in height. Raspberry has ovate leaves that are deeply veined and jagged around the edges. Leaves grow alternately up the spiny stems, displaying a compound formation with three to five leaflets. They are deep green, sometimes having a reddish tint around the edges. The undersides of the leaves are white with soft fuzz.

Flowers are small, delicate, and white with five tiny petals. The fruits are called berries, but in reality they are a cluster of a ton of minute drupelets, each drupelet containing an individual seed. When you chew a berry you will notice all the small seeds released onto your tongue. Each of these seeds came from an individual drupelet.

Blackberry can be confused with raspberry before its fruits start to turn deep purple. A key identifier is that raspberry fruits come off the stem slightly hollow, without the white, pithy receptacle. Blackberries will always come off with the receptacle still attached.

Leaves of raspberry are best gathered while the plant is in flower.

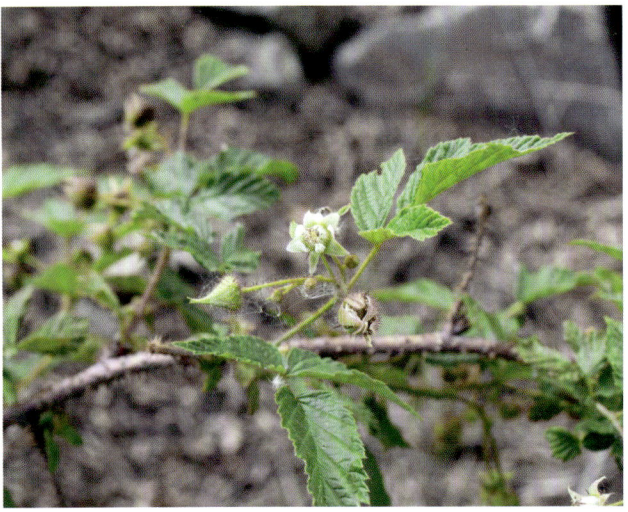
Stems have a reddish purple and white chalky hue to them.

Where, when, and how to wildcraft

Raspberry bushes are found all over the west, in yards, in the woods, near the water, and on the craggy hillsides of the mountains. They grow in partial shade or sunny places.

Leaves are best gathered in the early summer as the plant is flowering. Wearing gloves can be helpful when gathering the leaves because of the prickly stems. Pinch the flowers and leaves from the stems or clip with pruners. The stem can also

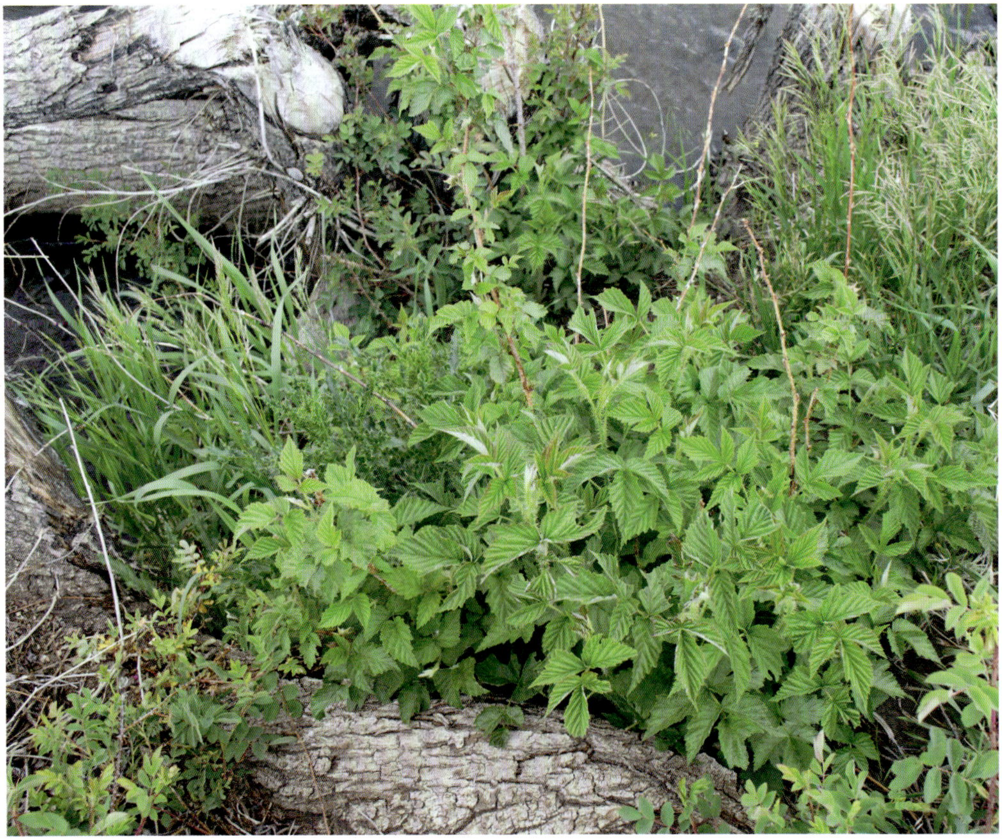

Prickly, shrubby, and a lover of rocky places, raspberry can be found across the mountain states, whether planted as an ornamental alongside a house or growing in the wilderness.

be clipped full of leaves and cut up along with or separated from the leaves.

Dry the leaves and flowers on a screen or loosely in paper bags. Once the leaves are dried you can easily crush them in your hand, or chop the leaves before drying. Stems and roots can also be used in medicine-making.

Berries are easiest to pick one by one. They ripen in mid- to late summer. Place them into a sturdy container that won't smash the delicate fruit.

Medicinal uses

Raspberry has a long-standing use among women for its astringent and tonifying effect on the uterus. It can be used for menses that seem to be excessive, for increasing muscle tone during pregnancy, and for assisting in uterine healing after birth by reducing swelling and bleeding. Raspberry leaf can bring relief for women suffering from morning sickness.

Being rich in nutrients and minerals like manganese, it is usually a component to my nourishing brews along with cleavers, catnip, and stinging nettles. The stems, leaves, and root clippings are astringent and can be beneficial in relieving loose stools. The fresh or dried fruit made into a syrup or honey also can be used to treat diarrhea in children and adults. The fresh berries can be a wonderful aid in tinctures, not just for their scrumptious taste but for their ability to help fight viral infections.

 Caution

Most herbalists are cautious using any herbs during the first trimester of pregnancy, and raspberry leaf is no exception, although it is revered and thought of as very safe during the second and third trimesters.

Future harvest

Make sure to spread out your leaf harvest between shrubs; do not strip any one plant of its foliage.

HERBAL PREPARATIONS

Tea
Hot infusion
1 ounce fresh or dried leaves, flowers, stems, fruit, or root
1 quart water
Drink 1–3 times a day.

Tincture
1 part fresh fruit
4 parts menstruum (75% alcohol, 25% distilled water)
Take 20–40 drops 3 times a day.

Vinegar
1 part fresh or dried leaves, stems, flowers, fruit, or root
3 parts vinegar
Take 1 tablespoon 1–3 times a day.

Oil
Infuse with fresh or dried leaves.

red clover

Trifolium pratense

PARTS USED leaves, flowers

The nourishing dense flowerheads of red clover are best picked just under the top leaves, so they too are part of the harvest.

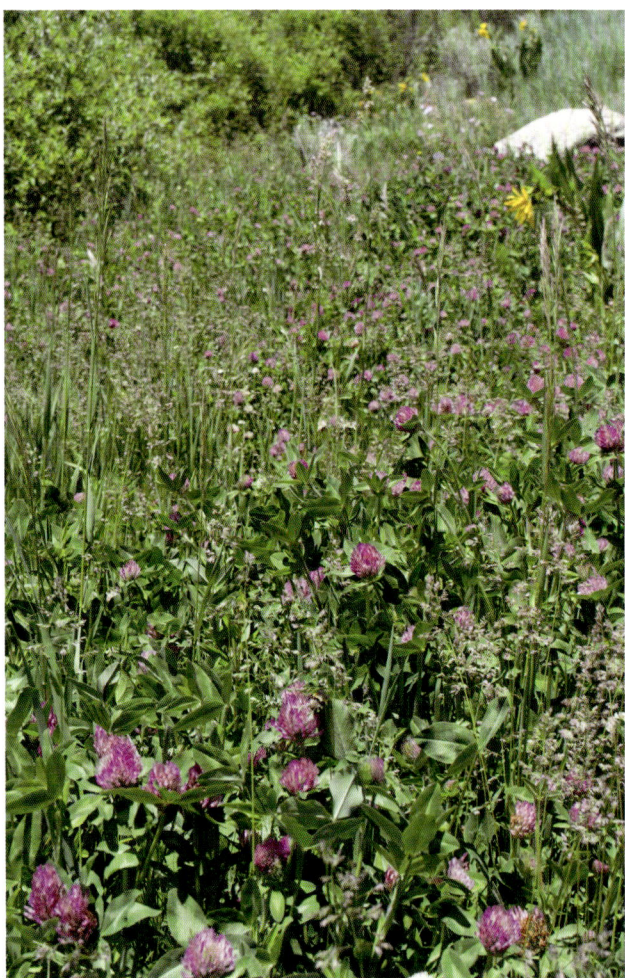

A pound of red clover can easily be gathered in the height of summer. Make sure you have adequate space for drying before you embark on such an endeavor. You do not want your red clover to mold as it dries, so circulation is necessary and important.

How to identify

Fields are dotted with the pinkish red, puffed flowerhead of red clover. The blooms consist of many small, tubular flowers that each hold a drop of sweet nectar. Leaves are soft and have three leaflets per stem, reminiscent of a shamrock, with each leaflet graced by a light chevron-shaped mark. The stem is hairy, and the leaves are arranged alternately along it.

Where, when, and how to wildcraft

The best place to find red clover is at the forest's edge, or in a meadow that is free of heavy cattle-grazing and far from pesticide-laden farms. Because red clover readily absorbs minerals from the soil, stay clear of polluted soils and do not harvest near old tailing piles from mines. The blush-red blossoms are part of late spring's overwhelming floral celebration and can be found through to the end of summer.

Pick a basketful of red clover blossoms and leaves on

a sunny, dry day; this will help the blossoms dry mold-free. Use your hands to pluck flowerheads, or bring a pair of scissors. Go for vibrant red flowers, not the ones turning brown, and pick the greenest leaves.

Medicinal uses

Red clover is primarily used for its blood-purifying agents, helping with swollen lymphs, skin ailments, and removal of toxins through the liver. Infused oil can be used to treat skin conditions, but true relief will come only from treating yourself with red clover internally as well. It goes well with amaranth, alfalfa, rosehips, cota, dandelion leaves, mallow leaves, and pineapple weed for a deluxe nourishing brew. It is highly regarded for its high content of minerals and nutrients. A tea, infused honey, oxymel, or a few drops of tincture can be easing to those dry, lingering coughs that need assistance in moving up and out.

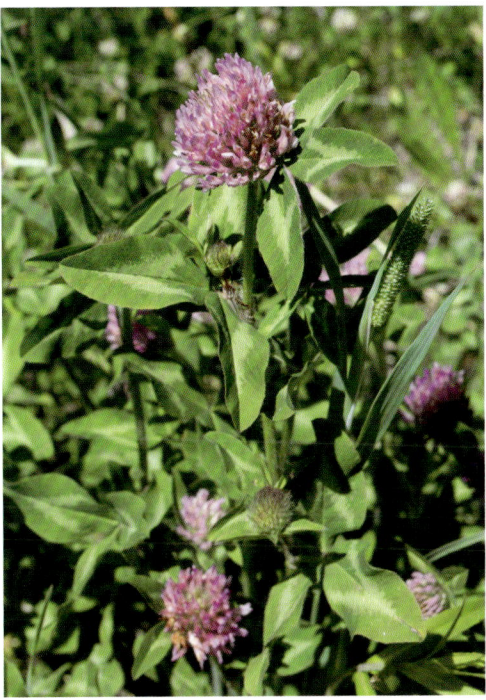

Gather the flowers right as they blossom, before they start to brown.

Caution

It is questionable whether you can use this herb in pregnancy due to its phytoestrogen content. Consult with a trained herbalist first.

Future harvest

Red clover is mostly known for being a weed, and a really hard one to eradicate, so don't worry about taking the flowering tops. Just make sure you are gathering in a clean, nonsprayed area, and stay away from soils polluted with nitrates, heavy metals, or pesticides.

HERBAL PREPARATIONS

Tea
Hot infusion
1 ounce fresh or dried leaves and flowers
1 quart water
Drink as needed.

Tincture
1 part fresh leaves and flowers
2 parts menstruum (75% alcohol, 25% distilled water)
or
1 part dried leaves and flowers
5 parts menstruum (60% alcohol, 40% distilled water)
Take 20–40 drops 3 times a day.

Oil
Infuse with fresh or dried leaves and flowers.

redroot

Ceanothus species
mountain lilac, New Jersey tea, buckbrush
PARTS USED roots, bark, twigs

Redroot combines well with a suite of other medicinal herbs,
in formulas that support the lymphatic system.

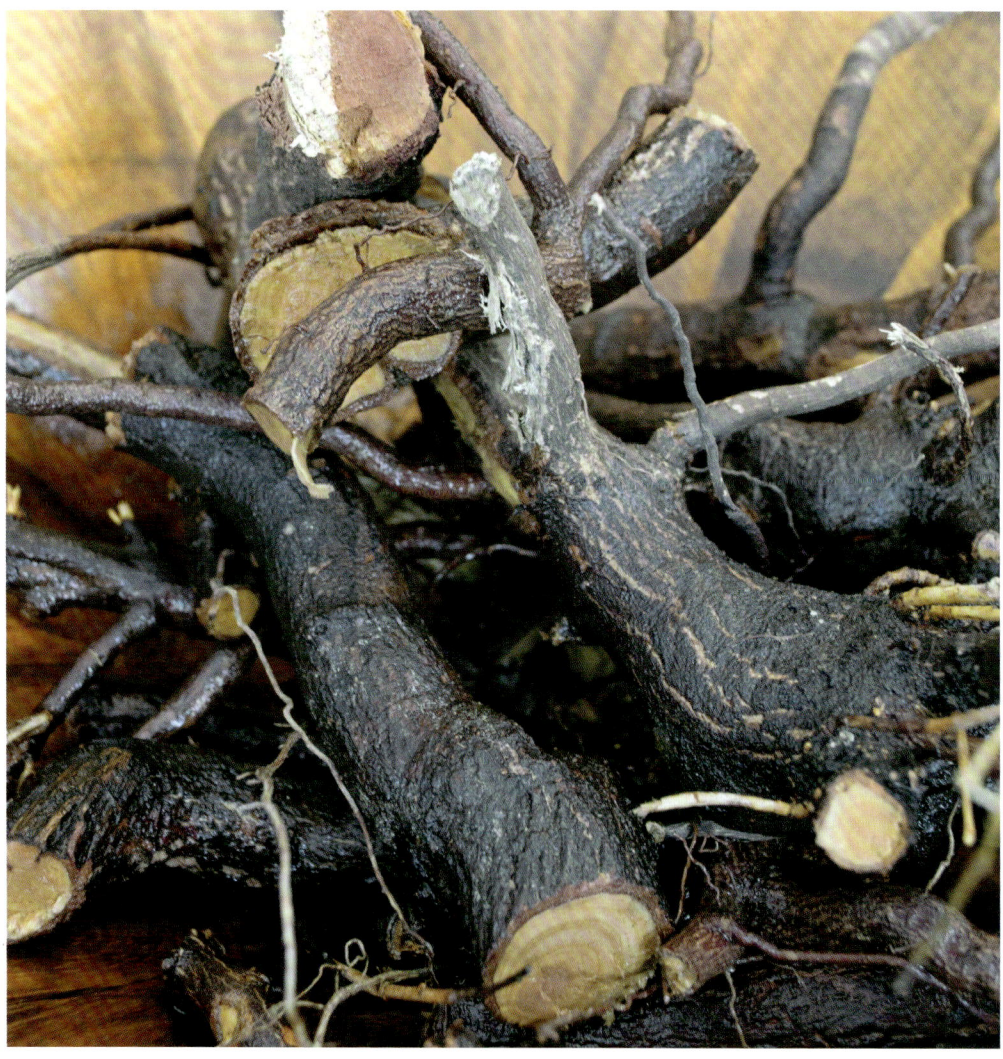

Notice the red freshly washed and sliced roots of redroot.

How to identify

Redroot has an alternative common name of mountain lilac for good reason. This small shrubby bush does have a faint resemblance to our ornamental lilacs. The five-petaled white flowers bloom on clustered panicles. Each petal has a spoon shape to it, curving upward. The thick and shiny leaves have three prominent midveins that go from the petiole to the top of the leaf. The bark is red and smooth, sometimes with thin spine-like projections from the stem that need to be minded.

The native species we have most commonly in the west are *Ceanothus fendleri* and *C. velutinus*, which is much more aromatic and has sticky leaves.

Where, when, and how to wildcraft

Redroot is found growing through rolling foothills of the mountain west and into the alpine forests. Harvest the root in fall or early spring. Be mindful of where you are gathering and whether there is enough for you to dig up roots. If not, twigs and bark are always an option. Bring a sturdy shovel and shears when you go out to harvest ceanothus.

This strong, woody root must be cut while fresh; if attempted once dried, you will cry with frustration. Use hefty loppers or clippers to chop the roots into pieces for drying or use immediately for tincturing fresh.

Medicinal uses

Redroot is a drying, stimulating herb that helps the flow of the lymph system. This is especially useful in illness and during recovery. It works best when combined with herbs that are also targeting your symptoms and combating the infection or virus. It can be used with osha and balsamroot for the onset of any inflammatory condition of the respiratory system. If there is a cough that is full of mucus, horehound can be a useful addition, helping to expectorate what is in the lungs. If it is a dry cough, try adding in mallow or plantain infusion. For a sore throat tincture or spray, combine redroot with Oregon grape, cottonwood buds, or alder.

Future harvest

Look to harvest redroot where the roots have already been disturbed, as they can be very difficult to obtain from the hard, rocky soil it prefers.

HERBAL PREPARATIONS

Tea
Hot infusion
3 tablespoons fresh or dried root, bark, or twigs
1 cup water
Decoction
1 ounce fresh or dried root
1 quart water
Drink 1 cup 3 times a day.

Tincture
1 part fresh root
2 parts menstruum (90% alcohol, 10% distilled water)
or
1 part dried root
5 parts menstruum (60% alcohol, 40% distilled water)
Take 5–10 drops several times a day.

Oil
Infuse with fresh or dried root.

rose

Rosa species

PARTS USED leaves, flowers, flowerbuds, hips

Rose is subtly familiar to our DNA. It gives us that nourishing connection, like the oxytocic flush you feel when you walk in the woods alone. Rose offers that to most people in a small little dose, like an aromatic sigh that makes us relax.

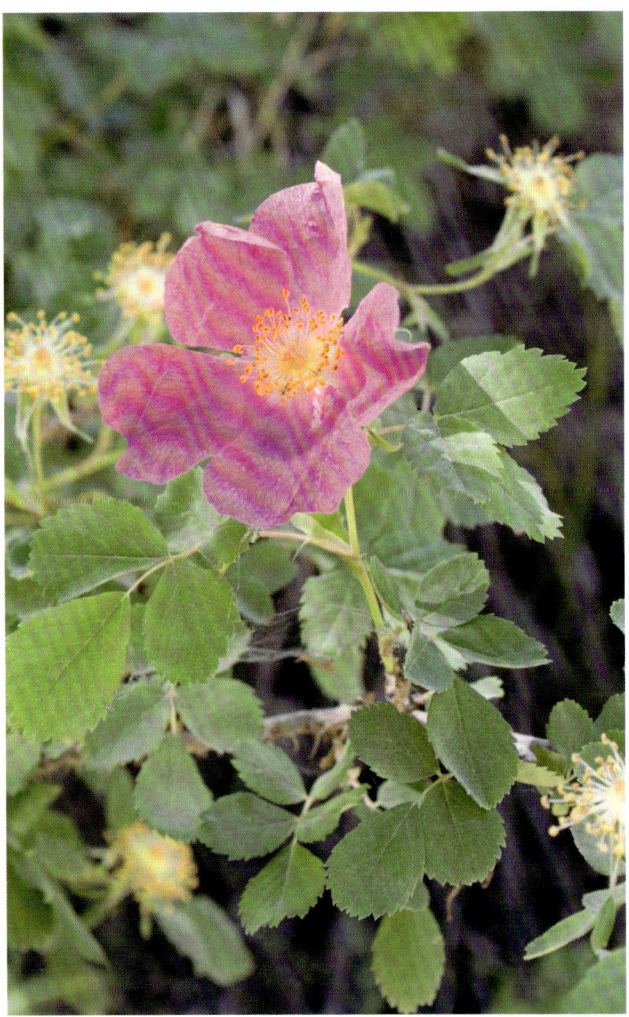

The fragrant petals of rose can be made into heart-supporting remedies such as elixirs, syrups, tinctures, teas, and hydrosols.

How to identify

The fruits of wild rose are called rosehips; when ripe they are deep red, round, and plump. Thorny thickets are recognizable throughout the year, thanks to either the lingering red rosehips or the heavenly scented flowers. Flowers range in size and color but are always a shade between white and dark pink; they have five petals, five sepals, many stamens, and a deep yellow center. Leaves grow alternately along the stem as pinnately divided leaflets. Each leaf has one to four pairs of leaflets, with a single leaflet at the tip. All leaflets are ovate in shape and serrated.

Where, when, and how to wildcraft

Roses can be found in many areas of the mountain west, along waterways, on craggy mountainsides, or at the edges of willow, cottonwood, and conifer forests. Rosebuds and the flowers that follow can be gathered as soon as you see the

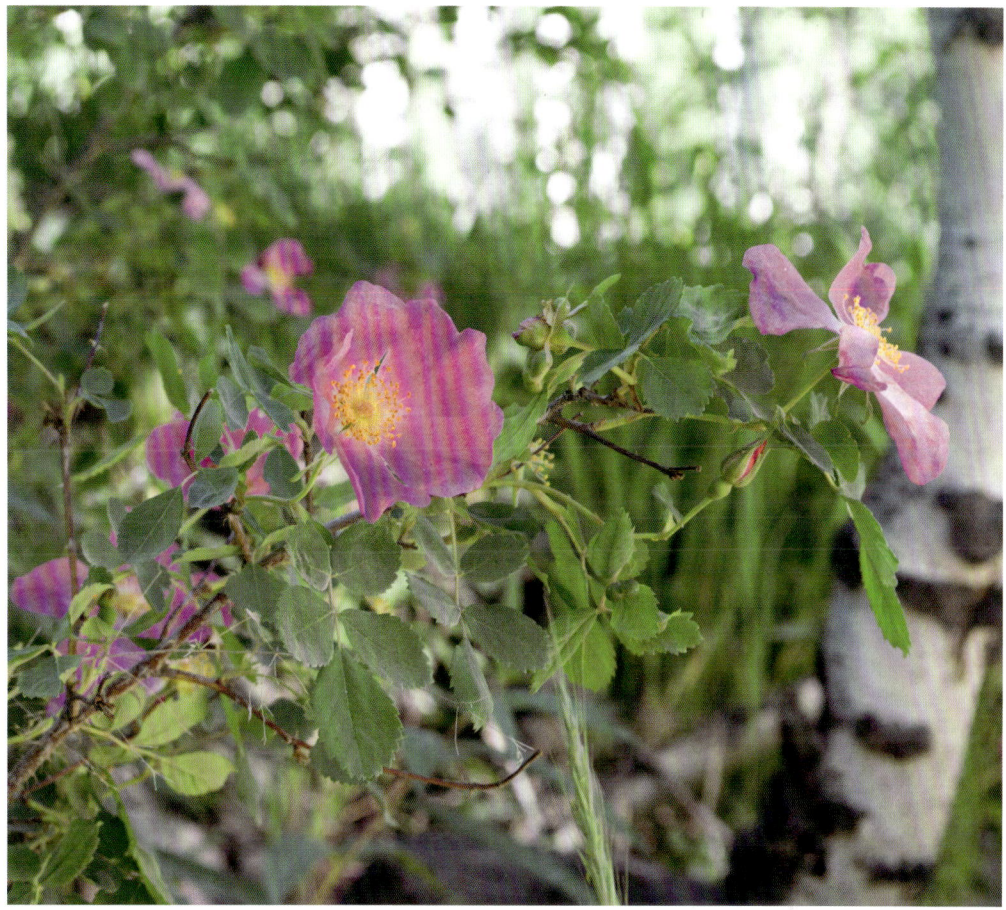

Gather just the petals from the flowering wild rose to give a chance for the ovary to turn to fruit.

pink petals swelling inside the green sepals. Rosehips can be gathered into the dark days of winter and are usually one of the only fruits remaining.

Bushes will have flowering roses and budding flowers at the same time. Rosebuds can be plucked and dried. Rose petals can be picked off individually by gently pinching all five petals from the calyx. Be sure to gather on a dry, sunny day, which will provide you with the most aromatic flowers. Rosehips can be munched on at any time (see caution). They are definitely best after the first few frosts. Frost helps to sweeten up the tangy flavor and soften the flesh.

Medicinal uses

Something is so comforting and familiar about the aromatics of rose. For most people, it relaxes the unneeded tension of the body, acting as an emotional stabilizer. It is the first remedy I reach for when someone needs the spark back, or could use an herb that feels like a mother's embrace.

Rose has a cooling effect on an over-worked liver or digestive tract. It can help soothe irritable bowel or leaky gut by astringing and healing the mucosa tissues; it combines well with mallow leaves or root.

Make a hot or cold infusion of rose petals or rosebuds, using a pinch of petals or three

Hydrosol

A hydrosol is the aromatic essential oils of a plant, captured through condensation and infused in water. Making a hydrosol is as simple as heating an herb in a covered pot of water. To do this, however, you need the right setup: a pot large enough to contain the herb, the water, a bowl, and another bowl or a brick to use as a pedestal; some ice to create the condensed steam; and a lid that can be turned upside down while still fitting snugly enough to contain the vapors. The upside-down lid should have a concave shape to it. This lets the hydrosol run down to its center and drip into the bowl that is propped up out of the water. Place the ice on top of the upside-down lid. I find it easiest to use leak-proof bags of ice, so you can pour out the water as it melts and refill the bags with ice.

Heat the herb water to a simmer and keep it covered for 30 minutes to an hour before you slowly lift the lid to check how much hydrosol has been collected. When lifting the lid, make sure to tilt it in such a way that the water condensation runs off into the bowl of hydrosol. Don't lose a drop!

Keep hydrosol stored in the refrigerator, or add 25% alcohol to make it shelf stable.

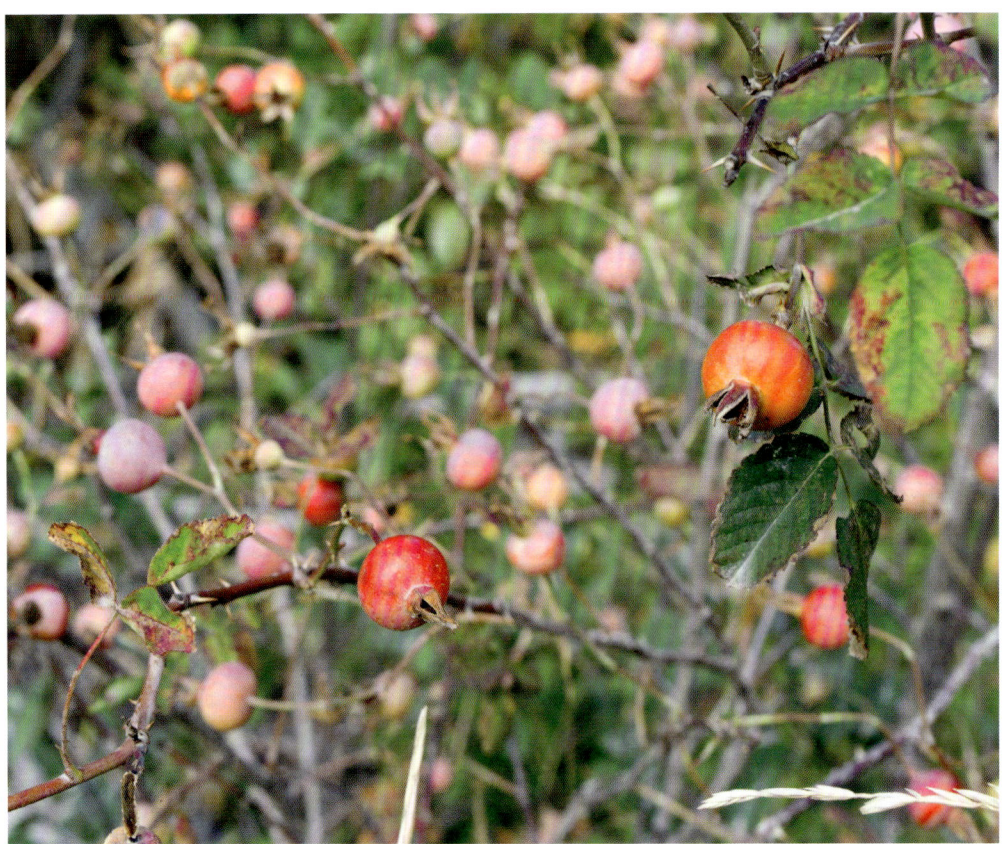

Large rosehips beginning to ripen. After a frost they will be perfectly soft.

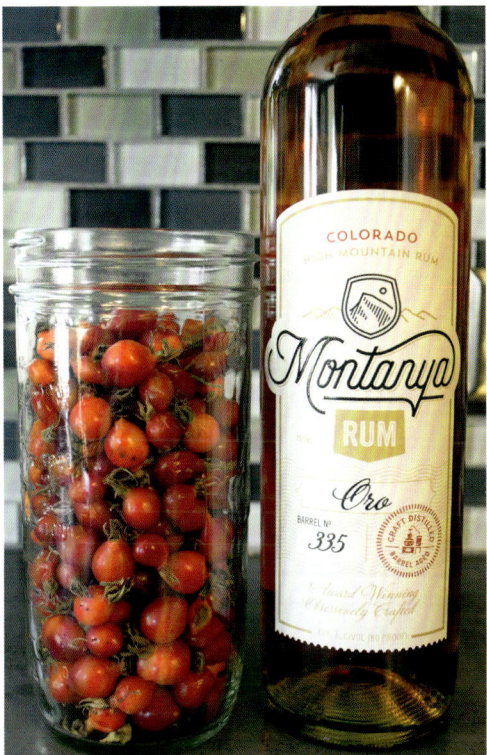

I highly suggest not only supporting your local distilleries, but creating a rosehip liqueur to enhance syrups and other concoctions.

The petals of rose infused into oils like coconut or jojoba are perfect for facial creams and serums. To capture the fragrance and a lovely light pink color, infuse your oil multiple times with fresh or dried petals.

⚠ Caution

The very fine hairs attached to the seeds inside rosehips can irritate the throat or digestive tract, causing diarrhea in some cases. I find that when I carefully strain the rosehips out of infused honey or tea, I am not bothered. Alternatively, slice open the hips and scrape out the seeds and hairs before eating or preserving.

Future harvest

Harvest wisely through the seasons—taking all the roses leaves behind no hips.

to five buds per cup of water. The hips are high in vitamin C and are a great addition to teas during cold season or to a nourishing brew of herbs that are mineral- and vitamin-rich, such as raspberry leaf, red clover, horsetail, and globemallow.

Rose petals, and the hips after they have been hit with a frost, are lovely infused into honey. This honey can sweeten tinctures or be dolloped into teas. An elixir, or tincture of rose petals or rosebuds steeped in brandy and honey or glycerin, is excellent for cheering up a dreary mood brought on by heartbreak or stress.

HERBAL PREPARATIONS

Tea
Hot or cold infusion
2–3 tablespoons fresh or dried petals, flowerbuds, hips, or leaves
1 cup water
Drink as needed.

Tincture
1 part fresh petals, rosebuds, or hips
2 parts menstruum (75% alcohol, 25% distilled water)
or
1 part dried petals, rosebuds, or hips
5 parts menstruum (60% alcohol, 40% distilled water)
Take 30–60 drops 3 times a day.

Oil
Infuse with fresh or dried petals and rosebuds. Repeat with fresh or dried petals and rosebuds 2–3 times for stronger fragrance and color.

---

sagebrush

Artemisia tridentata
PARTS USED leaves, stems, flowers

Be sure not to mistake sagebrush for your culinary sages, which are Salvia *species.*
Though both can be used in smudge bundles, they taste nothing alike.

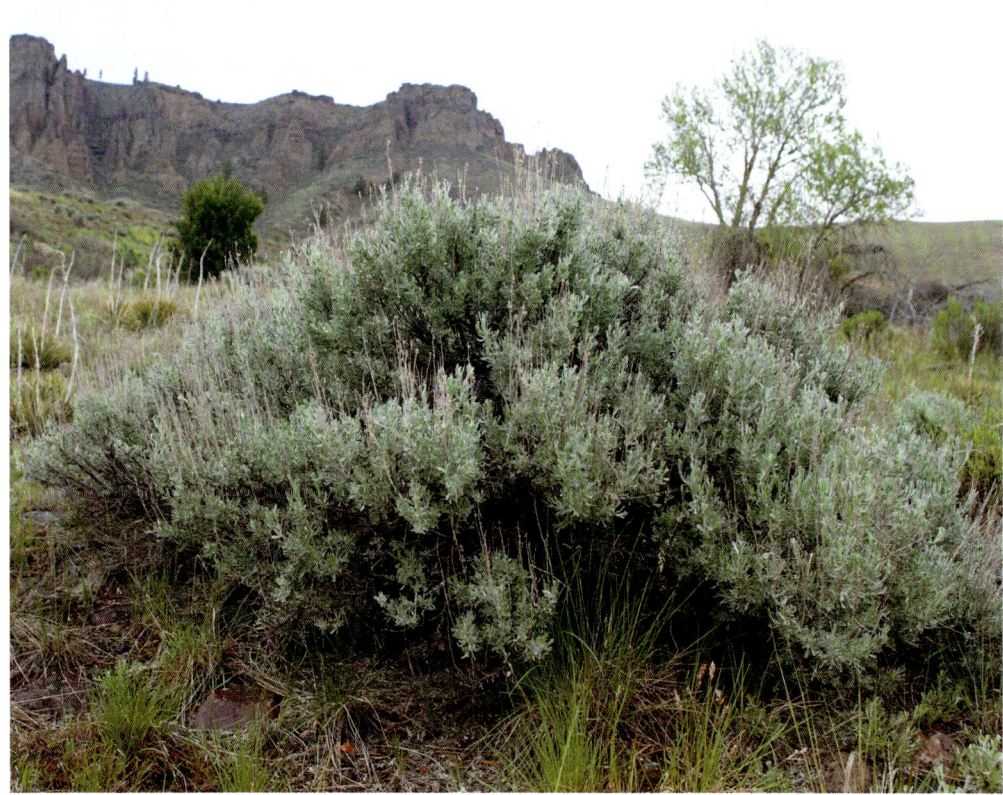

Gather bits and pieces from each sagebrush you walk past when harvesting.

How to identify

Artemisia tridentata is a woody shrub that grows widely throughout the west, in varying sizes, depending on variety and the location. Higher altitudes allow for smaller plants reaching 2–4 feet, whereas the big sagebrush of Wyoming at lower elevations can be two or three times the size of those that dwell in the mountains of Colorado.

Artemisia tridentata derives its name from its trident-shaped leaves. They are a soft, silvery green and have three prongs at the tip of

Smudge Bundles

Burning herbs for ceremony is a long-standing tradition in many cultures. It helps to ground energy, clear space, and purify the air. Most widely seen are sage bundles, which use either *Salvia* or *Artemisia* species. Smudge sticks can include many fragrant herbs, such as sagebrush, *Grindelia*, sweet clover, and juniper. Aromatic roots such as osha and balsamroot can be burned after they are dried. Sweet grass is often braided into long, thick strands for future igniting.

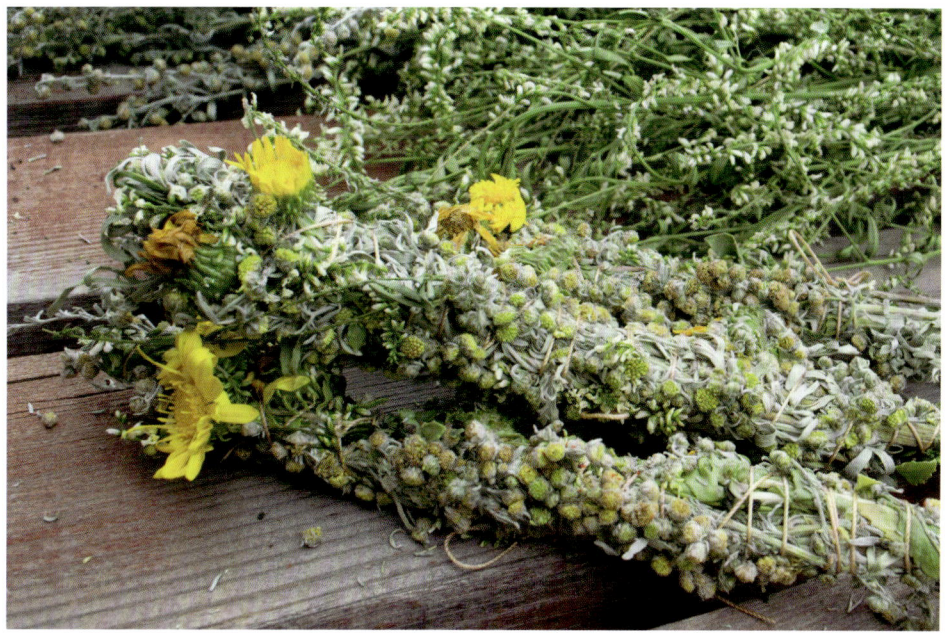

Bundling *Artemisia tridentata*, *Melilotus albus*, and *Grindelia squarrosa* into smudge sticks for burning.

each. Leaves grow alternately in clusters along the woody branches. Twigs of young sagebrush are silvery and pubescent. As the plant ages the bark starts to shred away in long pieces. The rounded, yellow flowers grow in heads along a spike-like inflorescence that sticks up higher than the sagebrush bush itself.

Where, when, and how to wildcraft

Artemisia tridentata is one of the most iconic sagebrushes of the mountain west. Look for it all over the Rocky Mountains at varying elevations and in the desert lowlands. The powerful scent of sagebrush can be smelled all the way through winter as the tops poke through the snow. The best time to gather is throughout the summer, and especially when the rains are plentiful. Try to go out and gather after the rains have subsided for a few days. Harvest on a dry, sunny day when you can smell the fragrance of sagebrush.

Medicinal uses

Artemisia tridentata is a strong aromatic, bitter, and warming herb. A cold infusion makes a lighter sipping aid that can help to calm a sour stomach or stimulate digestion. A hot infusion is much more warming and can be of assistance when viruses creep in, revving up the fever, breaking up stuck mucus, and aiding in expectoration.

Picking fresh sagebrush or adding dried herb to a pot of simmering water can be hugely beneficial as an inhalant for bronchial or throat infections. The antimicrobial aromatics are diffused through the steam and inhaled into the places they need to be active. The stimulating aromatics of sagebrush also make it useful as an emmenagogue, which means it will help to bring on stagnant or late menses.

For topical use, sagebrush can be extracted in alcohol, apple cider vinegar, or oil. It can also be made into a hot poultice to be applied to the chest as a compress for bronchial relief, and to inflamed or painful joints. It is very effective in salves for fungal or bacterial infections, and for use in sprains and strains formulas.

Long-standing use of sagebrush is to pick it while in bud in order to bundle it up into a smudge stick. This can be combined with other aromatic herbs such as juniper, other artemisias, grindelia, sweet clover, and more. Smudging can help to clear the air, both physically of airborne pathogens and energetically.

The fresh or dried herb can also be added to the hot rocks of a sauna for increased sweating and stimulation to the mucous membranes.

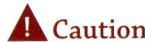 Caution

Avoid in pregnancy.

HERBAL PREPARATIONS

Tea
Hot or cold infusion
1 teaspoon fresh or dried leaves
1 cup water
Drink 1 cup 3 times a day.

Tincture
1 part fresh leaves, flowers, and stems
2 parts menstruum (75% alcohol, 25% distilled water)
or
1 part dried leaves, flowers, and stems
5 parts menstruum (60% alcohol, 40% distilled water)
Take 10–20 drops 3 times a day.

Vinegar
1 part fresh or dried leaves, flowers, and stems
5 parts vinegar
Take 1 tablespoon 1–3 times a day.

Oil
Infuse with fresh or dried leaves, flowers, and stems.

Future harvest

There is a lot of sagebrush—seas of it, in fact—however, that doesn't mean you have a license for clear-cutting. *Artemisia tridentata* takes a long time to reach the growth you are seeing. It's a woody, long-living shrub, with some varieties having a lifespan that may exceed 150 years. Respect it as you would an elder.

Saint John's wort

Hypericum species
Saint Joan's wort
PARTS USED leaves, flowers, flowerbuds

The bright yellow flowers turn menstruums a brilliant and unexpected ruby.

How to identify

Saint John's wort, *Hypericum* species, have bright yellow flowers that consist of five petals and many long stamens bursting from the center. Leaves and flowers are covered in a sticky red resin, which will stain fingertips—or your mother's white leather couch. If you pick a leaf and hold it up to the sun, you'll see it is perforated with tiny little holes. Leaves grow opposite and are oblong in shape.

Hypericum perforatum is invasive in some states of the west, with advisory to not even plant the seeds in certain counties. We have a native species, *H. scouleri*, which is much more dainty and slim, unlike *H. perforatum*, which is more branched.

Where, when, and how to wildcraft

Find *Hypericum perforatum* growing around the Front Range of the Rockies and in lower elevation zones. The native species *H. scouleri* can be found in wet, riparian areas of the west or even drier meadows.

Gather when the plant is in full bloom or when the buds are just starting to open. This should be in midsummer, but varies between elevations. Pick off the leaves, flowers, and flowerbuds and use fresh for best extraction of medicinals.

Medicinal uses

Saint John's wort is helpful with nerve injury or nerve pain, such as neuralgia, sciatica, and pains in the coccyx. Injuries with inflammation, convulsion, spasm, redness, heat, and shooting or sharp needle-like pains can be lessened by Saint John's wort.

The infused oil is great for rubbing on bruises and trauma areas. It can help heal deep wounds from inside out. Use as a wash

Our native species of Saint John's wort *Hypericum scouleri*.

or liniment on a wound to encourage healing at the deepest layer. It is useful for skin conditions, burns, radiation burns, ulcers, skin tags, boils, and carbuncles. It can be beneficial for fibromyalgia, rheumatism, and paralysis.

The oil blends well in a salve along with cottonwood or aspen buds and species of *Grindelia* and *Mertensia*. This salve can be used for just about anything the skin needs healing from, like minor burns, sunburn, cuts, scrapes, and itchy or chapped skin. Include the oil as an ingredient to enhance a handmade sun block. The addition seems to extend the time you can be in the sun without burning.

Saint John's wort blends well with other herbs to help lift the spirits or calm anxiety. Try blending for teas or tinctures with herbs such as hawthorn, pineapple weed, skullcap, or rose.

Caution

If you are taking any medications, it is best to consult with a healthcare practitioner, such as an herbalist or doctor, before using Saint John's wort, as it can have drug interactions. Though rare, phytophotodermatitis can happen when Saint John's wort is taken internally.

Future harvest

Harvest our native species with tender love and care. The invasive species can be clipped more readily. Still, no need to pull it from the ground unless you are asked to by a rancher.

HERBAL PREPARATIONS

Tea
Hot infusion
1–3 tablespoons leaves and flowers, flowerbuds
1 cup water
Drink 1 cup 3 times a day.

Tincture
1 part fresh leaves and flowers, flowerbuds
2 parts menstruum (75% alcohol, 25% distilled water)
or
1 part dried leaves and flowers, flowerbuds
5 parts menstruum (60% alcohol, 40% distilled water)
Tincture of fresh Saint John's wort is best, but dry can be used as well. Take 20–40 drops 3 times a day.

Oil
Infuse with fresh flowers, flowerbuds, and leaves to make the preferred rich red oil. If harvested at its peak and dried well, the dried herb can be infused in oil and will turn it a light shade of reddish brown. Try fogging the herb first by covering it with alcohol overnight before adding oil to your jar.

shepherd's purse

Capsella bursa-pastoris
shepherd's heart
PARTS USED leaves, stems, flowers, seedpods

*A spicy and circulatory medicinal herb, shepherd's purse is a weed
that can spare an overharvest for its blood-stopping (styptic) properties.*

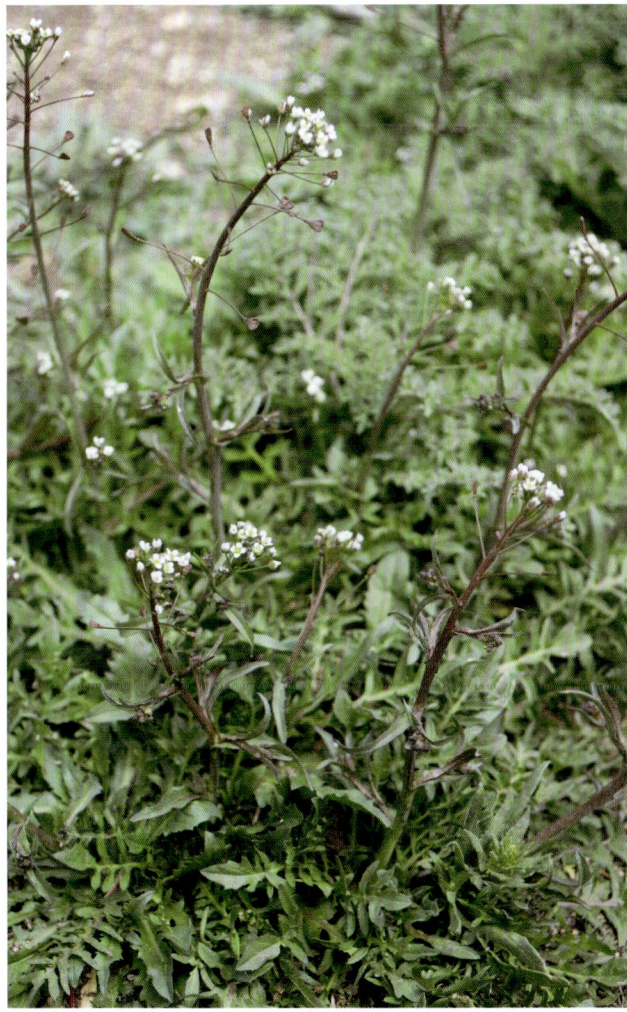

Find shepherd's purse growing as a weedy plant, taking up space
in abandoned fields or unkempt yards like mine.

How to identify

Shepherd's purse has distinct
basal leaves that have jagged
teeth on the margin that point
outward and upward, not downward like the dandelion. Basal
leaves are generally between 2
and 4 inches long and form a
rosette around the thin flowering stalk. Some small-toothed
leaves may be seen clasping the
stalk alternately; these are lanceolate or oblong. Flowers are
small with four white petals in
an X-shaped pattern, clustered
in loose racemes. The seedpod
(silicle) is what gives shepherd's
purse its name: it resembles a
heart-shaped pouch.

Where, when,
and how to wildcraft

Shepherd's purse is an invasive
weed that can be found in full to
partial sun, taking up space in
disturbed soils. Find it in parks,
along trails, or in abandoned
lots. The basal rosette of leaves
waits beneath the snow cover.
Once the snow melts, shepherd's purse can be spotted and

gathered in late winter or early spring. The seeds of the next generation germinate in the cool nights of autumn, so fresh young green leaves can be found again each fall.

Harvest the leaves right away in the spring before the plant sends up a flowering stalk; this is when they are most tender and full. Shepherd's purse will be in flower and seed by the first days of spring in lower elevations and will run its course by early summer when the days really begin to heat up. Gather the whole plant, stems, leaves, flowers, and seedpods.

Medicinal uses

Shepherd's purse is an astringent, spicy, pungent-flavored herb of the mustard family. It has been used to stop bleeding in acute situations such as external cuts and scrapes, and in more serious conditions, such as hemorrhaging after giving birth. It also acts as a diuretic and can help with laxity in the kidneys or bladder.

Shepherd's purse can be used to promote circulation in the body, when used internally as a tincture and externally in oil. It has anti-inflammatory properties that make it useful for arthritis or gout. The fresh poultice can be used to bring heat and circulation to an injury, for chronic pain, or for a deep chest cold.

Caution

Not for use during pregnancy, and should only be used postpartum once the placenta is out. Not recommended for people who have thyroid deficiency.

Future harvest

No worries. Shepherd's purse is an invasive medicinal that will always cover ground in the mountain west.

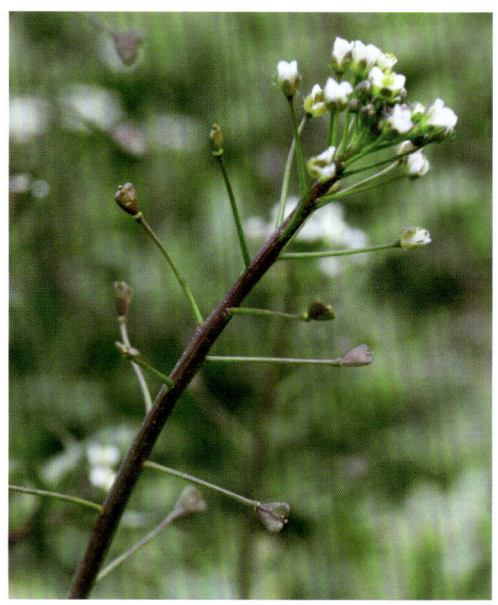

The seedpod of shepherd's purse is a two-chambered silicle that is shaped like a heart.

HERBAL PREPARATIONS

Tea
Hot infusion
1–2 tablespoons fresh or dried leaves, stems, flowers, or seedpods
1 cup water
Drink 3 times a day or as needed.

Tincture
1 part fresh leaves, flowers, seedpods, and stems
2 parts menstruum (75% alcohol, 25% distilled water)
The tincture of shepherd's purse tends to lose a good bit of its potency after a year or so. Best to make it in small amounts, then make a fresh batch each year. Take 20–40 drops 3 times a day.

Oil
Infuse with fresh or dried leaves, flowers, seedpods, and stems.

Siberian elm

Ulmus pumila
PARTS USED bark, leaves

The slippery infusion of Siberian elm is hydrating from the inside out.

How to identify

Siberian elm is a deciduous tree that can grow up to 60 feet tall. It has lofty branches that make the crown of the tree rounded, providing much shade. The leaves are toothed around the margins, and pointed at the tip, giving them an elliptical shape. They grow 1–2 inches long and are arranged alternately along the grayish silver branches. The branches can have a sort of zig and zag to them where each leafbud forms. The bark of the mature trees is furrowed and dark gray in color. Small purple flowers appear before the leaves in clusters along the stem. The fruits are rounded and smooth with wings (samaras).

Where, when, and how to wildcraft

The bark of Siberian elm can be stripped from the branches, or use the smashing-branch technique. When you smash the branch with something hard like a hammer or a rock, the bark easily peels off from the core of the branch. Use this outer bark in your infusions, or dry for future use. The leaves can also be gathered and used for tea or oil infusions.

Medicinal uses

Siberian elm is one of our superb demulcent trees of the west. Like its much-reputed relative slippery elm (*Ulmus rubra*) its bark can be peeled for an infusion of some seriously slick tea.

If constipation has a hold on you, making a Siberian elm tea or ingesting capsules filled

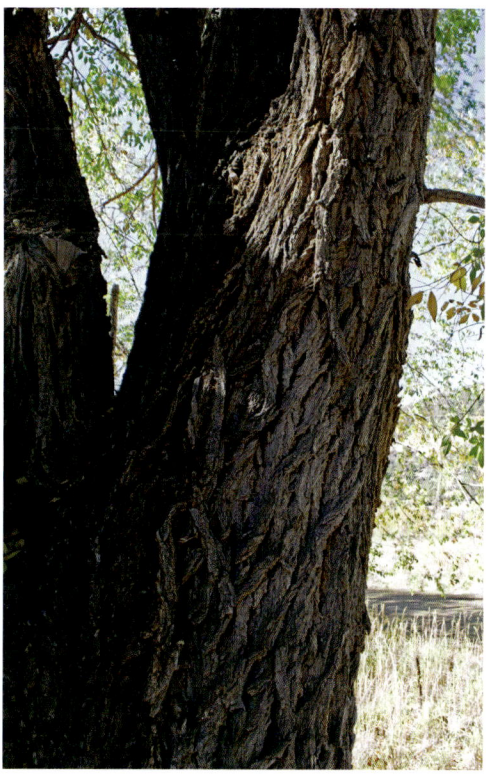

Siberian elm trees have rough and deeply furrowed bark.

with the powder of the bark can help with bowel movement. The demulcent properties coat the intestinal lining, aiding in moving out dry, hard stools. Drink about 1 teaspoon per cup of water at least 3 times a day. If it is diarrhea that is causing distress, a tripled dose of the bark can also be used to firm up stools and calm the inflammatory response in the bowel.

The mucilaginous properties of Siberian elm are also beneficial in any gastrointestinal complaints, such as ulcers, inflammation, or leaky gut, as it helps to lubricate and protect these membranes. For those who are sick or nauseous and having a hard time keeping substances down, a tea or porridge of Siberian elm can do the trick. For a porridge, use about a teaspoon of powdered or well-shredded bark per cup of broth. Easily absorbable, nourishing foods are excellent for convalescence.

Creating a poultice with the bark of Siberian elm can be cooling and very drawing. This can be used on boils, weeping wounds, burns, ulcers, or abscesses. Let the poultice crisp up and dry out.

When dryness is affecting you in any sort of way, a drink of Siberian elm tea will be one of your best plant allies. It can be very productive for dry, raspy coughs, or moistening nostrils made crispy from the arid winters.

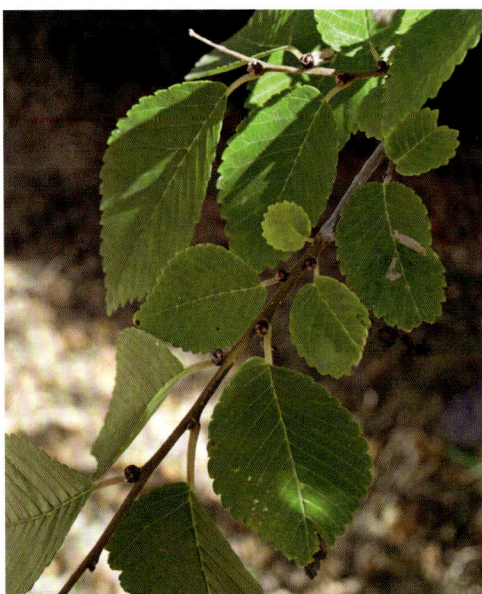

The young twigs and branches of Siberian elm can be harvested and peeled or snipped into pieces for drying.

Demulcent

When an herb is considered demulcent, or mucilaginous, it gets slippery when wet. These herbs create a sliminess that is super-nourishing to our mucous membranes, helping to soothe sore throats, dry coughs, irritated intestines, and digestive disorders such as acid reflux and ulcers. In the dry west, demulcents should be consumed in some form very often. These herbs are best extracted as hot or cold infusions. Cold water infusions best preserve the active constituent mucilin.

⚠ Caution

Consult with a physician if you are taking medications absorbed through the gastrointestinal tract, as Siberian elm can either slow or extend the absorption rate, due to its mucilaginous nature.

Future harvest

Siberian elms are a weedy tree of the west. They have come in as invaders and are generally not welcomed by ranchers and city officials. When working with trees, it's always best to harvest by pruning the branches of the tree. However, if you are trying to manage the spread of the tree, whole young trees can be cut down and the bark completely utilized. They will spring right back up!

HERBAL PREPARATIONS

Tea
Hot or cold infusion
2 tablespoons fresh or dried bark or leaves
1 cup water
Drink as needed.

skullcap

Scutellaria species

PARTS USED leaves, stems, flowers

Skullcap soothes and calms the woes of the anxious mind.

How to identify

A small, humble plant of the mint family, skullcap has opposite leaves and a square stem. The flowers are purple with a long neck that curls up into two lips. A white stripe is on the bottom lip of the flower. Our most common species regionally are marsh skullcap (*Scutellaria galericulata*) and Britton's skullcap (*S. brittonii*), which both offer great medicine. The species most commonly used from the wild, *S. lateriflora*, is not common in the mountain west.

Where, when, and how to wildcraft

Gather skullcap only if you find it in utter abundance. It is a dainty, marsh-dwelling plant, or can be found in moist meadows of the mountains. Find it growing alongside mints and willows on creeksides. The exception to this is Britton's skullcap, which tends to grow on drier rocky slopes.

Clip or pinch the top half of the plant, leaving behind plenty of foliage for the plant to survive. Never take the tops

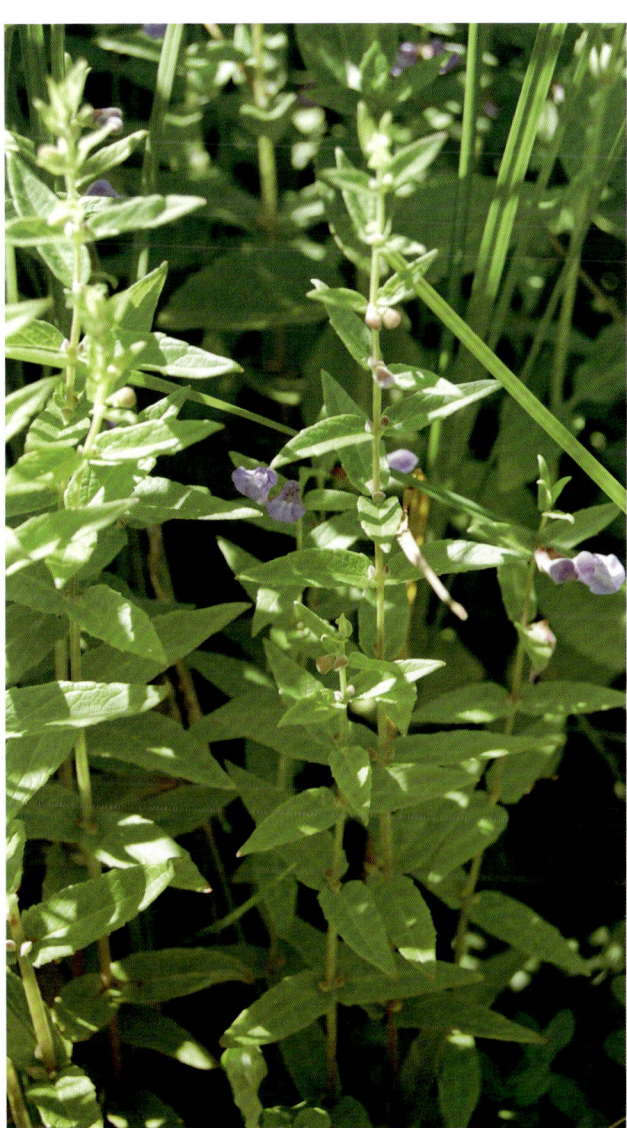

Find precious stands of skullcap in the mountain west and harvest with absolute gentleness and care.

off all the skullcap growing in an area. Leave flowers behind to propagate.

Medicinal uses

Skullcap is one of my favorite herbs to calm a rush of anxiety, nervousness, or to take the edge off a moody day that has you all sorts of tangled and dismayed. Skullcap is cooling, bitter, and calming in the best ways. It helps stressed-out parents with their coping skills, bringing them down from the mayhem of the day. It may sound like magic, but it's just a simple herb with a profound and delightful influence on the nervous system.

Mix with blue vervain (*Verbena* species), rose, and *Abies* species for a blend that can help nourish the person burning the flame at both ends, with no stop in sight. It is a cooling, nervine herb that can also be beneficial for menopausal hot flashes or night sweats. Think of skullcap for blending into formulas needed for sleep, where it can be useful in combination with hops or valerian.

Skullcap can be used as a tea, tincture, vinegar, or bath soak. Heck, I have even told the nonstop-stressed-out moms to throw it in with their French-pressed coffees.

Future harvest

Be super-careful with harvesting skullcap, as it can easily be pulled from the ground and should not be. Clip only the tops and tread with care around the habitat it dwells in.

HERBAL PREPARATIONS

Tea
2 tablespoons fresh or dried leaves, stems, and flowers
1 cup water
Drink as needed.

Tincture
1 part fresh leaves, stem, and flowers
3 parts menstruum (75% alcohol, 25% distilled water)
or
1 part dried leaves, stems, and flowers
5 parts menstruum (60% alcohol, 40% distilled water)
Take 20–40 drops 3 times a day.

Oil
Infuse with fresh leaves, stems, and flowers.

skunkbush

Rhus trilobata
squawberry, lemonadeberry, three-leaf sumach
PARTS USED leaves, stems, fruit

The tart berries of skunkbush make a pink-lemonade drink
that can soothe urinary tract infections.

How to identify
Skunkbush is a lower-growing shrub, ranging from 1 to 8 feet in height. The foliage
can look like miniature, shiny oak leaves;
however, they differ greatly in that they are
compound, with three leaflets, each leaflet
having margins with rounded lobes. When
rubbed, they emit a sweet skunky odor,
hence the common name. Fall foliage color
is a vivid red. Berries are technically drupes,
containing only one seed each. They turn
bright red when ripe and are coated with
a super-sweet-and-sour oily resin.

Where, when, and how to wildcraft
Skunkbush can be found among cottonwoods, scrub oaks, and sagebrush in rocky
soil. Berries start ripening in July; prime
gathering is when the berries are bright red
and glistening with the sticky resin. Gathering can continue on some bushes until the
leaves are as red as the berries. Bushes that
receive more water or shade tend to retain
berries the longest.

Clip off the bunches of berries or grab
handfuls from the bush. Their resin will coat
your fingers. I can never hold back licking my
fingers while collecting the drupes. The leaves
and stems can be gathered and dried on a
screen mesh. They can be cut into smaller
pieces or saved whole.

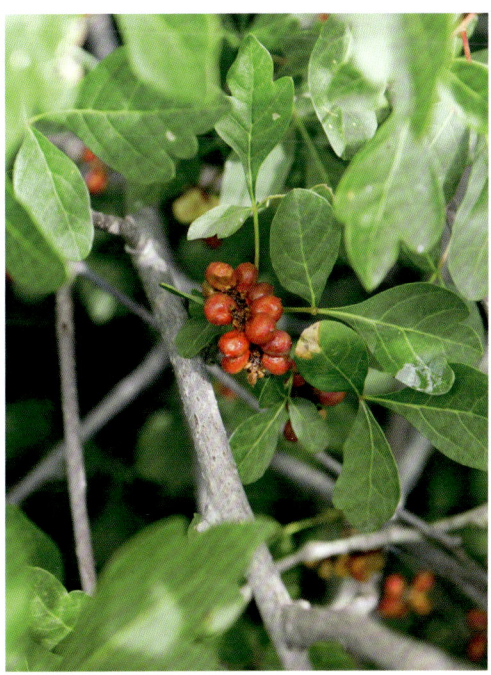

The small red, clustered berries of skunkbush are
coated in a sweet-and-sour resin that will coat
your fingers until they are licked or washed clean.

Medicinal uses
Pick apart the clusters of resinous drupes
and add about ½–1 cup of drupes per quart
of lukewarm or cold water. Hot water can
destroy the sweet-and-sour flavor of *Rhus*
species. Let this infusion sit for 4–8 hours.
Poured over ice, it is a great beverage for
overheated summer days.

This tart skunkbush tea can be helpful in easing bladder infections or irritation to the ureters. If you have recurring bladder infections, try freezing your infusion in ice-cube trays. Pop them out once frozen and store in a freezer bag, making enough to last until the following fall.

The berries can be extracted in vinegars for oxymels or sipping shrubs. Make an infusion in oil or glycerin from fresh or powdered dried leaves and stems. This is said to be good for sores around and inside the mouth, nostrils, or genital area. It helps to slightly disinfect and cool the sore while shrinking it.

⚠ Caution

If you have a known allergy to poison ivy, mangos, or cashews, then you may want to avoid this plant, as it is in the same family, Anacardiaceae. Poison sumac has white berries, not red.

Future harvest

Skunkbush is pretty abundant where it grows, and harvesting the berries is not a threat, as the plant spreads by sending out underground runners.

HERBAL PREPARATIONS

Tea
Cold infusion
1 ounce fresh or dried fruit
1 quart water
Steep for 4–8 hours and strain well. Drink as needed.

Vinegar
1 part fresh or dried fruit
2 parts vinegar
Take 1 tablespoon 1–3 times a day.

Oil
Infuse with fresh, or dried and powdered, leaves and stems.

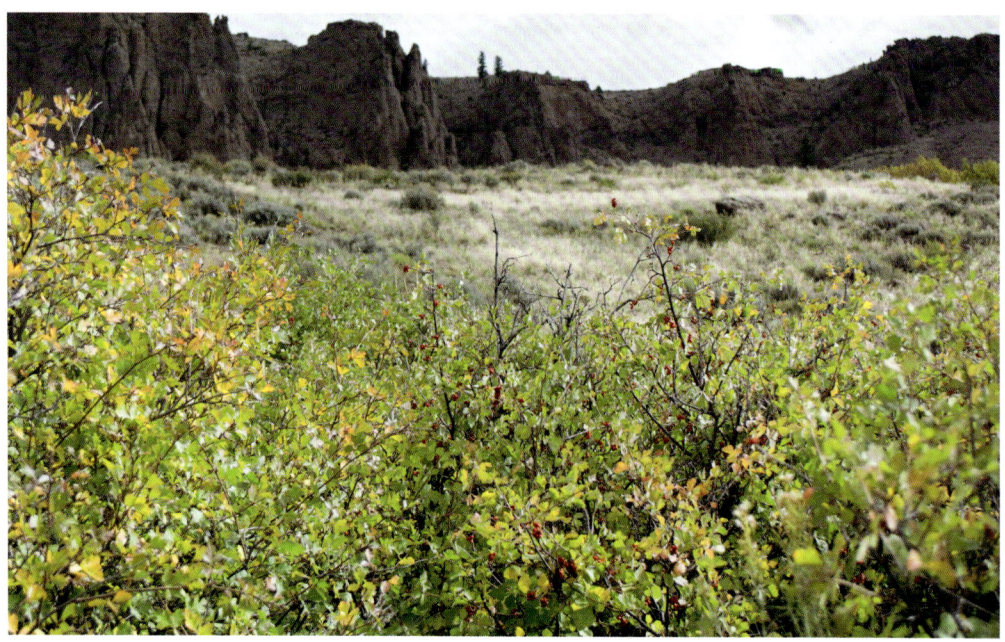

Get enveloped into a stand of skunkbush while searching for berries in late summer or early fall.

snakeweed

Gutierrezia species
escoba de la vibora, snakebroom
PARTS USED leaves, stems, flowers

Simmer freshly bundled snakeweed in a big pot of water,
and pour it into your bath before soaking your achy muscles.

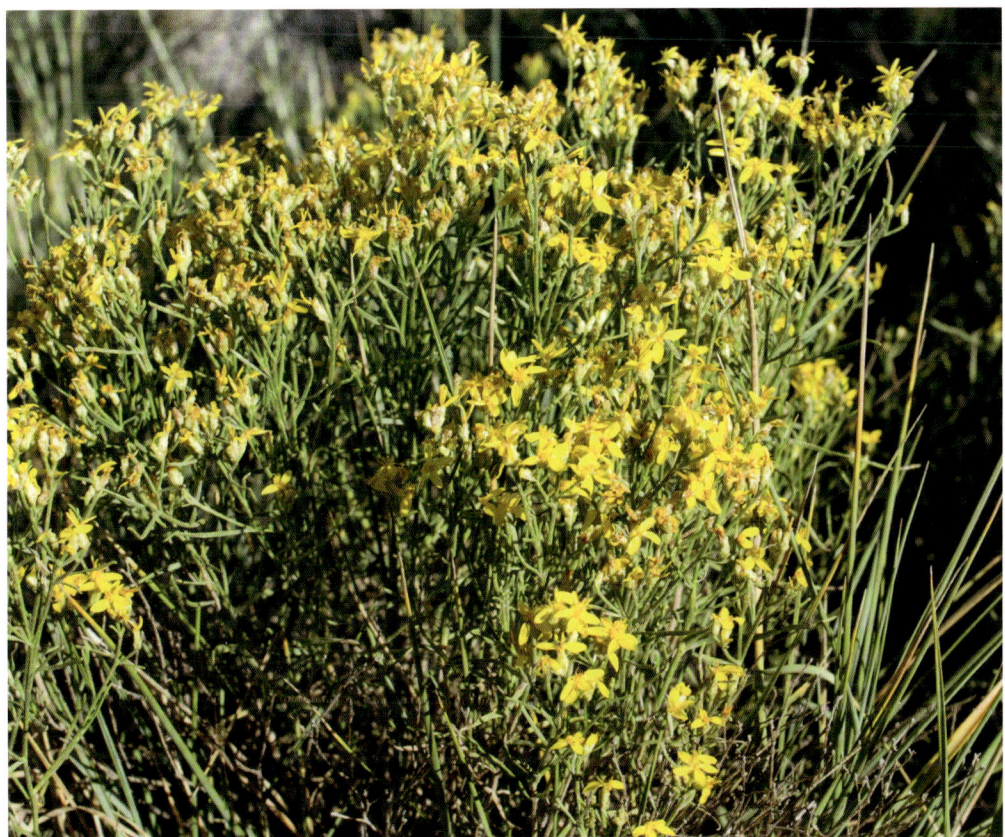

Early fall sets up with a golden sea of wildflowers—chief among them snakeweed. Harvest while it is in full bloom. It's a member of the sunflower family, with flowers composed of rays and discs.

How to identify

Snakeweed is a small yellow-flowering plant that blooms in late summer and through fall. It grows in clumps, with many branched stems, and looks like fluffs of gold. These fluffs contain many small citrus-piney-scented flowers. As a member of the Asteraceae, it has both ray

Bath Soaks

The idea of taking the time to soak in a tub is often overlooked, but its benefits are undeniable, especially when medicinal herbs are part of the magic mix. Bath soaks can be made a variety of ways. They may include salts or a giant pot of tea. They can be used for easing sore muscles, promoting relaxation and sleep, or to relieve the feeling of sickness.

Salts can be blended with dried herbs, fresh herbs, essential oils, and tinctures. Essential oils and tinctures can be dropped and mixed into the salts, to add the aromas and health benefits of the herbs. When using fresh herbs, chop them up finely, mix the herbs with the salt, and lay them out on a sheet or in a bowl, letting the herbs dry together with the salt. The salt will absorb the fragrance of your herbs and help them to dry. Salts to use are Redmond, Himalayan, Epsom, and other sea salts.

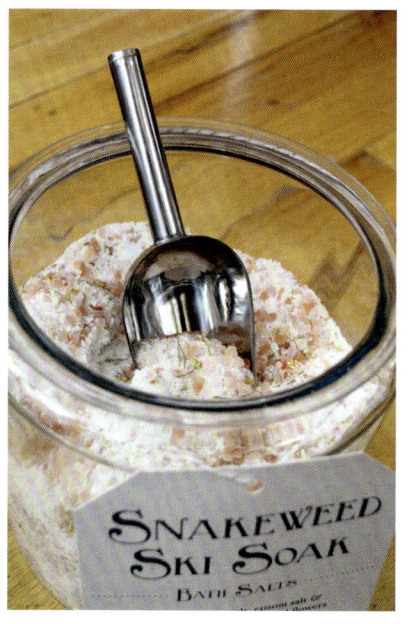

A mix of Epsom salt, Himalayan sea salt, and the flowers of snakeweed.

Combine herbs such as snakeweed, rose, pedicularis, conifers, artemisias, yarrow, or sweet clover to treat yourself to muscle-relaxing bliss. These herbs blend well in bath salts or soaks. Herbs can be put into a large pot of water and infused or decocted like a giant batch of tea. Strain well before adding this to your bathtub. Use 2–4 ounces of herbs per pot of water.

and disc flowers, about three to eight per bunch at the top of each stem. The leaves are slender and grow alternately along the stems. Snakeweed can look similar to two genera—*Ericameria* and *Chrysothamnus*—that are commonly known as rabbitbrush. Snakeweed is much smaller, however, and both rabbitbrush genera lack ray flowers.

Where, when, and how to wildcraft

Late summer and early fall is a yellow time of year for the flowering plants. In parts of the southwestern Rockies, fields are covered by a variety of glowing golden herbs such as snakeweed, rabbitbrush, and gumweed (*Grindelia* species).

I take clippers and grab half of the cluster of stems and clip a few inches up from the ground. While still fresh, I gather a small bundle in my hands, fold it back and forth, then tie it with string. These bundles can be used fresh, or lay them out on wire mesh for a few days to dry.

Medicinal uses

Snakeweed can be used as a bug repellent, especially good for no-see-ums. Liniment preparations extract the aromas that are repel bugs. Also oil infusions can be created for relieving bug bites.

Bundles can be used for bath soaks when sore achy muscles are slowing you down. A favorite in the apothecary is the Snakeweed Ski Soak, which is perfect for after the big snowstorms that leave the skiers and riders sore to the bone. It is a blend of salts and dried herb.

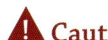 Caution

Snakeweed is not recommended to be taken internally, so do not consume. If you have an allergy to sunflower family plants, it is best to avoid it.

Future harvest

Do not rip the snakeweed from the ground. Bring clippers and snip at the base.

HERBAL PREPARATIONS

Tea
Sitz bath decoction
4 ounces dried or freshly bundled leaves, stems, and flowers
1 gallon water

Liniment
1 part fresh flowers, leaves, and stems
2 parts menstruum (75% alcohol, 25% distilled water)
or
1 part dried flowers, leaves, and stems
5 parts menstruum (60% alcohol, 40% distilled water)

Oil
Infuse with fresh or dried flowers, leaves, and stems.

Solomon's plume

Maianthemum racemosum

PARTS USED roots

The root of Solomon's plume can help the healing of connective tissues, bringing back some of the lost elasticity.

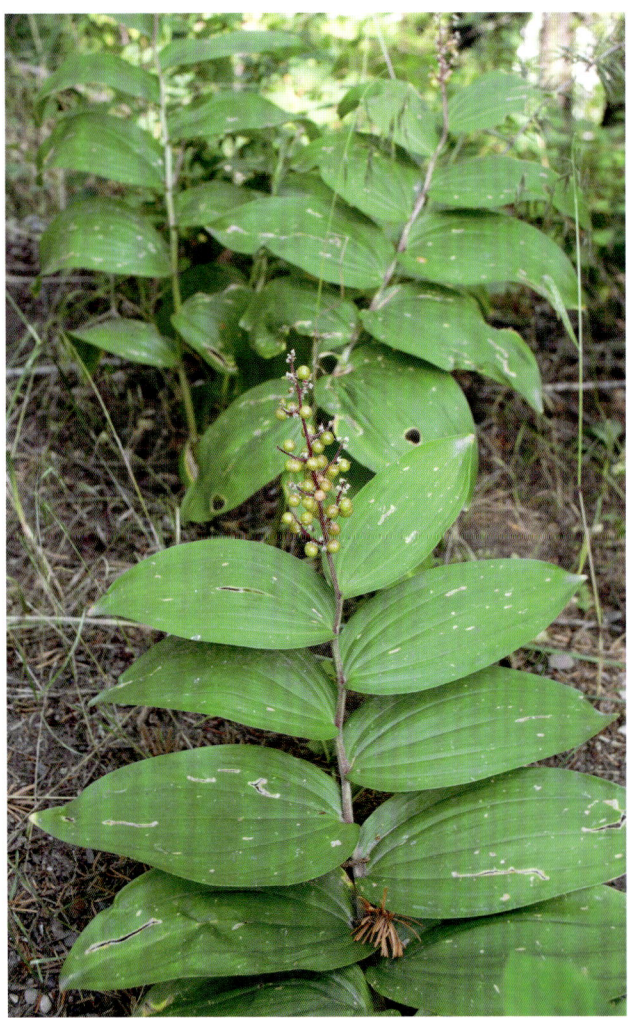

Maianthemum racemosum with unripe berries. Harvest the roots at this stage of growth or wait until the berries have turned red and start to fall off.

How to identify

The two species of false Solomon's seal we have in the western states are both called a variety of common names. All can be confusing to discuss because of the word "false" that tends to be in the common names of some *Maianthemum* species, such as false Solomon's seal. For the sake of simplicity, I call this species Solomon's plume (*M. racemosum*) and the smaller species starry Solomon's seal (*M. stellatum*). Solomon's seal (*Polygonatum* species) grows in the eastern United States, and many herbalists use all three of these plants interchangeably as medicine.

Solomon's plume is the bigger of the western maianthemums. It can reach heights of a few feet and arcs over the bigger it gets. The leaves grow alternately along the stalk, which zig-zags at each leaf junction. Leaves are a deep bright green, long, and smooth in texture, with parallel veins.

The flowers grow out in multiple inflorescences at the tip of

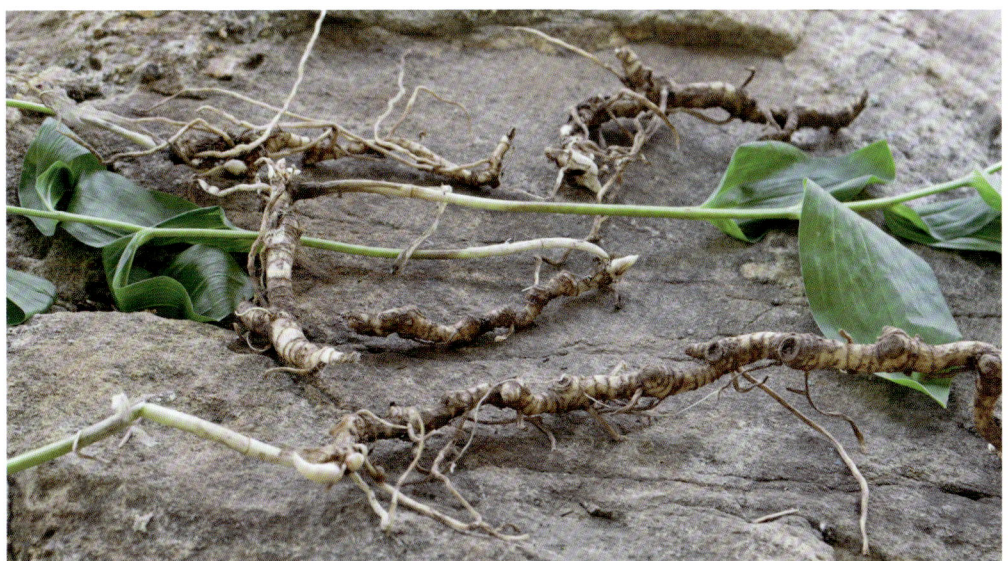

The jointed root of *Maianthemum racemosum*. Take the top joint along with the stalk and replant this into the ground, along with any other starts you see coming off the root. This helps to spread and thicken your nature garden, increasing growth for future harvests.

the plant, making it weigh down even further into an arch. Flowers are white and look like little starbursts. The immature fruits are greenish and red-speckled, maturing into solid red berries.

The roots are long and slender with little knuckles at each place where a plant has grown the previous year. They grow rhizomatously and have little rootlets growing alongside.

Where, when, and how to wildcraft
Find Solomon's plume in the rich forests of the mountain west. It prefers to stay in the shade of the trees. The roots of Solomon's plume can be gathered at the sign of first growth in spring, and in the fall after the berries have fallen. Harvesting the rhizomes of Solomon's plume or the roots closer to the surface is more sustainable than taking the entire plant. Carefully dig around the base of a mature plant until you come upon one of its rhizomatous runners. If you are gentle, this will tend to lead to another small leafy

sprout. Cut off the root between the sprout and the mother plant, taking this as your medicine. Then, leaving at least a few inches of root attached to the sprout, replant it. This allows you to harvest from one plant without taking too much life force, while simultaneously propagating another, which can help increase the population.

Medicinal uses
Where Solomon's plume really shines is in helping to heal fascial injury or joint immobility. An example of this would be joint pain from lack of synovial fluid, which causes dry, inflamed joints, with a lot of friction—noisy joints. The root of Solomon's plume seems to work by vitalizing the sinews and fascia, adding fluid, lubricating and moistening connective tissues. It can help strengthen loose ligaments and heal micro-tears that happen in tendons and ligaments, keeping them from becoming inflamed and dried out. The roots are good

for broken bones and bruising and can help relax and loosen tight tissues.

The fresh roots are preferred for use in oil extractions for massage oils and salves, also for alcohol extractions for internal or external use.

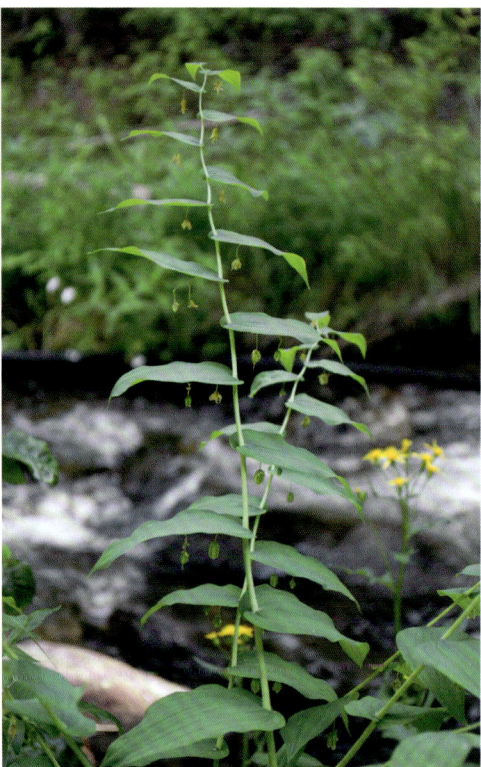

Twisted stalk (*Streptopus amplexifolius*) can be a lookalike to Solomon's plume, but the berries or flowers of twisted stalk hang under each leaf, as opposed to on the end of a dangling inflorescence.

It is a cooling, demulcent, and expectorant herb. This can be beneficial for coughs that need some hydrating and mucus moved out of them. It blends well in cough formulas with cherry bark and grindelia.

Future harvest

Solomon's plume grows more spaced out and is a bigger plant than starry Solomon's seal; therefore, harvest only when large areas have plenty growing. Replant the roots, as described earlier, for sustainable harvest.

HERBAL PREPARATIONS

Tea
Hot infusion
1 tablespoon dried or freshly chopped root
1 cup water
Decoction
1 ounce fresh or dried root
1 quart water
Drink 1 cup 3 times a day.

Tincture
1 part fresh root
2 parts menstruum (80% alcohol, 20% distilled water)
Take 20–40 drops 3 times a day.

Oil
Infuse with fresh or dried root.

spikenard

Aralia species
wild sarsaparilla
PARTS USED roots

When too much smoke has been inhaled over a long or short period of time,
spikenard can be beneficial in helping to clear the lungs of the heavy mucus.

How to identify

The two spikenard species of the mountain west can be partly distinguished by size. *Aralia nudicaulis* is a much smaller and daintier shrub than the bushy outward growth of *A. racemosa*. The leaves of both species are compound leaflets with a broad, ovate shape. The leafless flowering stalk grows from the base of the plant, separate from the leaf stems. The inflorescence is composed of a rounded compound umbel, with each umbel hosting 20 to 50 small white blooms. Each flower has five reflexed petals with five stamens projecting outward. The berries ripen to a deep purple. The roots are long and cream-colored and have many thin rootlets attached.

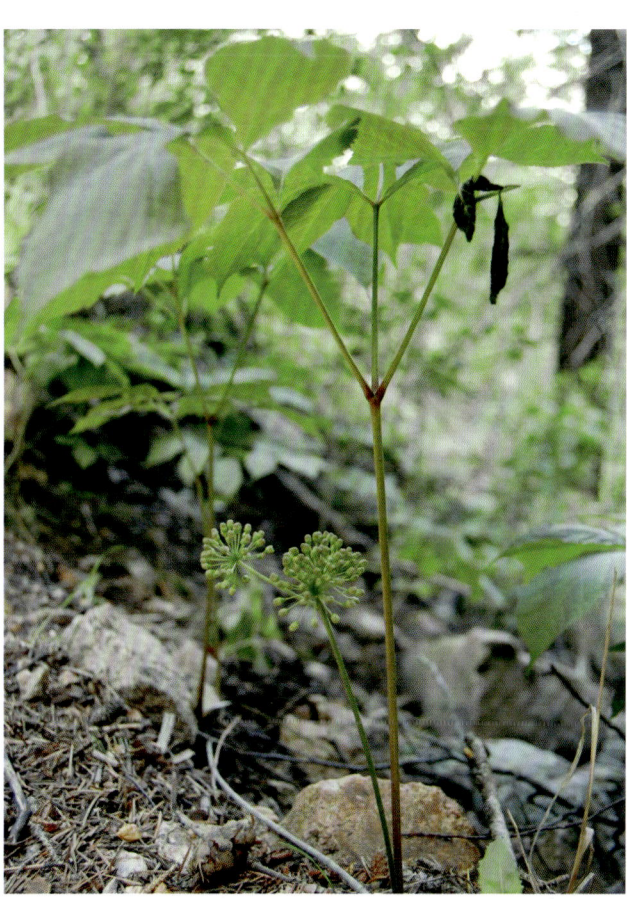

Our native spikenard *Aralia nudicaulis* does not grow very tall and can be found in patches.

Where, when, and how to wildcraft

Even though this plant grows minimally in the zone we cover in this book, it is worth mentioning. *Aralia racemosa* can be found growing in southern to southwestern Utah and can be found in parts of southern Colorado and the Front Range. In Arizona, New Mexico, and California you can find it much more frequently.

Aralia nudicaulis can be found on the Front Range of the Rockies in Colorado and Wyoming, in northwestern Montana, northern Idaho and Washington, and up into Saskatchewan and Alberta. *Aralia nudicaulis* grows in wet, rocky drainages or areas where moisture is harbored in the high elevations. Gather the roots in the spring and fall.

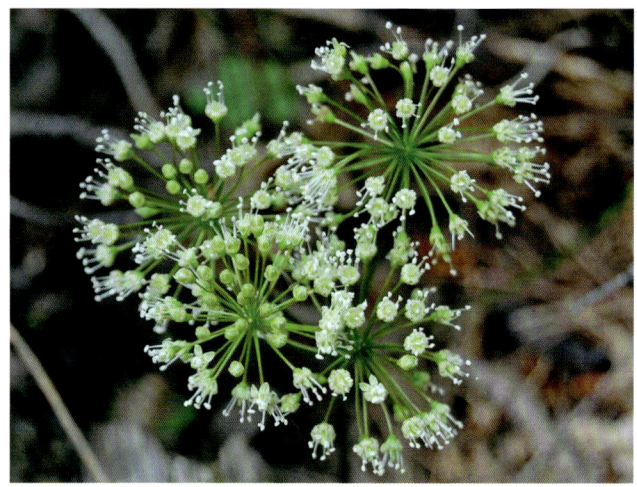

The beautiful umbel of *Aralia nudicaulis*.

Medicinal uses

Spikenard is a warming, drying, pungent, and oily root that I use most for lung conditions that are aggravated by dusty dirt or smoke. This can be beneficial for either smokers themselves, those affected by secondhand smoke, or victims in the vicinity of raging forest fires. Use the root for people who have begun to quit smoking as it acts as an expectorant and can help to rejuvenate the lung tissues.

It is also useful for the initial stages of a cold or respiratory virus. It infuses well into honeys and can be blended with herbs such as osha, grindelia, cherry bark, or elderberries and -flowers.

Spikenard can be administered internally as a tea or tincture. The root can be infused into oil for use as a chest rub. Try it along with yarrow, yerba mansa, and fir.

Future harvest

Spikenard is a rare plant to stumble upon in the wild. It is a relic species left over from the last ice age. Respect it as one of our elders. If you happen to find a large stand, take only a minimal amount and carry on.

HERBAL PREPARATIONS

Tea
Hot infusion
1 tablespoon dried or freshly chopped root
1 cup water
Decoction
1 ounce dried or freshly chopped root
1 quart water
Simmer for only 20 minutes to preserve the aromatics. Drink 1 cup 3 times a day.

Tincture
1 part fresh root
2 parts menstruum (75% alcohol, 25% distilled water)
or
1 part dried root
4 parts menstruum (60% alcohol, 40% distilled water)
Take 20–40 drops 3 times a day.

Oil
Infuse with fresh or dried root.

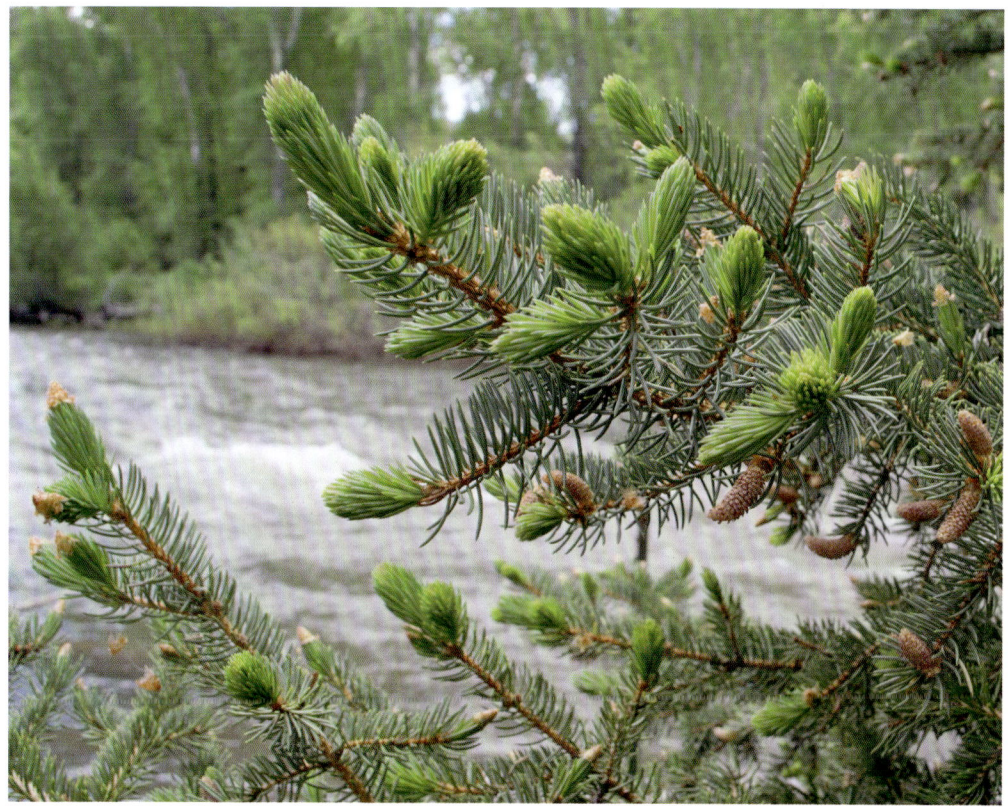

Picea species
mountain spruce
PARTS USED twigs, needles, resin

Careful while walking under the poky branches of spruce—these tricksters seem to always steal my hat.

The young, tender, and oh-so-flavorful tips of blue spruce.

How to identify

Spruces are tall evergreen trees, rising between 70 and 125 feet in height. Blue spruce (*Picea pungens*) and Engelmann spruce (*P. engelmannii*) grace the Rocky Mountains between 2000 and 12,000 feet. These species can be hard to tell apart, though there are a few distinguishing factors. Blue spruce will be seen growing slightly lower in elevation, while Engelmann's can be found in higher forests. Both trees grow in a symmetrical triangular shape. Each species has branches that are loaded with short prickly needles, but Engelmann's needles are much more flexible and not as sharp. Engelmann's has smaller cones that don't exceed 2 inches or so, while blue spruce has longer cones that will grow to at least 4 inches. The needles of both species have a blue-green or silver cast to them. Some say that Engelmann spruces have more of a camphor smell to the needles, while needles of blue spruce have a more pleasant lemony scent.

Where, when, and how to wildcraft

You will find spruces in mixed conifer forests at higher elevations. Engelmann's is most common throughout the mountain west, while blue spruce is primarily in Colorado, Utah, and Wyoming. The tips of spruces can be gathered in spring. Look for the brown covering at the ends of the branches. This covering is a casing around the young tip. Gather when these are plump and just beginning to blow off, but pick spruce tips with or without the brown casing—roll the tip between your fingers and let the casing carry off in the breeze. Tips are best gathered while the needles are tightly packed, but they are still good when the tip reaches an inch or so long.

Needles, twigs, and resins can be gathered any time of year. Find an old conifer forest full of spruces or look to neighborhood trees to easily gather plenty. Taste each tree as the flavors can vary, especially if you happen to be in a mixed forest of both Engelmann and blue spruces.

Medicinal uses

High in vitamin C along with a host of other vitamins and minerals, the spruce trees can be a veritable winter's harvest. The fresh needles can be infused for tea to help ease chest colds, or a large pot of decocted fresh twigs and needles could be poured into a hot bath to ease aches and pains. Create a steam inhalation or just make your house smell good with a decoction of spruce simmering on the stove. Keep the pot at a low rumble to create steam to help increase humidity in a dry house during the winter months. Spruce is ideal for chest colds. Add some usnea lichen to the pot with the spruce twigs and inhale the vapors and steam for about 10 minutes, several times throughout the day.

Infused syrups, honeys, vinegars, and alcohols are preparations that can inspire you to blend spruce into other formulations. Having a multitude of pleasant-tasting extractions can be beneficial when combining herbs. Spruces, especially in the spring, have a sweet yet bitter citrus flavor that complements numerous herbal flavors, as well as stimulating the digestion.

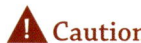 Caution

For some, when used in an excessive amount, conifer resin can be irritating to kidneys. Do not use spruce in pregnancy.

Future harvest

Spruce tree branches grow slowly, and harvesting the tips slows the growth of the branch even more. Luckily spruces like to grow close together, making it easy to gather tips from many trees, merely pruning nature's garden. Do be conscious of young trees, leaving them be and harvesting only from the older giants that can spare a light trim.

HERBAL PREPARATIONS

Tea
Hot infusion
3 tablespoons fresh needles and twigs
1 cup water
Drink as needed.

Tincture
1 part fresh needles, twigs, or resin
2 parts menstruum (75% alcohol, 25% distilled water)
Take 20–40 drops 3 times a day.

Oil
Infuse with fresh or dried needles, twigs, or resin.

starry Solomon's seal

Maianthemum stellatum

PARTS USED roots

Living in a ski town, I see my fair share of injured friends. Starry Solomon's seal is my go-to for helping repair their torn tendons and ligaments.

How to identify

Starry Solomon's seal (*Maianthemum stellatum*) is much smaller than Solomon's plume (*M. racemosum*) and grows more prolifically throughout the shaded woodlands of the mountain west. It has slender, bright green leaves that grow alternately up the arched stem. The stem zigs and zags between each leaf and grows only to about 6 inches or more from the ground. The flowers are delicate white stars that sit on the end of the stem in a raceme. These white flowers will turn into berries that are at first green with red stripes, eventually turning a solid red.

The roots are creamy-colored rhizomes with tiny rootlets that hang off the sides. They are crooked and run in all sorts of directions. Knuckles form at each point where a shoot has grown in previous years.

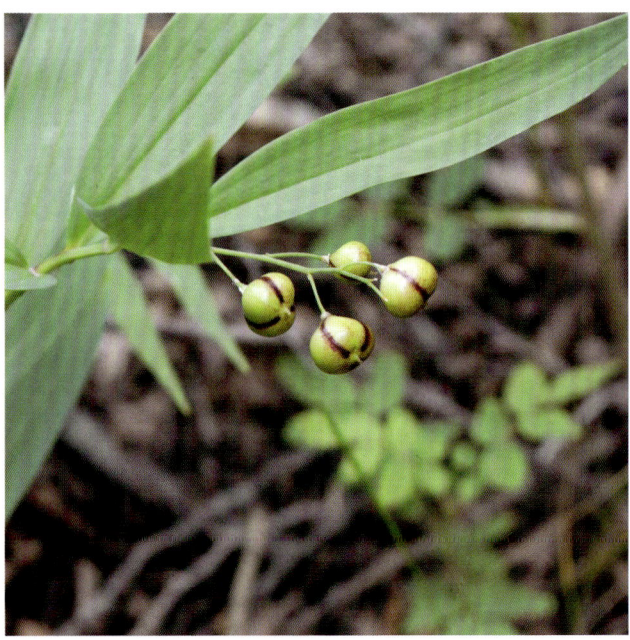

A much daintier species than *Maianthemum racemosum,* the berries of *M. stellatum* have stripes of deep scarlet before they turn to a solid shade of red.

Where, when, and how to wildcraft

Maianthemum stellatum can be found in dense stands under cottonwood, aspen, and scrub oak groves, or in coniferous forests. Find it settled close to a source of moisture, near creek beds in sheltered forests and damp canyons.

Harvest before the plant flowers in the spring or after the plant has begun to turn brown and dry to the ground in late summer or early fall. Dig up the little rhizomatous roots carefully, disturbing only a little bit from each large stand, then move to a new spot. Leave enough of each plant's root behind so it can regrow.

Harvest this species similarly to *Maianthemum racemosum*. Carefully dig around the base of a mature plant, until you come upon one of its rhizomatous runners. If you are gentle, this will tend to lead to another small leafy sprout. Cut off a piece of the root from in between the sprout and the mother plant, taking this as your medicine. Then, leaving at least a few inches of root attached to the sprout, replant it. This allows you to harvest from one plant without taking too much life force, while simultaneously propagating another, which can help increase the population.

Wash the roots, cut them into small pieces for drying, or use fresh for tinctures and oils.

Medicinal uses

Starry Solomon's seal and Solomon's plume can be used for the same applications and in the same manner. They are both my favorite herbs to use for increasing flow to the fascial layer. Use the roots in tinctured extractions or teas for people who have musculoskeletal injury, tears, or breaks.

Maianthemums have an action on the synovial fluids, helping to keep them more fluid and lubricated. It is called for when the joints or ligaments have a creaky feeling, such as cracking when you bend your knees

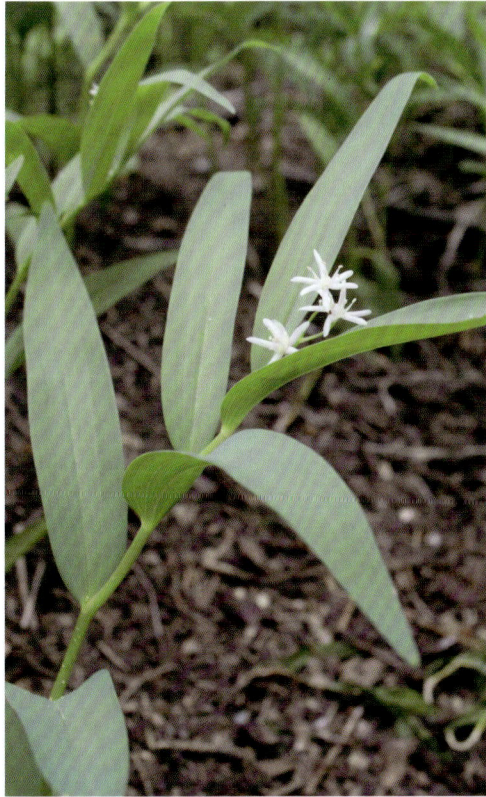

The star-shaped flowers of *Maianthemum stellatum* gave rise to its specific epithet and the common name of starry Solomon's seal.

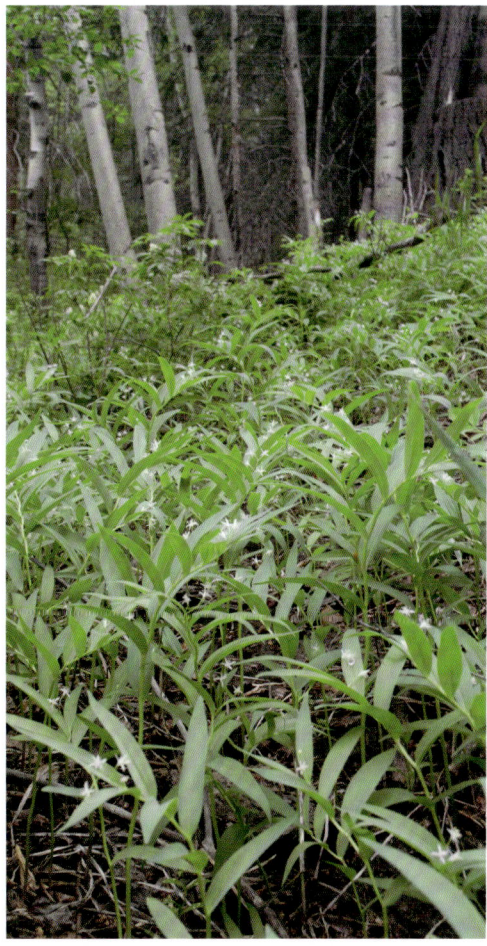

An abundant stand of starry Solomon's seal, as far as the eye can see, in an aspen forest.

or rotate your wrists. It helps old frozen injuries that need more stimulation to get things moving.

Oil extractions can be added to salves for those who, because they put themselves out there in the extreme environments of the mountains, tend to strain and sprain or bash and crash more easily.

The roots are also used to calm pelvic inflammations of the uterus, prostate, and ovaries.

Future harvest

Although stands of starry Solomon's seal can be found in many places, walk these places with care, as they are host to large mycorrhizal communities and ecosystems. Replant the roots for sustainable harvest, as described earlier.

HERBAL PREPARATIONS

Tea
Hot infusion
1 tablespoon chopped dried or fresh root
1 cup water
Decoction
1 ounce fresh or dried root
1 quart water
Drink as needed.

Tincture
1 part fresh root
2 parts alcohol (80% alcohol, 20% distilled water)
Take 20–40 drops 3 times a day.

Oil
Infuse with fresh or dried root.

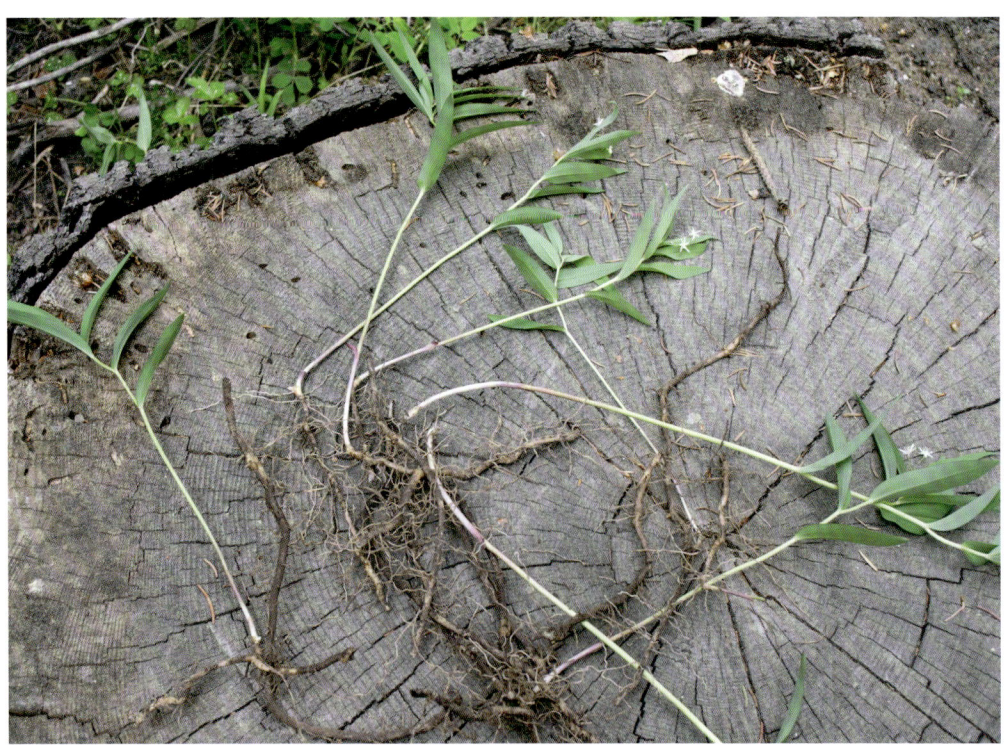

When harvesting starry Solomon's seal, clip the long running root from the ground and replant about an inch of the root head. This will help propagate the plant.

stinging nettle

Urtica species
nettle
PARTS USED leaves, seeds, roots

*It isn't officially spring until I have gathered stinging
nettle shoots with my bare hands, enjoying every sting.*

How to identify

Living up to its common name, stinging
nettle can be identified simply by brushing
up against it. The stinging hairs can be seen
running up the stem and all over the leaves.
Technically known as trichomes, the hollow
stingers hold formic acid and histamine,
among other substances, which produce a
stinging burn upon contact with skin. The
unpleasant feeling can last for hours and create small welts, depending on how sensitive
you are. *Urtica dioica* is the most prevalent
species of the mountain west.

So before you go grabbing a plant thinking it's a mint, take a peek at the stem and
underside of the leaf. If you see hairs, handle
with care. Stinging nettle leaves are opposite
each other and lanceolate, with serrations
around the edges forming a pointed tip.
Stems are square, thick, and can stand up to
about 10 feet, though in lowland areas 3–5
feet is more usual. Flowers are little and hang
in clumpy strands that dangle from the tops
of the plant. Once they start turning to seed,
the weight makes the plant bend over.

Where, when, and how to wildcraft

Stinging nettle likes to be near some moisture, shade, and disturbed soils. Look near
creeks, rivers, or wet fields. Reddish tops of
the stinging nettle emerge first in the spring.

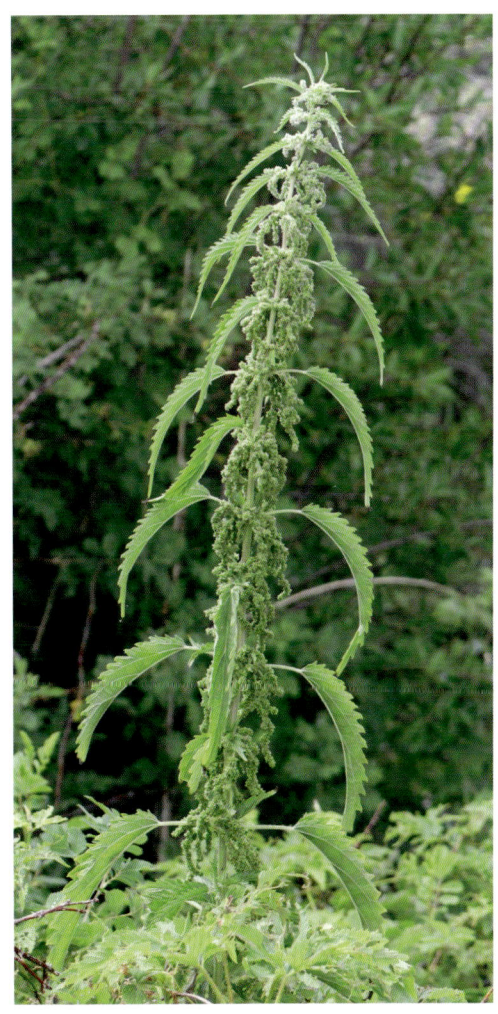

Clip the overflowing seeds of stinging nettle while
they are still young and green. Dry for later use.

Gather stinging nettles throughout the spring and into summer, *before* they start to flower. Gather seeds in the fall.

Depending on your threshold for lingering stings or your agility level, you may or may not want to wear gloves. Wearing gloves and using pruners makes harvesting stinging nettles much more efficient and less painful. If you are in for the gamble, try pinching the stem of the plant with your thumb and index finger. The trick is to reach under the leaves from the bottom up, avoiding the opposite direction of the hairs.

A quick natural remedy to the stings, should any irritation result, is the juice from stinging nettle itself! Carefully roll up a stinging nettle leaf in the same direction that the hairs are growing. This way you can cautiously use your fingers without being stung. After it is rolled up, fold in half and chew it up, then spit the green poultice out on to the itchy area. Or simply roll, fold, and squeeze between your fingers to get some juice out, if the whole chewing thing is too much.

The reddish new shoots are the most nutritious and my favorite to dry for tea. Gather them when the plant is still young, snipping off 1–6 inches of the tender stalk. Snip the heavy, hanging seed strands in late summer and early fall and dry them.

Medicinal uses

I value stinging nettles for their deliciously nutritious use in the kitchen and as an all-around fabulous medicine. Rich in calcium, iron, magnesium, vitamins, and protein, it is a robust herb to have in the cabinet.

Make a fresh cup of tea with the reddish green tips in the spring. I eat the infused herb once I am done sipping. A blend of stinging nettle, raspberry, alfalfa, and rosehips is a very supportive tea during

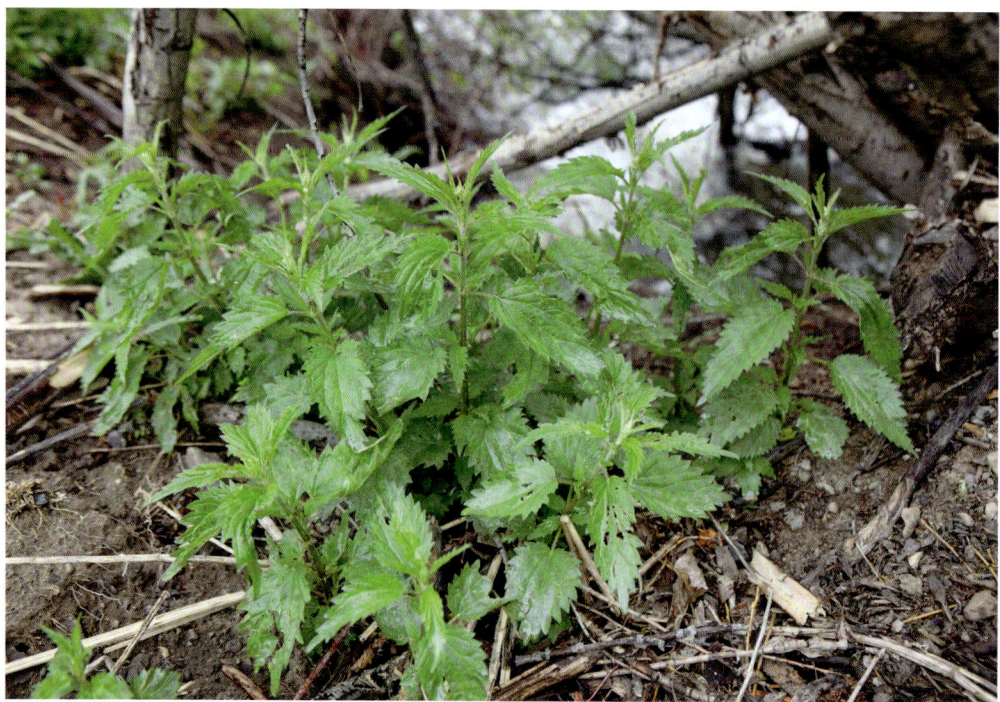

The time to gather stinging nettle tops is while they are still short, vibrant green, and not flowering yet.

pregnancy. Stinging nettle leaves can help to move uric acid out of the system, relieving symptoms of gout and rheumatism. They also provide relief from allergies and asthma. Stinging nettle is nourishing to the blood, bones, joints, and skin. It can be helpful with restless leg syndrome due to the presence of essential minerals like magnesium.

Stinging nettle root has been reported to increase the growth of hair. I like to use the root and the leaves infused into jojoba oil for a lovely hair and beard oil. Blend in Douglas fir tips for their citrusy aroma. Add argan oil for its hair-replenishing benefits and rosemary essential oil, which has an affinity for treating damaged hair.

Infuse stinging nettle leaves or seeds into vinegars that can be used as a medicinal food. I love a spring blend of stinging nettle tips, chickweed, spruce tips, and wild onion bulbs. Add a dollop of honey and a little pepper to create a tasty oxymel. This can be used in culinary endeavors or for a medicinal sipping tonic.

Stinging nettle seeds are trophorestorative to the kidneys and adrenals. They can help people with chronic kidney issues.

Caution

Cystoliths begin to accumulate in the leaves after the plant starts to flower, and especially once they go to seed. This can be irritating to the kidneys or cause kidney stones to accumulate.

Future harvest

Gather only the tops of a stinging nettle plant once or twice a year. If digging the roots, make sure you are gathering from a large patch.

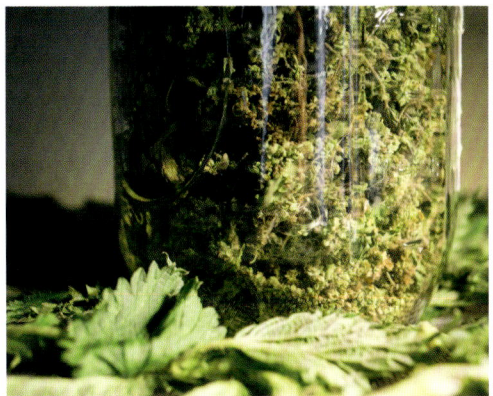

The seeds of stinging nettle, jarred from the previous fall.

HERBAL PREPARATIONS

Tea
Hot infusion
2 tablespoons fresh or dried leaves
or
1–2 teaspoons fresh or dried seeds
1 cup water
Drink 3–5 times per day.

Tincture
1 part fresh leaves, root, or seeds
2 parts menstruum (75% alcohol, 25% distilled water)
or
1 part dried leaves, root, or seeds
5 parts menstruum (60% alcohol, 40% distilled water)
Take 30–60 drops 3–5 times a day.

Vinegar
1 part leaves, root, or seeds
4 parts vinegar
Take 1–2 tablespoons 1–3 times a day.

Oil
Infuse with fresh or dried root or leaves.

Rhus species
lemonadeberry, sumach
PARTS USED fruit

Gather up all the sumac berries you can find in late summer for a cooling, tart, pink-lemonade drink high in vitamin C.

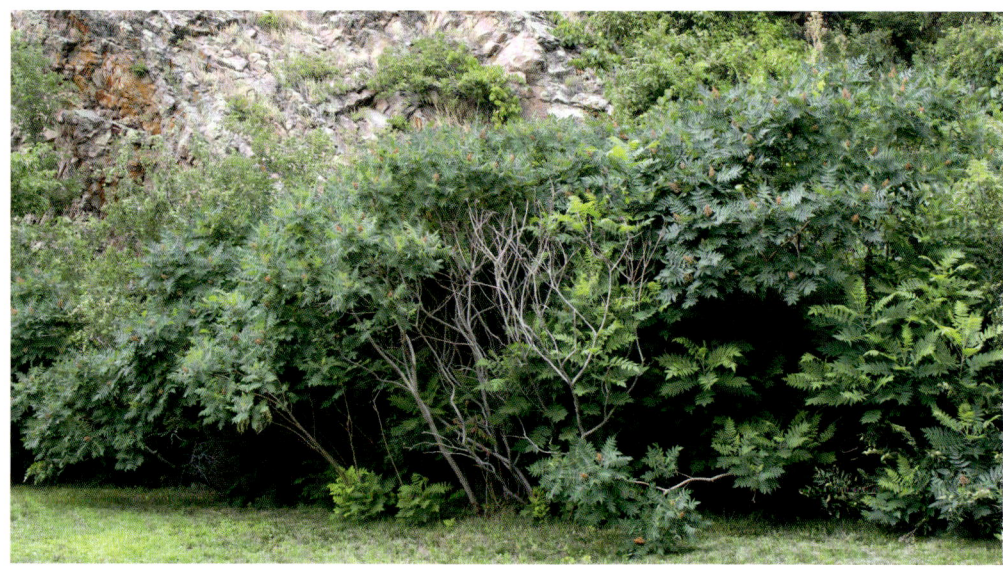

Rhus species are usually found in a stand or grove-like formation, with a cluster of slender trunks.

How to identify

Smooth sumac (*Rhus glabra*) is far less common in the wild than its sibling, skunkbush (*R. trilobata*); it is more often found as a tree-like ornamental shrub in western towns, forming thickets with plants averaging 7–9 feet in height. Its berries and twigs have a waxy coating, whereas those of staghorn sumac (*R. typhina*), another close relative, are covered with velvet-like hairs.

The flowers of smooth sumac are green or cream-colored, packed tightly in a spire that turns into maroon, semiflat berries—technically drupes, as each has only a single seed. Leaves are pinnate with nine or more leaflets. Each leaflet is serrated around the margin. The scent of sumac also tends to be distinctive, giving off a slightly sweet rank odor when touched.

Where, when, and how to wildcraft

You'll probably have better luck finding this plant around cities and neighborhoods. In the wild, look for it at lower elevations in the foothills. Gather the clusters in summer and fall when the berries are still sticky. As

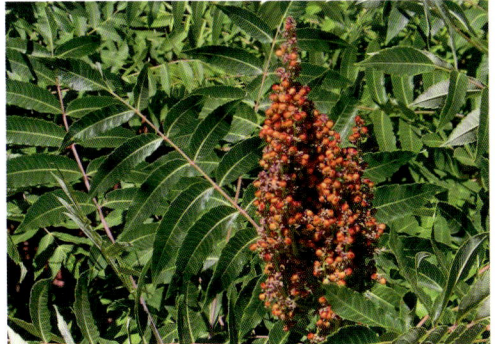

Smooth sumac (*Rhus glabra*) looks very similar to staghorn sumac at first glance; however, smooth sumac lacks the fine hairs.

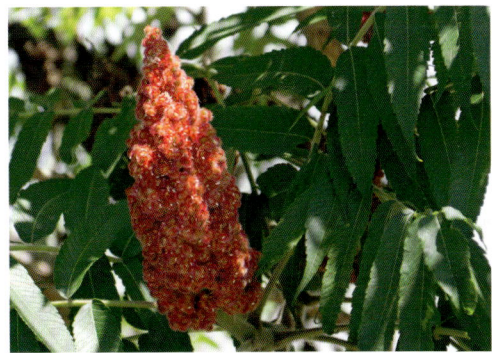

Notice the little hairs all over the flowering raceme and branches of staghorn sumac (*Rhus typhina*).

time goes on and rain showers rev up, the oils get washed away, leaving the fruit not as flavorful.

Clip off entire red spires loaded with berries. Clusters can be rinsed if they are cobwebby or full of debris, but this can decrease flavor, so it's better to just pick away any unwanted bits. The fruits can be separated off the stem and dried.

Medicinal uses

Cold infused teas can be made with the fruit of both *Rhus typhina* and *R. glabra*. Break up a few of the fresh spires loaded with berries into a quart or half-gallon jar and cover with cold water. Work your fingers around the fruits to release the resinous medicinal coating. Let this infusion sit for 4–8 hours. Strain well, especially if you are using *R. typhina*, as it has fine hairs that can be irritating to the throat and digestive tract. This tart beverage can be helpful in easing bladder infections or irritation to the ureters. If you struggle with bladder infections, try freezing your infusion in ice-cube trays. Pop them out once frozen to store in a freezer bag, making enough to last until the following year.

The tea is a lovely cooling tonic for overheated summer days. Fruit can also be extracted in vinegars for oxymels or sipping shrubs.

Caution

If you have a known allergy to poison ivy, mangos, or cashews, then you may want to avoid this plant, as it is in the same family, Anacardiaceae. Poison sumac has white berries, not red.

Future harvest

Clipping off the clusters of berries does no harm to this plant. Smooth sumac propagates through its underground runners, which is why you rarely see just one shrub.

HERBAL PREPARATIONS

Tea
Cold infusion
1 ounce fresh or dried fruit
1 quart water
Steep 4–8 hours and strain well. Drink as needed.

Vinegar
1 part fresh or dried fruit
3 parts vinegar
Take 1 tablespoon 1–3 times a day.

sweet clover

Melilotus species
melilot
PARTS USED leaves, flowers

The sweet and soft aromatics of Melilotus *species are best harbored in a tincture, used as a clearing facial spritz, or infused into a massage oil.*

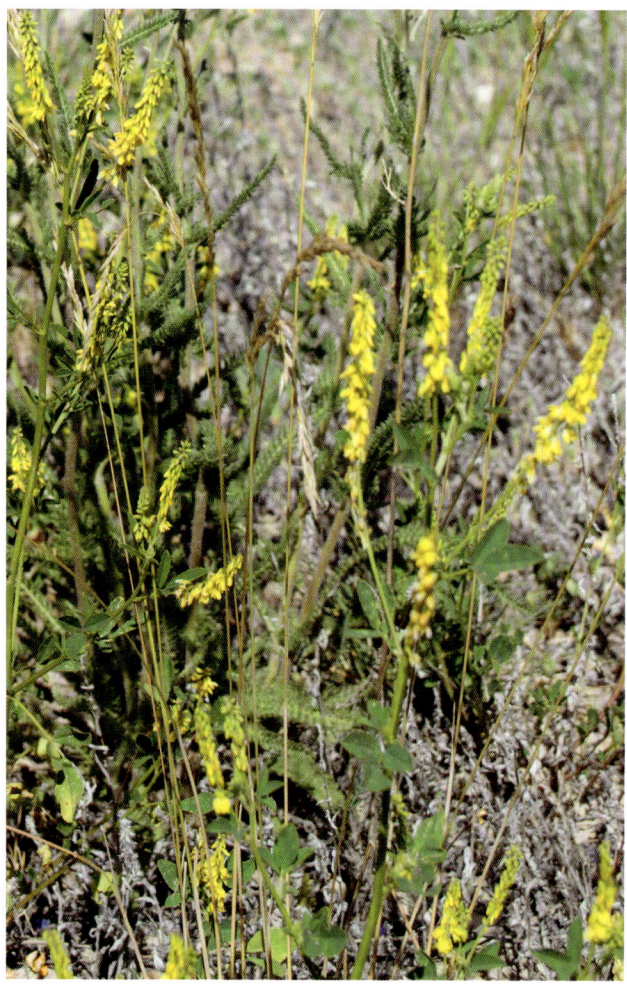

Sweet clover (here, the yellow-flowered *Melilotus officinalis*) covers the mountain states, lining roadways and cropping up in the fields with sagebrush, western blue flax, and yarrow.

How to identify

Sweet clover arises to various heights; it can be puny or quite tall. Leaves are alternate, light green, oblong, and serrated around the margins, with a trifoliate formation. Tiny yellow flowers of *Melilotus officinalis*— or white on *M. albus*—grow in slender spikes. Sweet clover resembles alfalfa before it blooms, but alfalfa's blossoms are usually purple and its leaves are serrated only halfway around the margin.

Where, when, and how to wildcraft

Sweet clover can be found in disturbed soils all over the mountain west. Some roads are lit up with the bright flowers for most of the summer. In drought, sweet clover can be one of the first inhabitants of a starved reservoir's shoreline. The shoots can be gathered along with the young leaves in spring. The entire plant can be cut at the base of the stalk once it is in flower or gone to seed.

Sweet clover is best to gather in the morning, once the sun has come up and evaporated any dew from the plant. Harvest on dry, sunny days. Gathering plants after rains while they are damp can cause them to mold, especially if the sweet clover is bundled before drying. It is best to spread the herb out on a drying rack immediately after collecting, or process it fresh right away.

Medicinal uses

As a tincture, sweet clover can be used topically or internally for inflammation and brings slight pain relief for muscular injury. Think of sweet clover when you are formulating tinctures, as it carries soft vanilla, cooling, and bitter notes.

Sweet clover, sagebrush, yarrow, and Saint John's wort infused into alcohol carries a beautiful fragrance. Combined with ⅓ distilled water or a hydrosol, it can be a wonderful smudging spritz or can be useful as a base for bug spray or a spritz-on deodorant.

For a massage oil I love a combination of yarrow, arnica, and sweet clover. It smells sweetly of a rainy day in the mountains and provides warming relief to an overworked body. It can release tension, clear trauma, move stagnant zones, and ease aches throughout the body. It smells heavenly and can be blended with many other herbs, like

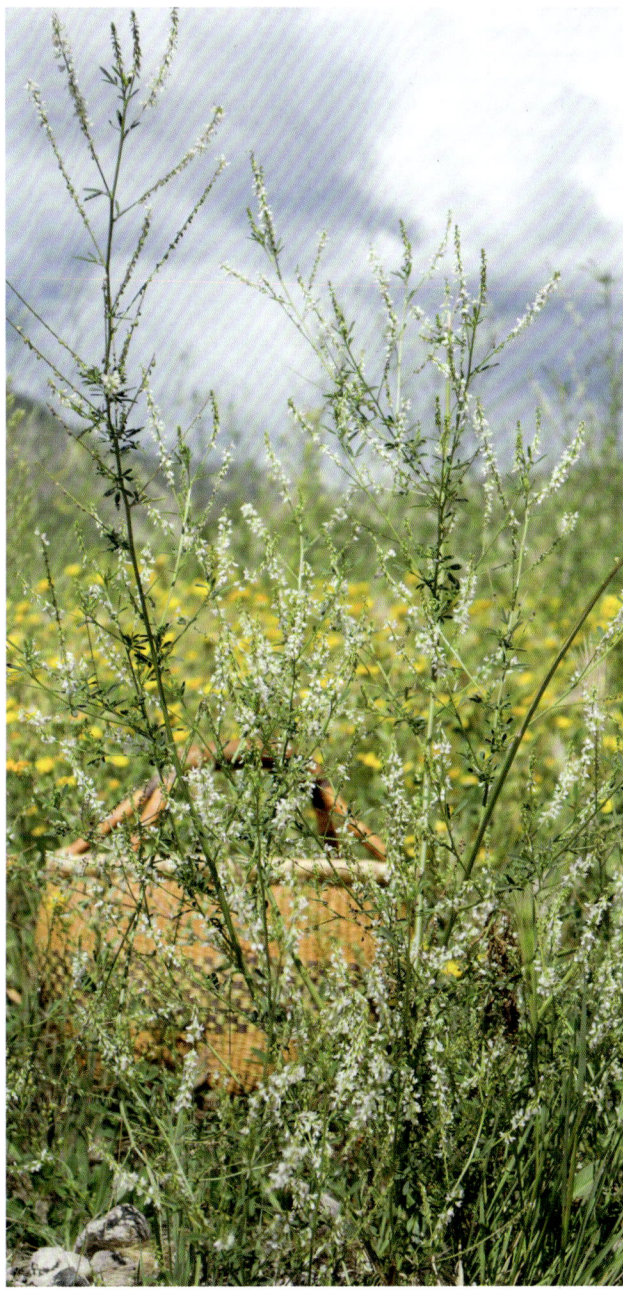

Melilotus albus has white flowers; it and *M. officinalis* can be used interchangeably.

goldenrod, Solomon's plume, cottonwood, violet, and hops for aches-and-pains salves or postinjury rubs.

I find an infused massage oil or spritz of sweet clover to work very well to help hold boundaries and clear space. It helps me not take on other people's stuff, which is supportive while working with clients.

Caution

Be careful not to confuse *Melilotus officinalis* with golden banner (*Thermopsis* species), a toxic plant with yellow flowers. Golden banner has similar young leaves. The fungal metabolites of moldy sweet clover can act as a profound blood thinner and have been known to poison cattle. Never use moldy herb!

Future harvest

Take as much as you want. Sweet clover is another plant that has made its way onto the invasive weed list. Be mindful, however, that as a plant that fixes nitrogen in the soil, this "noxious weed" may actually be trying to heal the soil from which it is growing.

HERBAL PREPARATIONS

Tea
Hot infusion
3 tablespoons fresh or dried flowers and leaves
1 cup water
Drink 1 cup 3 times a day.

Tincture
1 part fresh flowers and leaves
2 parts menstruum (80% alcohol, 20% distilled water)
or
1 part dried flowers and leaves
5 parts menstruum (60% alcohol, 40% distilled water)
Take 20–40 drops 3 times a day.

Oil
Infuse with fresh or dried flowers and leaves.

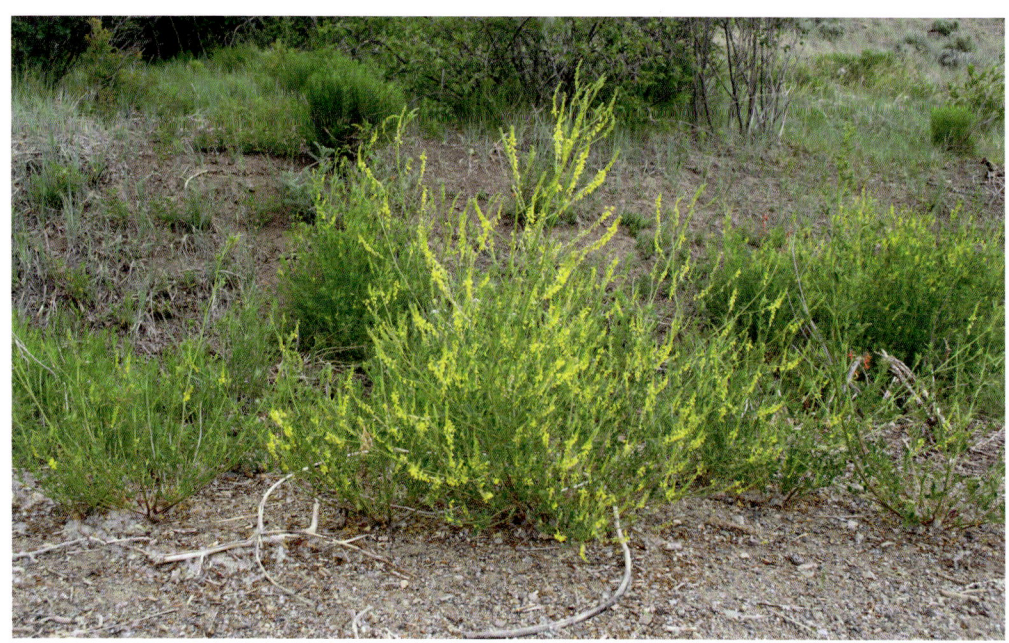

It is always best to gather sweet clover and other aromatic plants on a dry, warm, sunny day. The most scent is produced and released in the heat.

sweet grass

Anthoxanthum species
vanilla grass, holy grass, buffalo grass
PARTS USED blades

Braiding the blades of sweet grass on a late summer's day can be a soothing activity for the non-fishing partner who is patiently waiting for dinner to be caught.

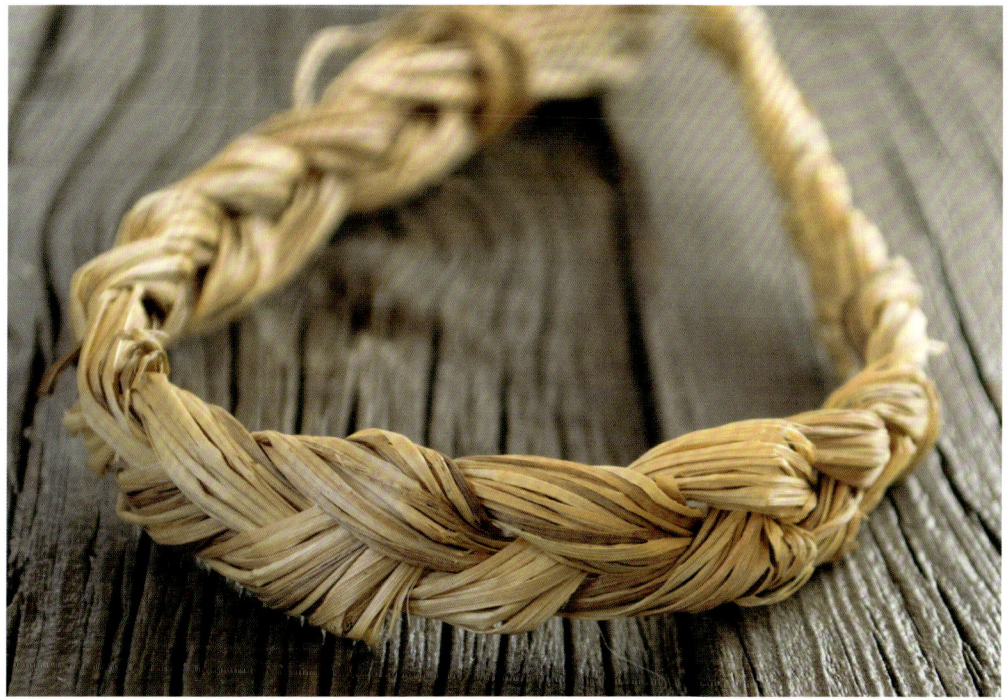

The traditional braid of sweet grass strands, often used as a smudge.

How to identify

A perennial grass with the sweetest smelling scent of vanilla, sweet grass distinguishes itself in many ways. Leaves are flat, shiny underneath, and either lack hair or have fine hairs on the surface of the leaf. The leaves grow alternately along the smooth, hollow stem. Flowers grow in spikelets with petalless flowers that are tinged with purple from the stamens. The rhizomes of sweet grass are long and grow in colonies. *Anthoxanthum odoratum* is an introduced species, and *A. hirtum* is our native sweet grass.

Where, when, and how to wildcraft

Anthoxanthum hirtum is our most common species of sweet grass. Harvest the sweet-smelling blades of grass in late summer or early fall while the scent is most aromatic and the color is still vibrant. Find it growing in wetlands, riparian zones, and marshes where clean, clear waters flow.

Make a smudge braid to be burned. Use scissors or clippers to snip the blades of sweet grass at the base to create bundles. With about 20 blades in hand, tightly secure the cut ends by wrapping another blade of grass around the bundle. If you create a loop at the end, you can fasten it around your toe or to a stick in the ground. Braid the vanilla-scented grass. Get creative and fashion a grassy loop for hanging to dry. Conclude with using another blade of grass to tightly secure the end of the braid.

Medicinal uses

Sweet grass is most often seen braided for use as a smudge. The smoke of sweet grass brings in good spirits and improves the energy of a space, honoring Mother Earth and all her creations.

A tea, however, can be lovely in cold blends, to help alleviate coughs and sore throats. Infused oil of the dried or fresh blades gives off a sweet scent that can be good for massage oil blends.

Future harvest

The stands of sweet grass may be affected by overdevelopment and agriculture in parts of the mountain west, leaving it with few places to inhabit clean waters. Become a caretaker and spokesperson for the wild plants and watersheds in your region!

HERBAL PREPARATIONS

Tea
Hot infusion
1 tablespoon freshly cut or dried blades
1 cup water
Drink 3 times a day or as needed.

Oil
Infuse with freshly cut or dried blades.

---

sweet root

Osmorhiza occidentalis
sweet cicely
PARTS USED roots, leaves, seeds

All parts of sweet root are full of a fennel-like flavor and can be added to formulas for their carminative aromatics.

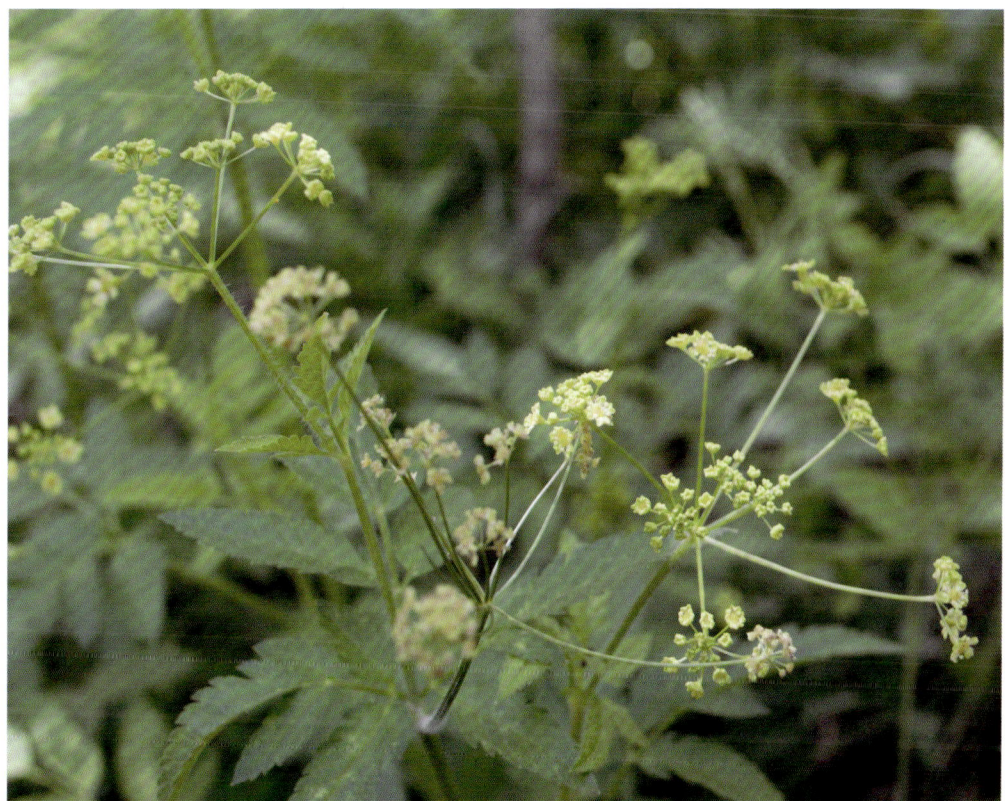

Flowers of sweet root are yellow; other species of *Osmorhiza* have white flowers and do not offer the aromatic root.

How to identify

Sweet root has mountain-hardy, lush green foliage. Leaves are compound in threes, pointed, and serrated. Some can be found along the stem, but many arise from the base of the plant. Older plants have many flowering stems, sometimes reaching 4 feet tall; younger plants may have only a few flowering stems and grow smaller, with more basal leaves.

Fire Folkin' Cider

Many herbalists around the world combine apple cider vinegar with super-spicy and aromatic herbs and vegetables to make a concoction traditionally known as Fire Cider, a name coined by Rosemary Gladstar in the 1970s. My version, Fire Folkin' Cider, is a spicy apple cider vinegar extraction to kick the crud out. Use it as an herbal sipping tonic in cases of sinus and chest congestion or at the onset of illness.

Try a combination of hot peppers, garlic, onion, ginger, turmeric, horseradish, wild mustard seeds, sweet root seeds, wild caraway, rosehips, stinging nettle leaf and seeds, and alfalfa leaves, along with a slice of citrus. Fill a glass jar and cover with vinegar. Let this sit for a week to a month, then strain and add honey to taste.

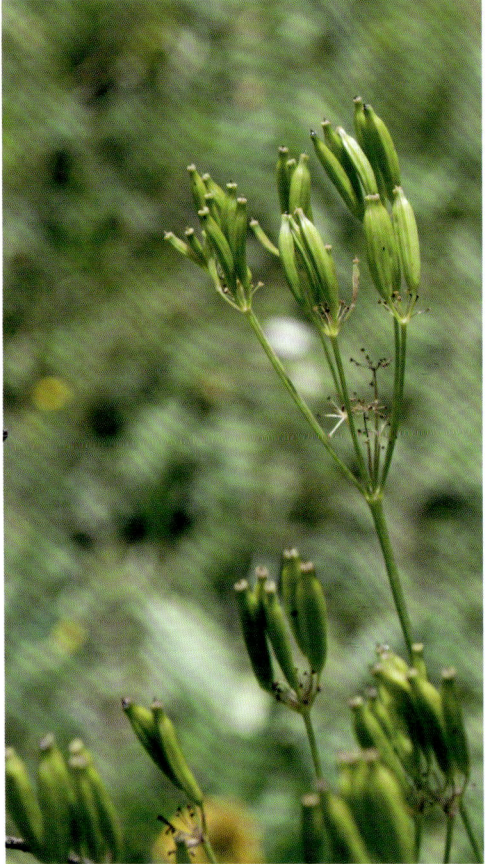

The elongated seedpods of sweet root can be picked fresh and eaten as a trailside snack. Add them to vinegars, honeys, or alcohol for an extraction of their fennel-like flavor.

Flowers are yellow, sometimes greenish, and hardly noticeable compared to the sizeable seedpod each becomes. Seeds are long, slender, smooth, dark green crescents that are dorsally flattened. Roots have a gray or brown surface and a light creamy-colored interior; they grow in what seems like a tangled intertwined mess of rhizomes and roots. The scent of the roots, as you might have guessed from the common name, is noticeably fragrant and sweet.

Where, when, and how to wildcraft

Sweet root dwells in higher forests, especially in mountainous terrain. It likes damp clean mountain soil and shade. It is an early-blooming flower, and the seeds ripen in early summer. Pick an umbel full of green seeds. I find these lose a lot of flavor later in the season and after they have been dried, so they are best enjoyed while fresh and early in the season.

Roots of older plants are more aromatic and can be smelled just as the root is uncovered. Leaves and flowers can be gathered as well. The scent will stay in your house for days after sweet root has been processed.

Medicinal uses

In a tincture, the root of sweet root offers an interesting fennel flavor with a tingle. It has been said to be beneficial for treating external and internal fungal infections.

The fresh seeds, leaves, and root can be used in making a spicy vinegar sipping tonic, traditionally called Fire Cider. To make your own, use the root or seeds very sparingly until you understand how much flavor they can impart.

Sweet root leaves can be used fresh or dried for an incredible flavoring, if you are one who likes a fennel flavor. The seeds are a carminative and can be used in formulas for upset stomach, and for some it can help to stimulate bowel movements.

Caution

This plant is in the Apiaceae, meaning it can have deadly lookalikes. Water hemlock (*Cicuta* species) roots are odorless, but poison hemlock (*Conium maculatum*) roots can have a sweet celery-like scent. Sweet root has very aromatic seeds, leaves, and roots. Always make sure you are 100% certain about the seeds you are consuming. The smallest amount of seed from the wrong plant could be fatal.

Future harvest

Since this plant spreads through its root system, it's not a threat to gather seeds. But be conscious of your surroundings. Take the whole plant only if sweet root is saturating the forest floor, and when harvesting the root, gather only from large stands. Rhizomes seem to transplant well. After harvesting, plant a few rootlets around the forest floor before you head home.

HERBAL PREPARATIONS

Tea
1 tablespoon fresh seeds, crushed, or fresh
  or dried leaves
1 cup water
Drink after meals as a carminative.

Tincture
1 part fresh root, leaves, or seeds
2 parts menstruum (75% alcohol, 25%
  distilled water)
or
1 part dried root
5 parts menstruum (60% alcohol, 40%
  distilled water)
Take 10–20 drops 3 times a day.

Oil
Infuse with fresh or dried root, seeds, or leaves.

Dipsacus fullonum

PARTS USED roots

*Teasel is an excellent remedy to have in the medicine cabinet
for helping to ease joint inflammations and musculoskeletal woes.*

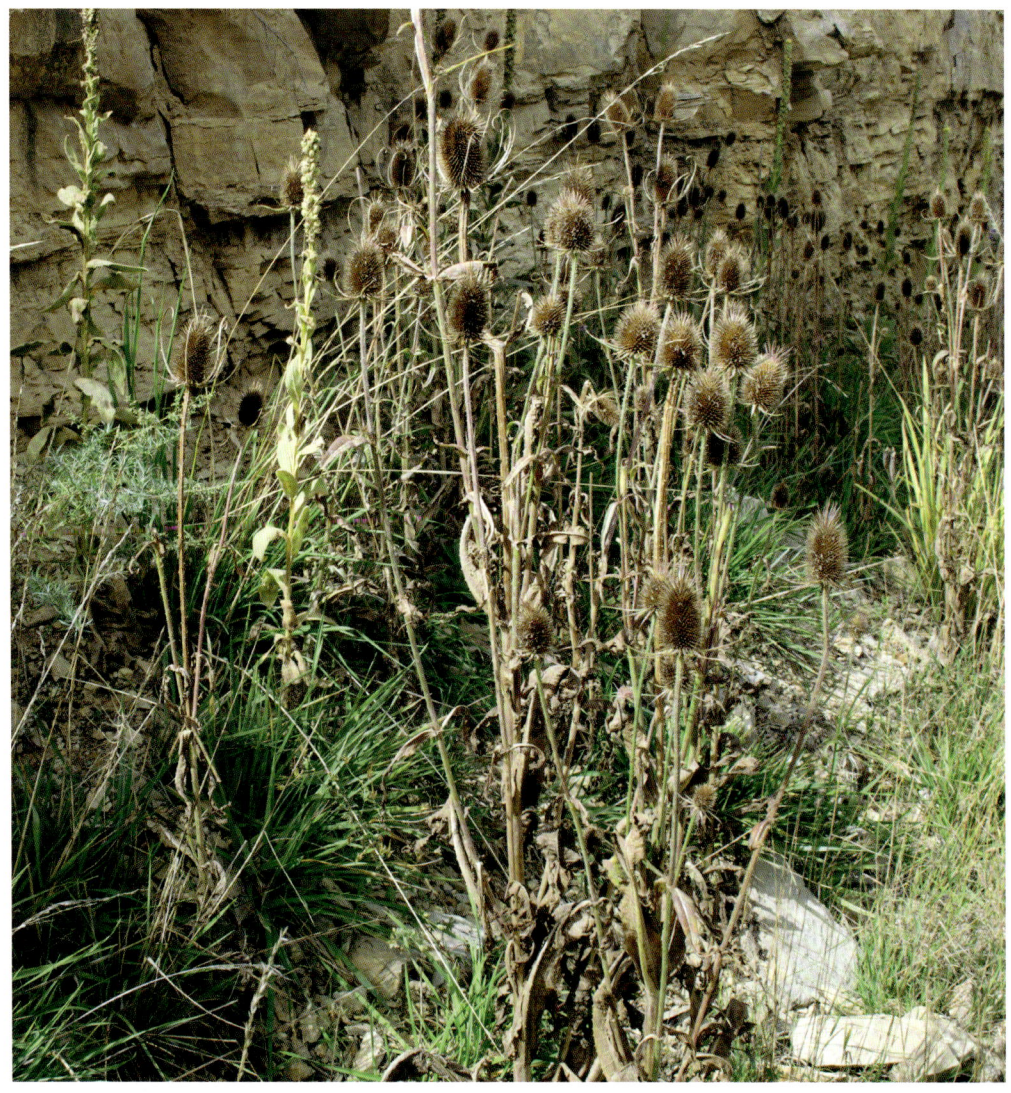

Teasel marks itself quite well with a tall dried stalk and poky seedhead. Dig roots in the spring and fall.

How to identify

Teasel is more noticable after it has died back and is left standing from the previous year. The tall brown afterlife of teasel looks like a gathering of dried microphone-shaped flowerheads, which used to host a bunch of tiny light purple flowers. It is an invasive monocarpic perennial, meaning that after growing as a basal rosette for one or many seasons, the purple flowerheads bloom once, then the entire plant dies back. Below ground, the growth is a spindly taproot with numerous tendrils.

Where, when, and how to wildcraft

Teasel can be seen lining roadways, irrigation ditches, and highways across the west. Find harvesting places that are well away from the industrialized world. Gather the root before the flowering stalk shoots up, which can be in the spring or fall. After the plant has flowered, the root becomes less medicinal.

Medicinal uses

A somewhat bitter-tasting plant, teasel has cooling and drying energetics. It can be used as an alterative in supporting the liver and also as a digestive aid.

Teasel can help ease aches and pains from inflammatory issues in joints and muscles. It has been used to help mend tears in connective tissues. Blending it with *Maianthemum* species, mullein root, and alder can help with structural alignment and the fluidity of connective tissue. It has been used to help those who have autoimmune responses or Lyme disease to cope with the various conditions that affect the musculoskeletal system.

Future harvest

This plant is a very tenacious, weedy species found throughout the west. It can handle heavy harvesting of the root.

HERBAL PREPARATIONS

Tea
Hot infusion
1–3 tablespoons chopped dried or fresh
   root
1 cup water
Decoction
1 ounce chopped dried or fresh root
1 quart water
Drink 1 cup 3 times a day.

Tincture
1 part fresh root
2 parts menstruum (75% alcohol, 25%
   distilled water)
or
1 part dried root
5 parts menstruum (60% alcohol, 40%
   distilled water)
Take 30–60 drops 3 times a day.

Oil
Infuse with fresh or dried root.

Usnea species
old man's beard
PARTS USED all

I gather usnea as I move through conifer forests in the winter on my splitboard, collecting the lichen and filling all empty spaces of my backpack with it while I hike up the skin track.

How to identify

Ever look at a tree and see a green stringy mass of fluff dangling from it? That could very well be a species of usnea, otherwise known as old man's beard. The tendrils of this lichen shoot out in all sorts of directions from the adhered part that meets the bark of the tree. The main identifying factor for usnea is the inner white thread you reveal when you ever so gently tug on either side of a single green strand or tendril— the green breaks apart and the white thread is beneath. If it does not have this thread, then do not use the lichen you found as medicine.

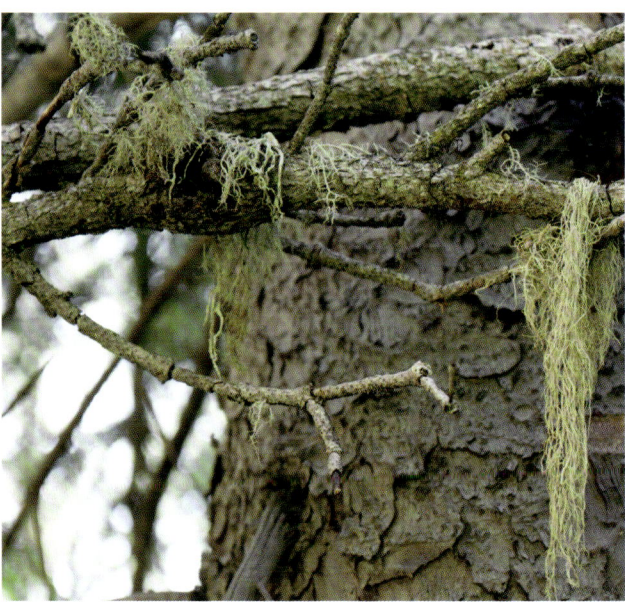

Usnea, a lichen, can be found growing in conifer forests. Pick only the pieces that have fallen to the floor.

Where, when, and how to wildcraft

Usnea is one medicinal that can be gathered all year long and during snow or rain, as long as you let it dry out after. My favorite way to gather is in the middle of winter. While heading to the top of a mountain, I can stop along the way and pick the little green fluffs of lichen lying on top of the snow.

Find usnea in conifer forests, growing on the trees. It may appear that the usnea is killing the tree in a parasitic way, but in fact it is helping the tree extend its life, by bringing in more oxygen. Usnea is a lichen that acts as the lungs of the forest. It is found at higher elevations where moisture hovers over the mountains.

Medicinal uses

Usnea has become a go-to herb for sinus and lung infections here in the dry mountainous region I dwell in. It is often combined with

Respiratory Steams

A respiratory steam is something more people should include at the onset of colds. The aromatic herbs of the steam help to break up mucus and open up the bronchioles, letting in more breath, making a gateway for other herbs to be inhaled.

Fill a pot with water, bring it to a boil, and then turn it down to a simmer. Add in fresh or dried herbs, such as pine or spruce twigs, usnea, osha leaves, or beebalm flowers. Drape a towel over your head and hover over the steaming pot, adjusting your position and the temperature under the pot so you do not get burned. Inhale and exhale for 5–20 minutes a few times a day.

Try extracting herbs into vinegar and using the vinegar in a boiling pot of water, a few tablespoons per pot. The vapors help to loosen mucus and can be helpful for heavy coughs.

Essential oils may be added to your steam, but do be cautious of adding too much camphorous-type oils, as they can burn the mucous membranes.

other herbs, such as osha, balsamroot, yerba mansa, spikenard, or redroot, to help ease respiratory infections. I often combine it in herbal steams for its antimicrobial and mucilaginous ways. Even though mucilage is not generally noted to release in a steam, it is still beneficial for the bronchioles. This is a remedy I have used effectively for years—is it the education of telling people to go home and steam their lungs and sinuses, or is it the true power of usnea? We like to give people who come into our shop dead conifer twigs loaded with usnea to take home and inhale in a pot of steam, and they come back feeling like the gunk has moved out of their lungs. Sometimes creating rituals and taking time for yourself can be more important than the actual herbs you are using.

Infused oil of usnea is great for wound-healing salves. Try combining it with cottonwood buds and Oregon grape for an outstanding ointment.

Future harvest

Do not rip usnea from the trees. It is alive and well, offering its gifts to the forest. There is always more than enough usnea on the ground. You can easily make an usnea ball in a short period of walking through the woods. Make sure to look for the white thread for correct identification.

HERBAL PREPARATIONS

Tea
Hot infusion
2 tablespoons usnea
1 cup water
Drink 3 times a day.

Tincture
1 part usnea
2 parts menstruum (60% alcohol, 40% distilled water)
Macerate this mixture and tightly cap it inside a clean glass jar. Place the jar in either a pressure cooker with a water bath for 1 hour, or place it in the dishwasher and run a full cycle. The heated atmosphere will help the alcohol better extract the medicinal benefits of usnea. Take 20–40 drops 3 times a day.

Oil
Infuse with usnea.

Arctostaphylos uva-ursi
kinnikinnick, bearberry, creeping manzanita
PARTS USED leaves

A creeping evergreen shrub that sprawls across forest floors, uva-ursi creates a peaceful place to sit and harvest beneath a canopy of trees.

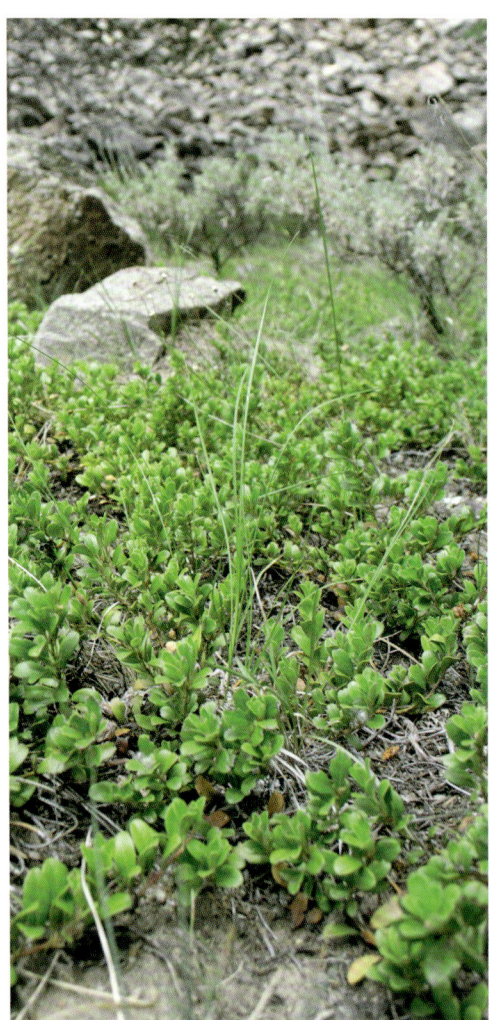

Find uva-ursi growing along the floor of mixed conifer forests or among sagebrush.

How to identify

Uva-ursi is an evergreen shrub that has a woody stem and deep green, thick, and waxy-feeling leaves. The flowers are little white nodding, urn-shaped bells that have a touch of pink around each tip. They fruit into red mealy berries that can be nibbled in late summer.

Where, when, and how to wildcraft

You find the trailing mats of uva-ursi on the forest floor under the conifers and aspens. It springs forth vine-like shoots that are covered in oblong leaves that grow alternately along the stem. Find it after the snow melts, and right up until the snow starts to cover the ground again. It can be harvested at any point of the year and used for its medicine. Clip pieces of the trailing stems and either allow the leaves to dry on the stem or pick them off to dry fully before storing in a glass jar. Fresh leaves are best for tincturing.

Medicinal uses

Where uva-ursi works really well is infections and inflammations of the urinary tract. It can also help relieve kidney and bladder infections. Its strong antimicrobial and astringent properties make it work fairly quickly. These same properties make uva-ursi leaves a great

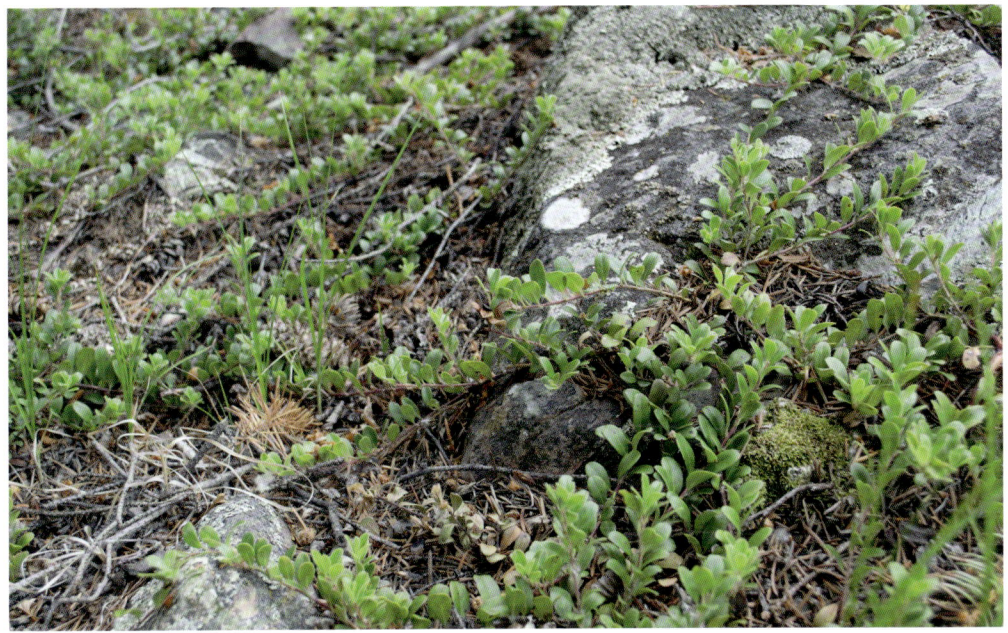

Clip trailing pieces of uva-ursi, gently pruning it from the floor of the woods.

addition when creating a sitz bath blend for postpartum healing or even hemorrhoids.

The tea can also be used as a wash for skin infections or wounds. Uva-ursi can be extracted into oil for bug-bite-soothing ointments or serums. It combines well with rose, plantain, and alumroot.

Smoking blends often contain uva-ursi; it is a common ingredient in Native American blends. I find it works well only in a pipe; otherwise, the herb needs to be finely ground so it can bind with herbs in rolled herbal smokes.

⚠ Caution

Prolonged use, longer than 3–7 days, can cause stomachaches and be overly drying. Uva-ursi can be used in moderation and in small doses during pregnancy, but not for longer than 3 days.

Future harvest

Uva-ursi is a primary groundcover in many areas of the forested west. It needs only to be clipped—never take the whole plant. Prune off only the long runners.

HERBAL PREPARATIONS

Tea
Hot infusion
3 tablespoons fresh or dried leaves
1 cup water
Drink 3 times a day while symptoms persist, but not for longer than 3 days.

Tincture
1 part fresh or dried leaves
2 parts menstruum (60% alcohol, 40% distilled water)
Take 20–40 drops 3 times a day.

Oil
Infuse with fresh or dried leaves.

Valeriana species
tobacco root
PARTS USED roots, stems, leaves, flowers

Stimulant or sedative? However you intend to use it, when you find a meadow of valerian, take a moment to lie down and drink in the scent of fairy dreams.

How to identify

The star-shaped flowers of valerian are a pleasure to behold and intoxicating to smell. In the Rocky Mountain states we have several different species of valerian; plants vary in size but otherwise have a very similar appearance. Valerian has basal leaves that are slender and spade-shaped at first, turning into lobed leaves as they mature. *Valeriana acutiloba* and *V. arizonica* are the smaller species. Medium-sized plants that grow in our region are *V. dioica*, *V. occidentalis*, and *V. sitchensis*. *Valeriana edulis* is our largest species and has the biggest root, but it can sometimes provide medicine weaker than the medium- or small-sized roots. Go on, smell—the more strongly aromatic the roots, the better. Their unique smell is quite stinky to some, but it has a sweetness that can make it alluring.

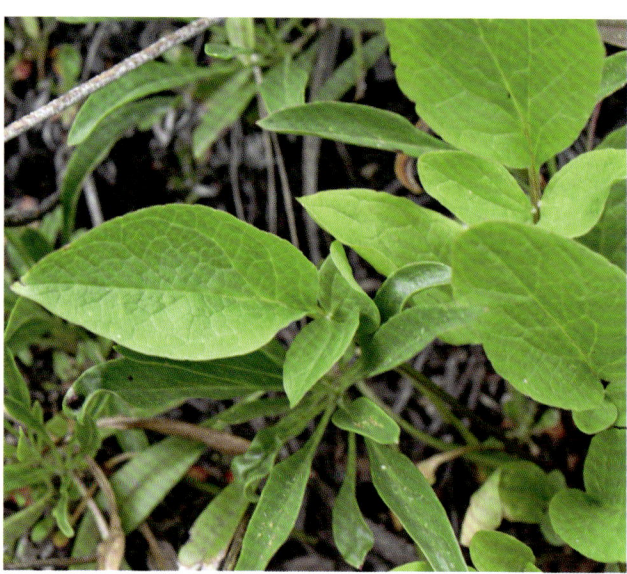

The leaves of *Valeriana* species are lobed or dissected.

Where, when, and how to wildcraft

Valerian is a mountain-dwelling plant that can be found in moist, rich lands such as alpine meadows, forests, and creeksides. The smaller species of valerian have little roots but provide a lot of foliage, which is better to harvest and utilize. The roots of the larger species can be harvested, and the whole plant can be used in extractions. The fresh plant material makes the strongest extractions, but the dried root and plant parts can also be used. The smell will stay strong for years in valerian root that has been dried and preserved well.

Medicinal uses

Valerian root has long been a traditional remedy for sleep. It has the ability to really knock you out for getting those Zs. Oddly enough, it can have the opposite effect on some people, giving them energy and keeping them restlessly awake. This seems to be most common in folks whose constitution runs on the warmer side. Try this herb by itself for the first time, to know how it makes you feel.

All parts of valerian can be a relaxing addition to menstrual-cramp formulas. It works as an antispasmodic to the muscles, is calming, and helps quell the pain a bit. The antispasmodic properties can be helpful, when taken in small doses, to calm coughing fits or intestinal cramping. In the musculo-skeletal system, valerian can be used to ease backaches or tensing, seizing muscles.

A tea of fresh or dried flowers has a pleasant floral flavor and relaxes the most anxious of beings. The aerial portions of the plant seem to have as strong a sedative and relaxing effect as the root; however, they seem to come with less of the stimulating side effect that valerian has on some people.

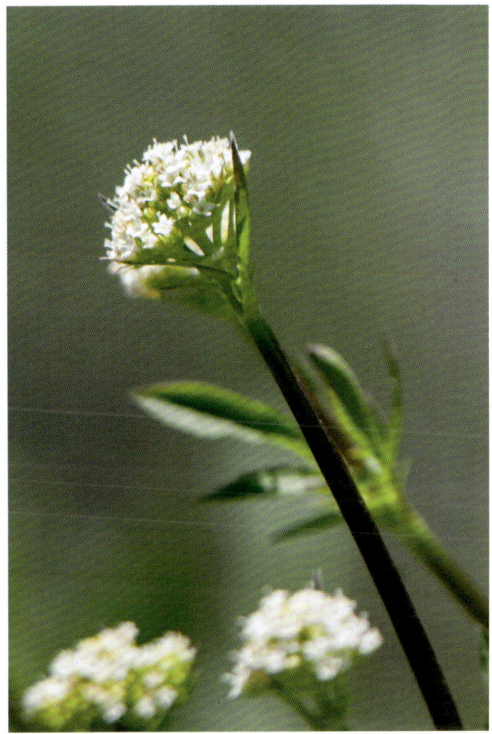

Valerian flowers just beginning to bloom.

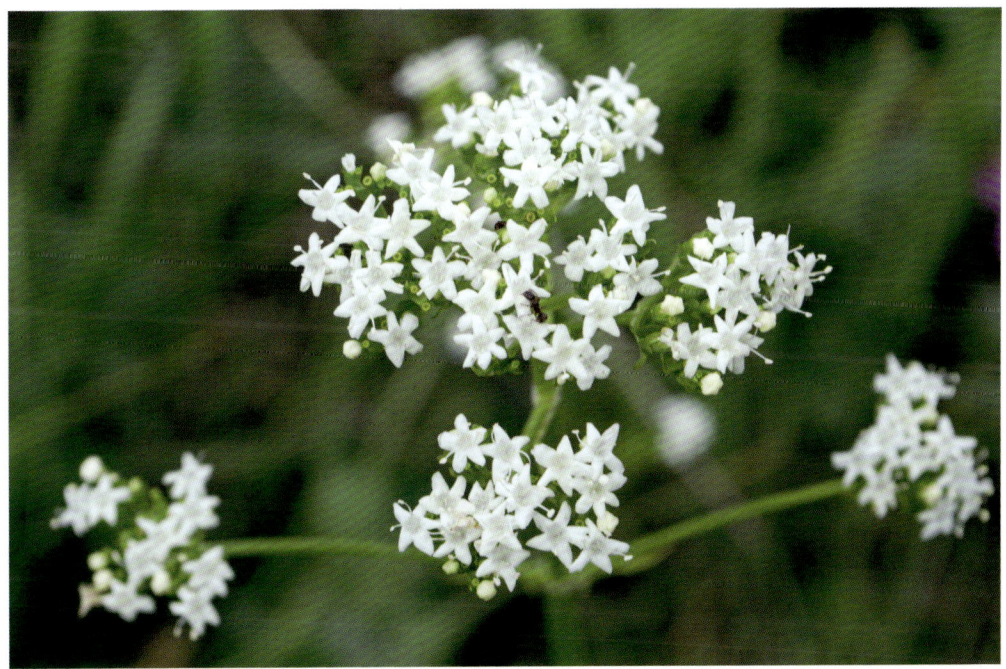

The star-shaped flowers of valerian have the sweetest fragrance. They are a lovely dried flower for tea.

⚠ Caution

For some people, valerian acts as a stimulant as opposed to a sedative. It seems to affect about 25% of people this way, so it is always best to use this with caution. Try the tincture or tea at some point when you are neither sleepy nor stimulated and see how it affects you before you commit to making this a regimen for sleep. Relying on valerian for long periods of time as a sleep aid has been shown to induce depression or lower energy in some people. Some experience a "hangover" or are groggy upon waking after taking too much or for too long a period of time. Not for use in pregnancy.

Future harvest

Be very mindful of this dear plant, as well as where you step when harvesting. It often grows in habitats with other sensitive species. Take roots only from places where a large quantity of valerian is growing.

HERBAL PREPARATIONS

Tea
Hot or cold infusion
1–3 tablespoons fresh or dried leaves, flowers, and stems
1 cup water
Decoction
3 tablespoons root
1 quart water
Drink 1 cup 3 times a day.

Tincture
1 part fresh leaves, stems, flowers, or roots
2 parts menstruum (75% alcohol, 25% distilled water)
or
1 part dried leaves, stems, flowers, or roots
5 parts menstruum (60% alcohol, 40% distilled water)
Take 20–40 drops before bed or upon waking.

Oil
Infuse with fresh or dried leaves, flowers, or root.

veronica

Veronica species
American speedwell
PARTS USED leaves, stems, flowers

One of my favorite creekside ingredients to add into nourishing face serums.

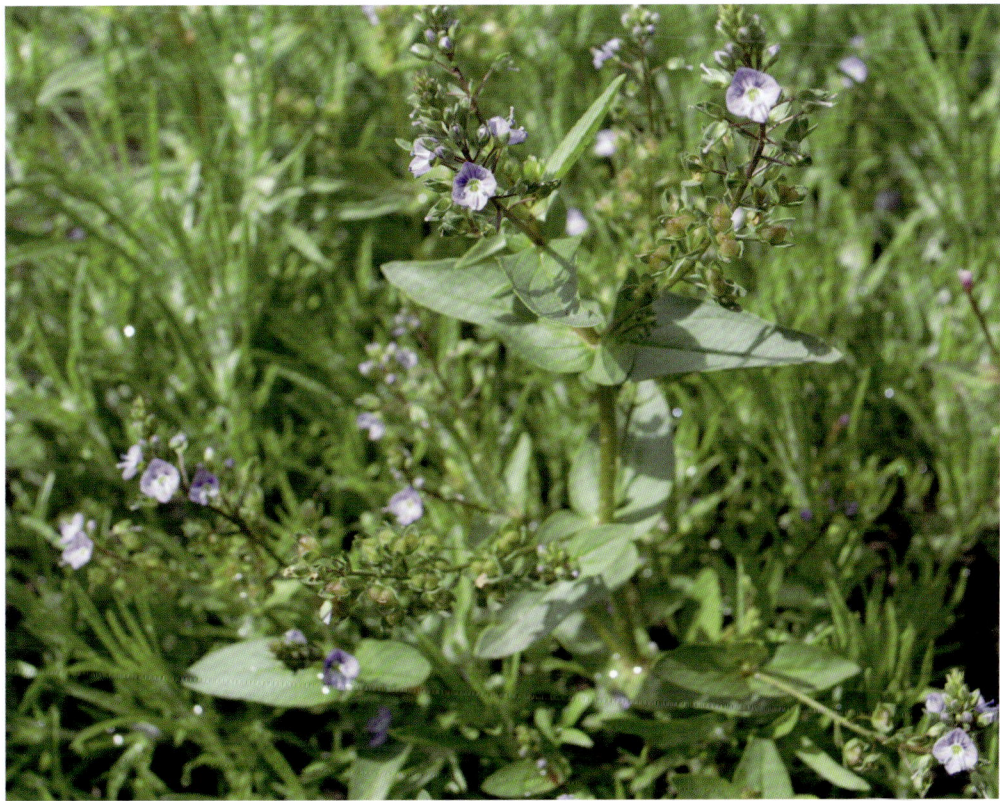
Find lots of veronica growing along the banks of rivers and creeks.

How to identify

Veronica is a creeping, matted plant that grows along and at the edges of creeks and rivers. Leaves are opposite, lanceolate, and serrated or entire around the margins. They are widest at the base, where they hug the stem closely. In early spring, young leaves have a reddish tint. Also, the rounded stem may be red, especially at branched junctions. Flowers grow on axillary racemes and are pale purple to blue, with four petals. Due to its opposite leaves, sometimes angular stems, and irregular-looking flowers, veronica can at first glance be confused for a member of the mint family.

Where, when, and how to wildcraft

Find *Veronica americana*, our more common species, growing alongside streams, bogs, or ponds, often with willowherb and wild mint as companions. Harvest only from clean waters, gathering the young tips, leaves, and flowers in spring or early summer. All species of *Veronica* have similar properties and can be used interchangeably.

Gather the young leaves from the aerial part of the plant. The stem and flowers can also be used. The plant can be cut into pieces and laid to dry on a screen.

Medicinal uses

Veronica has an affinity for helping skin disorders such as acne or eczema. Just the juice of the veronica plant can be used on itchy or eczema-like skin conditions. It is one of the wild herbs I use in my infused oil facial serum. Living in the high mountains, we need extra special ingredients to treat our skin, which is affected so much by our weather. We have to think about the intensity of the sun, wind, and dryness, and the fact that we dehydrate quicker than those at lower elevations. I blend elderflower, willowherb, veronica, and violets into jojoba-and-rosehip-seed oil for a luxurious facial serum that is scented with bergamot and rosewood. This light oil can be used to treat the face morning and night.

Veronica has been used historically in teas and tinctures as a tonic for the kidneys and for respiratory infections. It is high in vitamin C and can be brewed into a tea for a throat gargle or to expectorate coughs.

Future harvest

Leave this plant to do its job as a bank stabilizer and water purifier. Take only little aerial portions from the top of the plant.

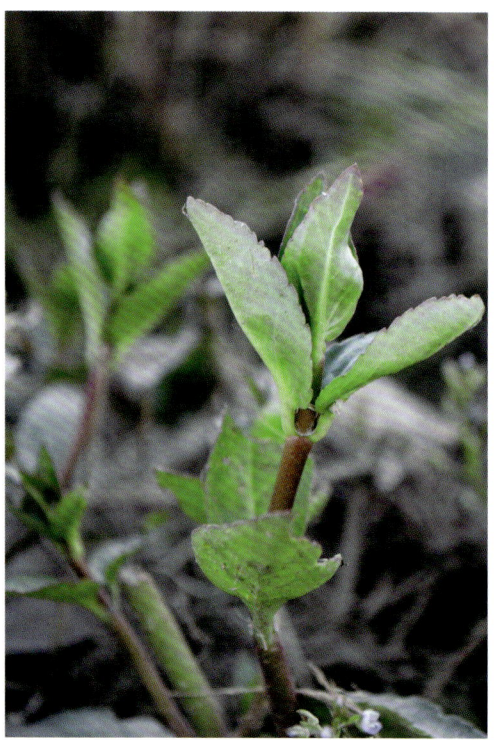

The opposite leaves of veronica can make it appear at first glance to belong to the mint family.

HERBAL PREPARATIONS

Tea
Hot infusion
1–2 tablespoons fresh or dried leaves, stems, and flowers
1 cup water
Drink 1 cup 3 times a day.

Tincture
1 part fresh stems, leaves, and flowers
2 parts menstruum (75% alcohol, 25% distilled water)
Take 20–40 drops 3 times a day.

Oil
Infuse with fresh or dried stems, leaves, and flowers.

vervain

Verbena species
PARTS USED leaves, flowers

When you feel like a candle burning at both ends, take a seat and blend yourself
a cup of tea, adding a small amount of vervain as a dried herb, tincture, or infused honey.

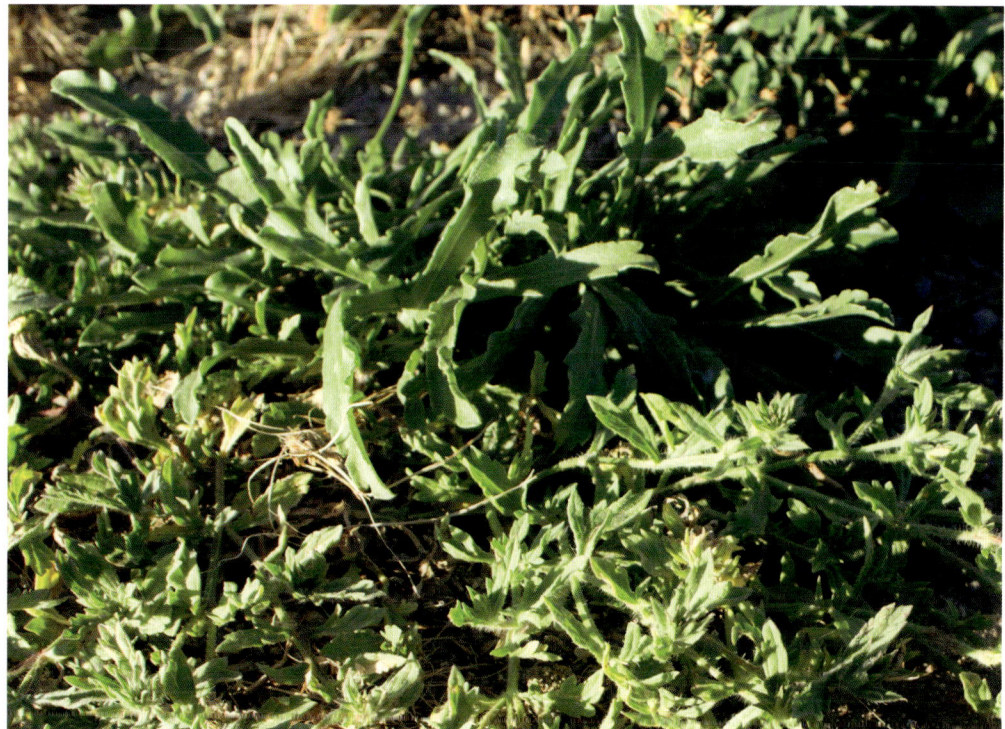

I kept cluelessly walking past prostrate vervain (*Verbena bracteata*), grumbling about how we have no vervains around here, until I recognized this ground-dwelling species as a very close relative of our blue vervains (*V. hastata, V. stricta,* and all the tall, erect species).

How to identify

Blue vervain is the name applied to the common taller species of the mountain states, *Verbena hastata, V. stricta,* and *V. macdougalii.* These perennial plants have square stems and could easily be mistaken for mints, but they lack any smell, and a taste would provide you with a bitter pucker. Rubbing the lance-shaped leaves gives you a sense of its rough hairiness. The leaves grow opposite or in a whorled fashion around the equally hairy stalk. Flowers are more of a purple-magenta than blue and grow in a slender spike atop the plant. which grows to 3–5 feet tall.

The smaller species, prostrate vervain (*Verbena bracteata*), grows low to the ground as a sprawling, branched mat. It is also a hairy plant with bluish purple flowers that peek out of the long, leaf-like bracts that form the dense flower spikes. The leaves are opposite and deeply clefted.

Where, when, and how to wildcraft

Gather vervain in late summer when the bluish violet flowers are starting to bloom. The tall vervains can be cut from midstalk, harboring the leaves and choice flowers that never blossom all at once. The roots of the taller species of vervain I do not use; others have spoken of it being nauseating. Dry the stalks by hanging or laying on a drying rack, then garble the leaves and flowers from the central stem, which can be discarded.

The sprawling shorter vervains, such as *Verbena bracteata*, can be gathered as whole plants, using the roots, stems, leaves, and flowers. Since these are hairy, low-growing plants, it is best to give them a rinse before drying. All species could use a good rinse, as the hairs trap all sorts of debris, like cobwebs, plant matter, and dirt.

Medicinal uses

When agitation is setting in from nervous exhaustion, restlessness, or sickness, vervain can be useful as a relaxant, sedative bitter-nervine that is also an antispasmodic, diaphoretic, and diuretic. This means it can help settle a nervous or upset stomach, while encouraging a sweat and the release of fluids to assist a fever, all while it is promoting deep relaxation, which can be great for the onset of any virus or cold.

Taken as a relaxing nervine, it can soothe frayed nerves in the overworked parent or college student. For those who feel like they are burning the candle at both ends, vervain can help dampen out one of the ends to provide rest and repair.

The tea or tincture can be taken at nighttime to help assist with falling asleep while soothing the overactive mind. A calming combination would be vervain, skullcap, and flowering valerian tops.

Caution

The hairs of *Verbena bracteata* are intense—strain teas well using a fine tea bag or coffee strainer. This is a plant that has been used as an emetic, to induce vomiting. Smaller doses are advised, or smaller portions for formulating.

Future harvest

Taking just the flowering tops and leaves will not harm the life of this plant.

HERBAL PREPARATIONS

Tea
Hot or cold infusion
1–2 tablespoons fresh or dried leaves and
  flowers
1 cup water
Drink 3 times a day.

Tincture
1 part freshly chopped leaves and flowers
2 parts menstruum (75% alcohol, 25%
  distilled water)
or
1 part dried leaves and flowers
4 parts menstruum (60% alcohol, 40%
  distilled water)
Take 10–20 drops 3 times a day or as needed.

Oil
*Infuse with freshly chopped or dried leaves
and flowers.*

violet

Viola species

PARTS USED leaves, flowers

The demulcent leaves and flowers of violets make lovely teas in the arid west.

How to identify

The common name is a bit misleading. Not only do these plants come in violet but also yellow (*Viola nuttallii* and *V. orbiculata*), white (*V. canadensis*), and blue (*V. adunca*). A plant that always seems to hug the soil it grows in, violet is found blooming from spring through summer. Flowers look complex: two matching petals arrange themselves on either side, another matched set radiates upward, and the fifth and largest petal points down. The fifth petal displays the most beauty, varying in its color and shape from the other four and having deep-colored stripes that radiate from the center. The thick leaves of violets are usually heart- or teardrop-shaped, and their distinctive veins give them an almost leathery appearance. The leaves have a mild wintergreen fragrance when crushed or chewed.

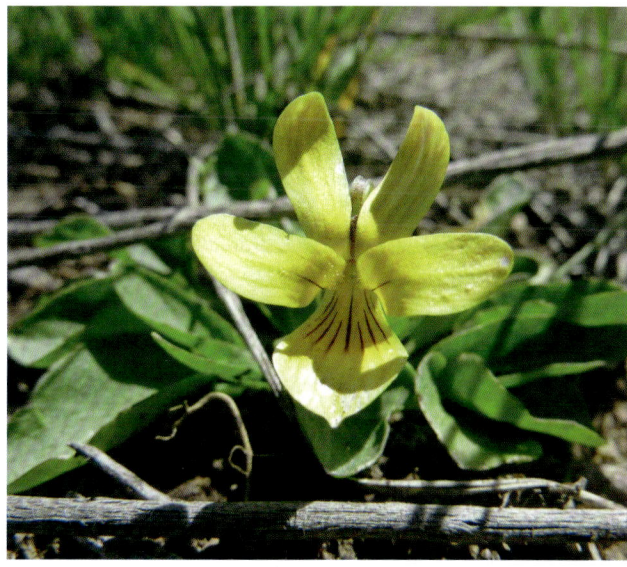

Colors vary by species. Find yellow, white, or purple violets blooming in the spring and still offering their demulcent leaves until the snow starts to flutter.

Where, when, and how to wildcraft

Shade-loving plants, violets are found on forest floors in the springtime. This is the best time to gather, while they are in flower and hosting tender leaves. In mountain valleys, summertime is best for gathering; you can find them in places ranging from sunny meadows to aspen groves.

It is best to use a pair of scissors or small pruners to gather leaves and flowers. Sometimes pinching the leaves can result in uprooting the entire plant. Some species are more elusive than others, so respect them all and gather only a few flowers and leaves from each plant.

Medicinal uses

Violet leaf and flower tea can be drunk daily for its demulcent properties that can greatly benefit those who are constitutionally dry and hold a bit of heat. The herb is cooling and moistening, which can be useful to

[243

expectorate a dry cough. Violet can be made into syrups or infused into honey to be used for sore throats or coughs due to dryness. The tincture or tea can be beneficial for lymphatic stagnation, where there is swelling of lymph nodes or spleen.

Used topically, the herb's demulcent properties can be soothing in formulas for dry skin or sensitive, sore, and raw areas. It can be useful on swollen glands and with lymphatic congestion. Violet-infused oil is another favorite ingredient to include in face serum, massage oils, or breast oils.

Future harvest

Violets are not very abundant in the mountain west. They grow in small groupings and could easily be overharvested. Please keep the whole plant in the ground. Harvest only a few flowers and leaves from each plant.

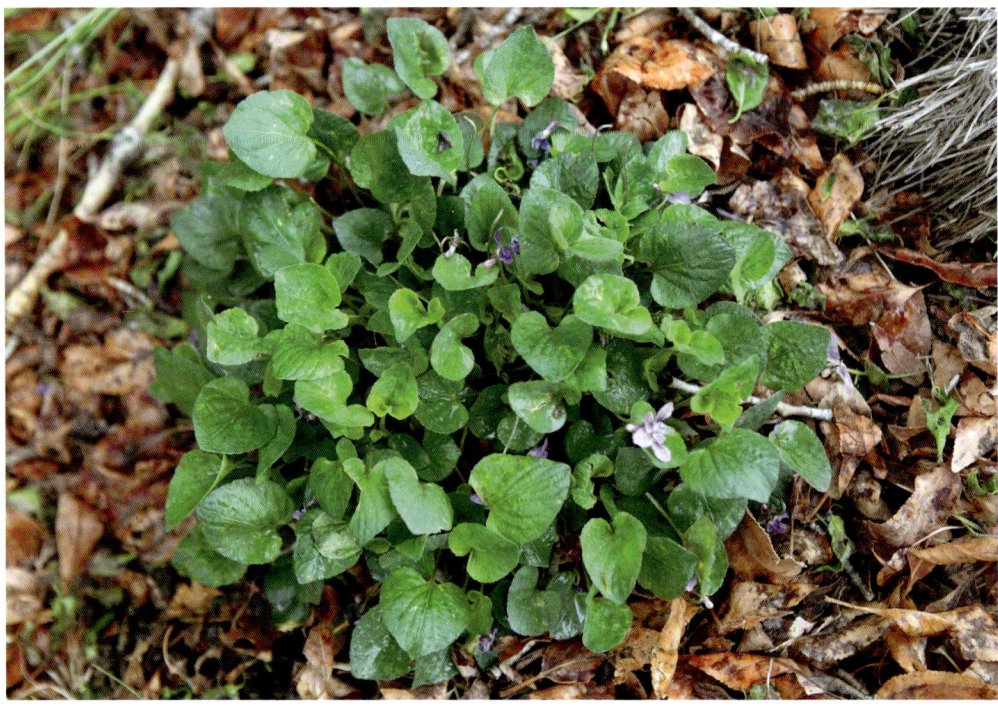

Violets, though tiny in the mountain states, can be found growing all over our damp, forested, alpine hills.

wild asparagus

Asparagus officinalis

PARTS USED roots

The nourishing demulcent root of wild asparagus gives sweet relief to wheezy lungs.

How to identify

It is best to scope out asparagus territory in the fall, when the plant looks nothing like the spring shoots. Look for the yellowed, branched plant, standing tall when all the other plants have died back. This perennial plant's woody stalk will be poking through snow, providing you with a perfect marker to the spot you should revisit once the snow melts in early spring. Shoots look just like their cultivated counterpart, although they may be a lot skinnier or sometimes giant. The tips are dark green when young, before the plant branches out and forms small green flowers. Inedible red berries are produced by the mature female asparagus plant, making the many-branched green asparagus look like an ornate Christmas tree.

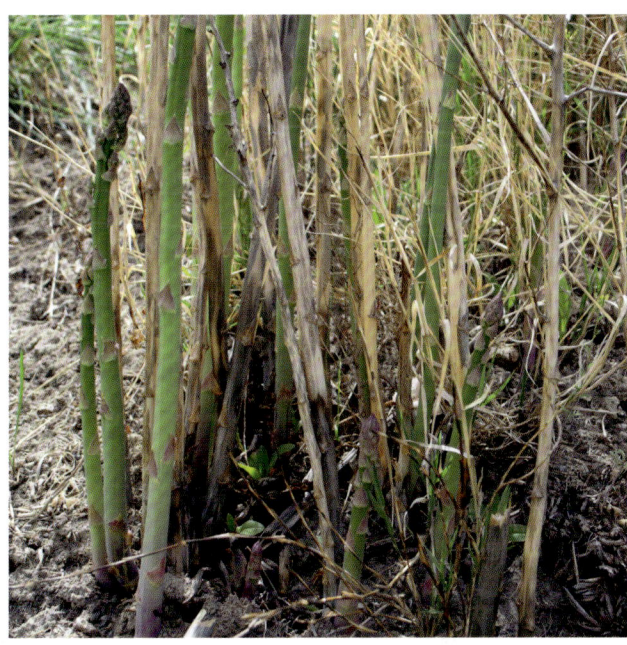

In the spring, dig the roots of asparagus as the tops of the shoots are emerging from the ground.

Where, when, and how to wildcraft

Asparagus needs water to thrive, so start by looking there. It also doesn't grow well above 7000 feet. Find tall, overgrown asparagus in midsummer when out fishing, or spot it growing in irrigated fields and ditches. The roots can be dug in spring or in the fall, when the plant has turned to brown, leaving its marking skeleton of branches.

Dig around a cluster of asparagus, loosening the soil, so the roots are easier to pull up. Wash well, as asparagus grows in damp and muddy soils. Chop up the root to dry for storage or use fresh in a tincture.

Medicinal uses

The root of the Asian species, *Asparagus racemosus*, called shatavari, has a long-standing use in Ayurvedic medicine as a reproductive tonic. I have used our locally common species, *A. officinalis*, for similar purposes, and have found it promotes cervical and arousal fluid production. This can be hugely helpful for vaginal dryness or tenderness.

Traditionally it has been used by southwest herbalists as a nutritive diuretic and in quantity as a gentle laxative. As with many demulcents, asparagus can be useful for respiratory conditions where there is wheezing present and the lungs seem to need to be moistened a bit.

Future harvest

Where asparagus is found at lower elevations, it is usually abundant around waterways, making harvesting roots no problem. Do respect the fact that you do not need to dig up the entire plant but can take just a portion of its roots and leave the rest behind.

HERBAL PREPARATIONS

Tea
Decoction
1 ounce fresh or dried root
1 quart water
Drink 1 cup 3 times a day.

Tincture
1 part fresh root
2 parts menstruum (75% alcohol, 25% distilled water)
or
1 part dried root
5 parts menstruum (60% alcohol, 40% distilled water)
Take 20–40 drops 3 times a day.

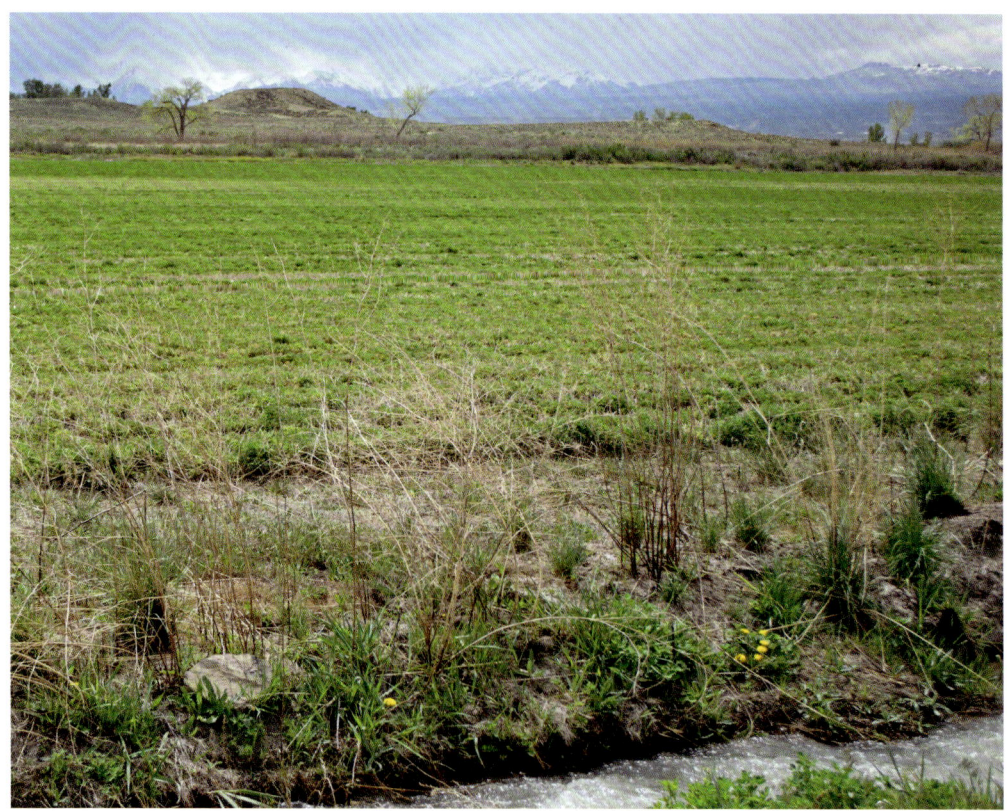

Come fall, asparagus are easily spotted by the trained eye. Look for the dead-branched plant, growing along irrigation ditches, creeks, or rivers. This is another time that the roots are harvestable.

Carum species
Persian cumin
PARTS USED leaves, flowers, seeds

The carminative seeds of wild caraway can begin to ease a disturbed stomach that needs help dispelling trapped gas.

How to identify
Caraway is usually a biennial plant, putting out basal leaves the first year and flowering in the second—and sometimes a third—year. Leaves of caraway look like a mix of carrot and yarrow; they are arranged alternately up the flowering stalk. The stalks grow 1–3 feet tall, putting forth white or pinkish flowers arranged as a flat-topped umbel. Stalks can be green, straw-colored, or purple-tinged; they stand tall from a small taproot that can be up to ½ inch thick. The seeds of wild caraway, technically achenes, are highly aromatic, crescent-shaped, slender, and brown, with linear ridges that are lighter in color.

Where, when, and how to wildcraft
Wild caraway can be found near water, in woods or open fields, at elevations up to 9000 feet. A spot where pastures are nearby is often a good area to look. Collect leaves and taproots in

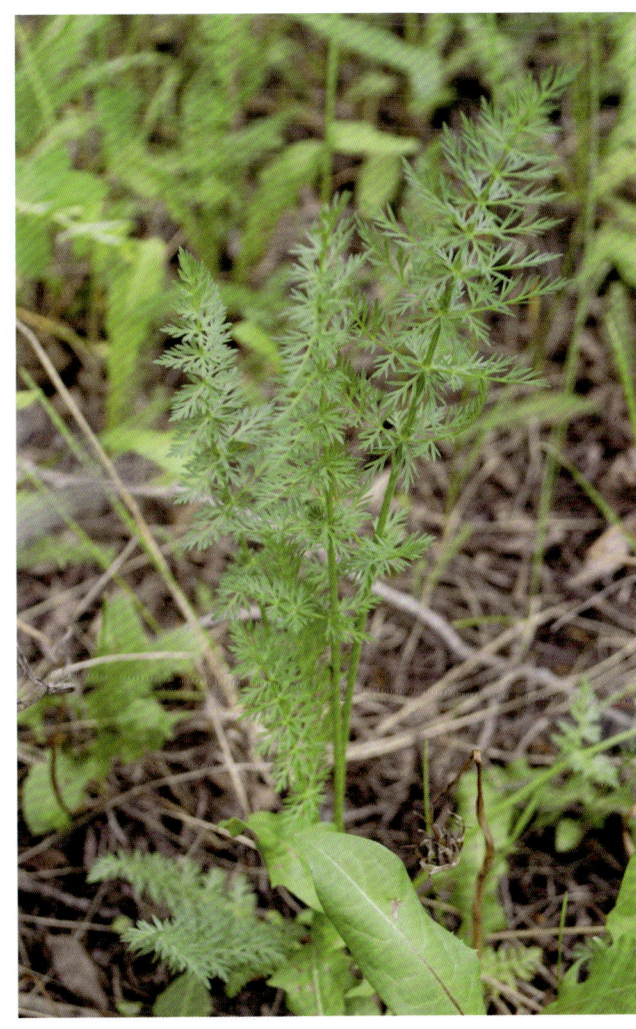

Pick leaves of wild caraway and add them into the carminative formulas you are blending for settling the stomach.

late spring and early summer. Gather flowers in summer, when present. Seeds are ready by late summer or early fall.

Collect the drying achenes directly from the stalk of wild caraway. Gathering can be easy in large areas; cut the stalk just under the umbel, or use your fingers to take achenes off the tops. Let the seeded umbels dry out for a few days in paper bags.

The fresh achenes can be tinctured. The leaves and flowers can be dried for use in teas. Roots can be chopped, dried, and stored for future use in decoctions.

Medicinal uses

Chew the seeds of caraway after meals for indigestion, bloating, or to dispel gas. Fresh

leaves and seeds can be tinctured for use in carminative or bitter formulations. Try adding the dried or fresh seeds to vinegar for Fire Folkin' Cider.

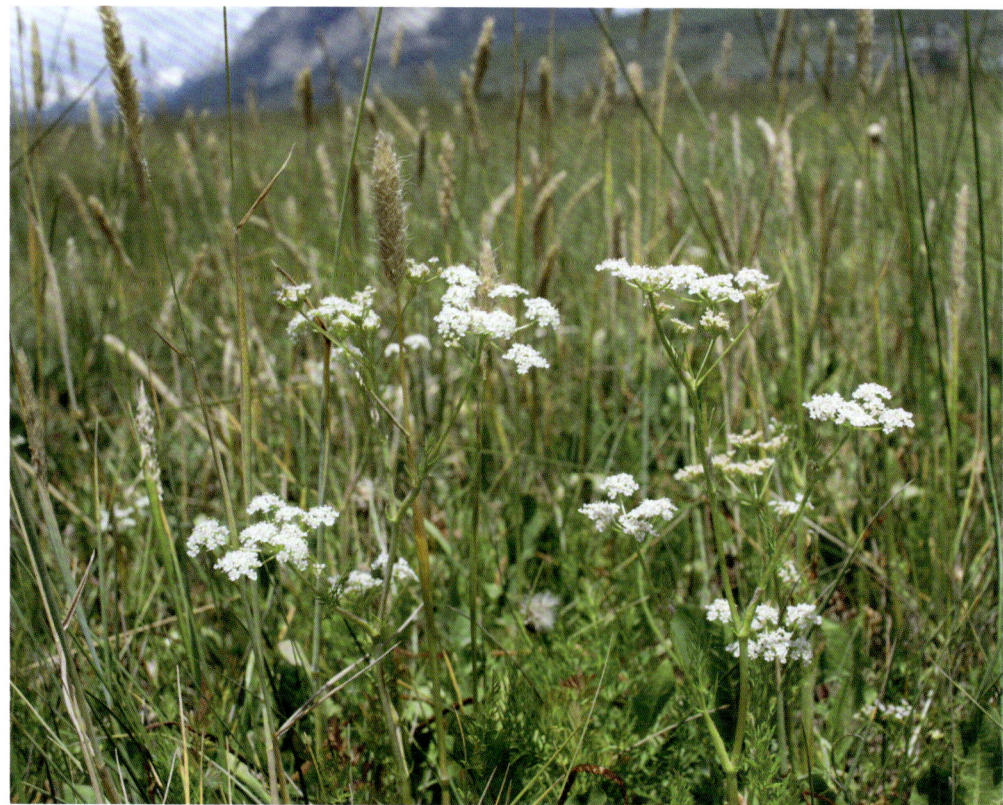

A culinary invader of the mountain west, wild caraway can be found growing throughout cattle pastures and into the nearby woods.

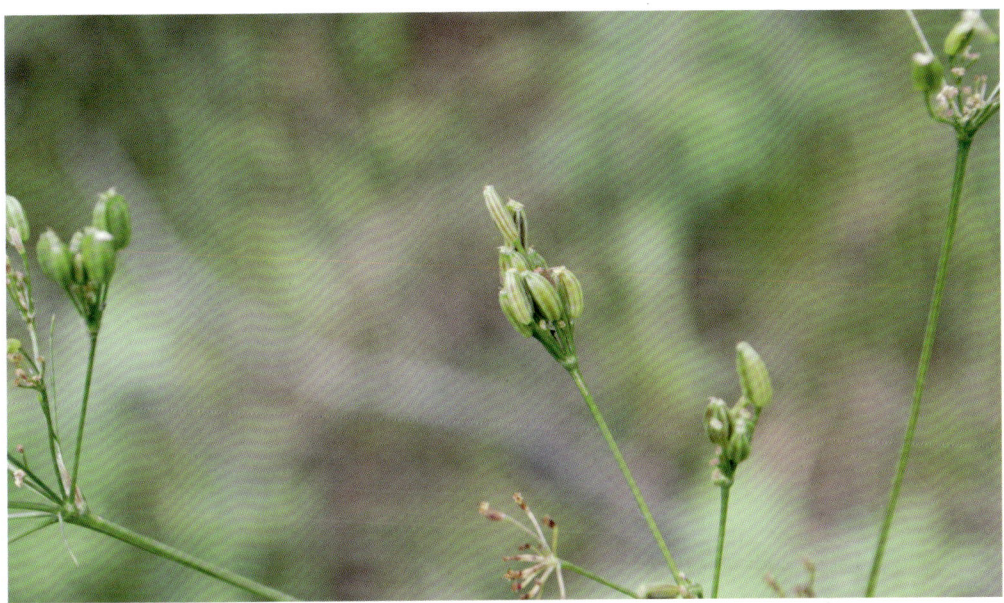

Always be 100% certain when harvesting the seeds of wild caraway. They can look similar to toxic plants of the Apiaceae, such as water hemlock and poison hemlock.

Dried flowers, leaves, and seeds can be used for making infusions, and the root can be used for decoctions. An infused oil of wild caraway can harbor fragrance and be used topically for skin conditions. An infused honey would also make a lovely addition to teas or remedies. All parts of wild caraway are useful when trying to calm a sour stomach.

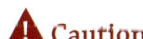 Caution

As with all members of the carrot family, it is important to be 100% accurate with your identification before harvesting. Both poison hemlock and water hemlock are deadly lookalikes to wild caraway. Always check your seed shape!

Future harvest

Wild caraway is a weedy plant that can handle harvesting of the leaves and seeds.

HERBAL PREPARATIONS

Tea
1 tablespoon fresh or dried leaves or flowers
or
1 teaspoon fresh or dried seeds
1 cup water
Drink 1–2 cups 3 times a day.

Tincture
1 part fresh seeds or leaves and flowers
2 parts menstruum (75% alcohol, 25% distilled water)
or
1 part dried seeds
5 parts menstruum (60% alcohol, 40% distilled water)
Take 10–20 drops as needed.

Oil
Infuse with fresh or dried leaves, seeds, and flowers.

Prunus species

PARTS USED bark, twigs, stems, flowers, fruit

Honey infused with fresh wild cherries is the best-tasting medicinal cough syrup.

How to identify

Quite a few wild cherry species grace the mountain west. Trees of chokecherry (*Prunus virginiana*) are most abundant along rivers and highways and in subalpine forests. In late spring, identifying can be easy. Look for shrubby trees with long, white, clustered racemes of flowers that hang from the sides of the branches. Find a good group of trees in flower and return to this prime spot to harvest cherries later in the summer.

Thin-trunked trees grow from a few feet to 10 feet tall; they tend to be hardier in the foothills and smaller and more shrub-like the higher in elevation they grow. Leaves are shiny green with a lighter hue on the underside; they are oval with little jagged edges and are arranged alternately along the stem. Bark ranges from gray to reddish brown, with horizontal lighter-colored air pores called lenticels. Fruit is a drupe, a berry with only one seed—the nut or pit, in the case of wild cherries. Berries ripen to an almost black color late in the summer.

Where, when, and how to wildcraft

Wild cherry trees grow near streams, along ditches, in canyons, and in conifer forests. Gather the flowers in spring when they are highly aromatic.

Beat the birds to the fruits when they are about a quarter inch in size and darkened to black, in late summer or early fall.

In order to use for teas and tinctures, twigs can be clipped into smaller pieces, bark can be peeled from larger branches, and flowering racemes can be plucked off the tree. Use pruners to trim twigs along with the flower spikes, and dry the flowers while they are on the twig. Lay them over a mesh screen or cloth sheet that gets adequate circulation above and below.

Medicinal uses

The spring-flowering twigs of wild cherry, the bark, and the fruiting stems all carry astringent, bitter, and cooling properties. They also provide a lovely flavor of cherry with a little bitter almond and sweet notes.

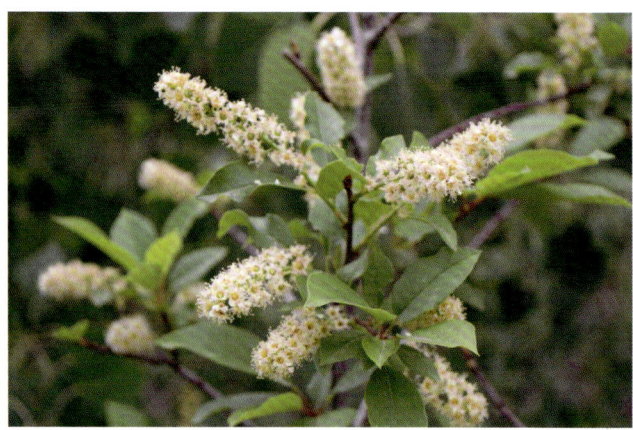

The blossoms of wild cherry fill small mountain towns with their lofty aromatics each spring.

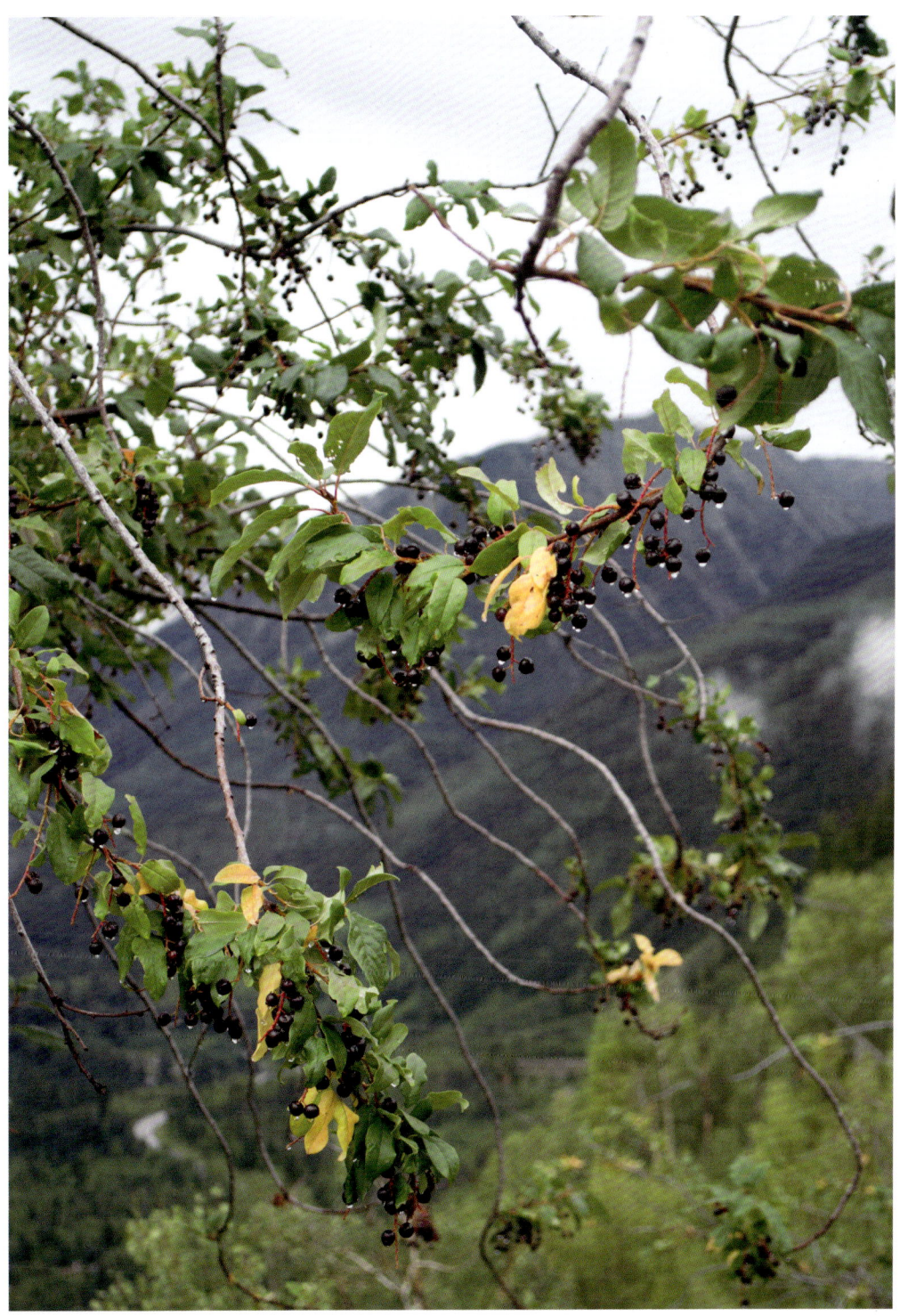

Wild cherry fruits can be harvested for use in cough syrups or honeys.

Teas can be made from fresh flowers or dried flowers, twigs, and bark. Cherry bark, flowers, berries, and twigs can be added to cough and bitter formulas, whether in a syrup, tincture, or elixir. Start your cough syrup with an infusion of chokecherries in honey. Wild cherry can help relieve diarrhea in children and calm a stomach experiencing food sensitivities.

The extracted aroma of wild cherry can enhance topical preparations. Infuse the plant parts into oils for use in cough rubs and lip balms.

Caution

A word of warning when using fresh cherry bark and twigs: due to the cyanide content of the fresh plant matter, it should be administered only in small and infrequent doses. Dried plant matter of wild cherry is of no concern.

Future harvest

Spreading your pruning of flowering twigs and a few branches among many trees will not threaten future harvesting.

Humulus lupulus

PARTS USED leaves, strobiles

The calming and sedative qualities of hops make it a nice tincture for long plane rides.

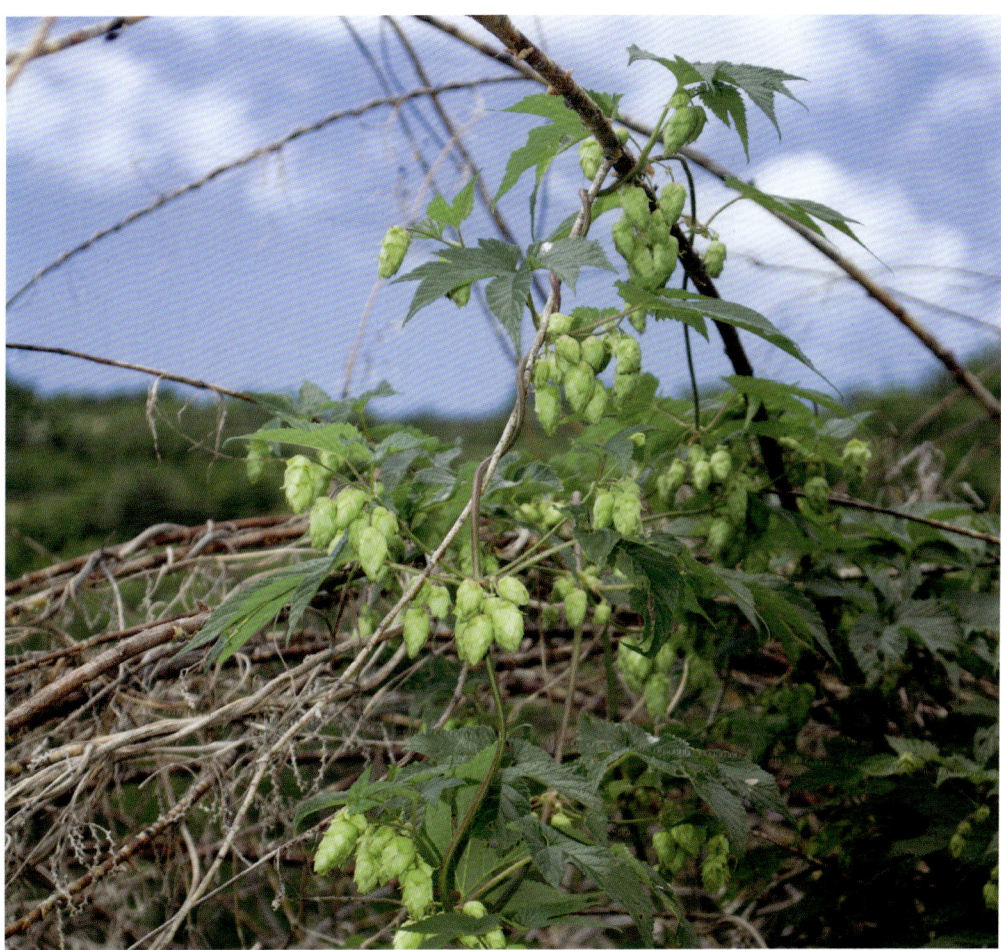

A stand of hops can live for many years, sourcing from a giant old root with many little rootlets.

How to identify

Wild hops grow from a creeping bine, not a vine, as plants do not have tendrils, suckers, or hooks, but instead use stiff hairs and a vigorous stem to climb bushes and other natural trellises. As a perennial plant it dies back in the fall and grows again the following year. Each year the bine will reach quite impressive lengths of 10–40 feet. Leaves are either heart shaped or have large lobes, usually three to five, and are finely toothed, growing opposite one another. *Humulus lupulus* is dioecious, meaning it has separate male and female plants. Both plants are needed for pollination. The female flowers, or strobiles, look like small, soft, green pinecones. The male flowers hang in loose panicles that grow 3–5 inches long.

Where, when, and how to wildcraft

Wild hops grows throughout the mountain west, and indeed North America, in open meadows, disturbed soils, and forest edges. Find them draping over fenced alleyways and sprawling over willows near a creek. Gather strobiles in late summer and early fall.

The strobiles are ready to be picked when they are highly aromatic and vibrant in color; get them before they dry out. Pick them from the stem and place in a paper bag to keep all the lupulin. A fine golden powder will be present on the strobiles or in the bag after harvesting; this resinous powder is the lupulin, the source of this plant's sedative and calming effect.

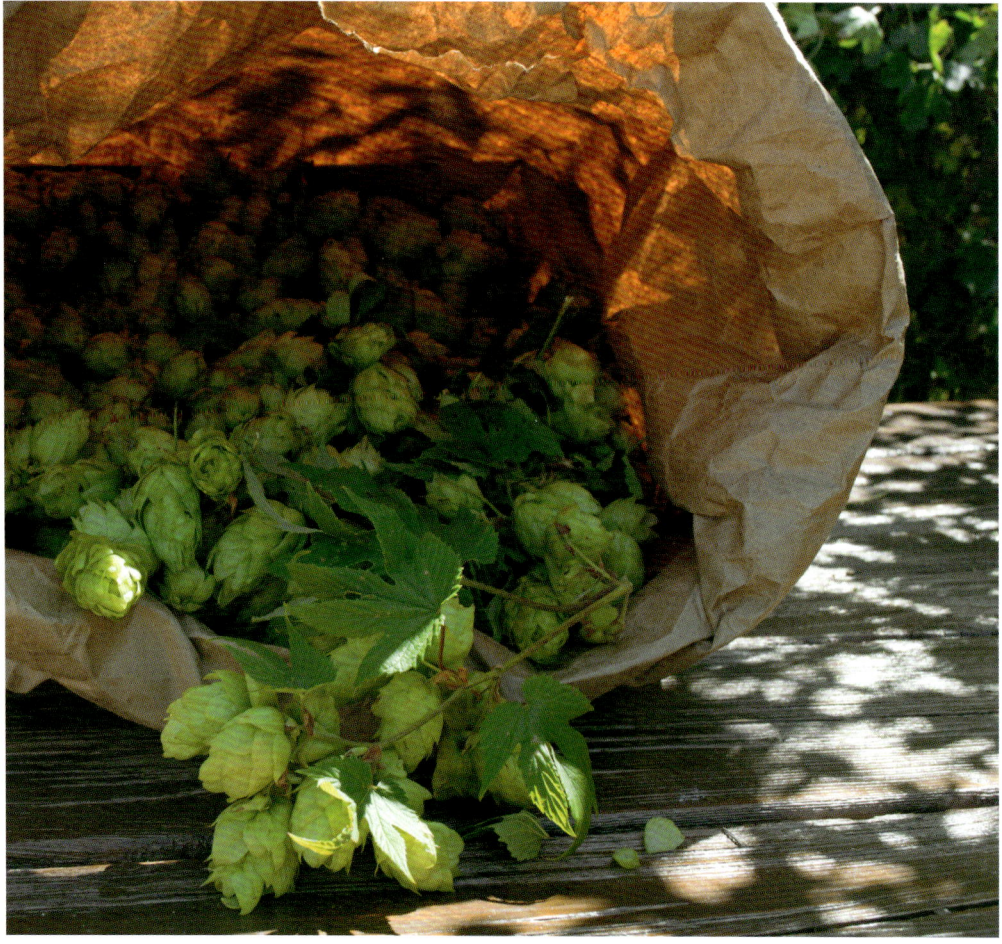

Gather hops strobiles while they are brilliantly green, sticky, and highly aromatic. Don't wait until they start to brown.

Medicinal uses

Wild hops strobiles are highly aromatic and antimicrobial with a citrusy, bitter taste. This herb is calming to anxious nerves and can ease digestive cramping or discomfort. It can help soothe the intolerable feeling of having a fever, relax the body, and remedy minor aches and pains. Hops has an affinity for mellowing the feeling of butterflies in the stomach that may be brought on by a slew of emotions—love, anger, jealousy, or angst.

Taken as a tincture or tea it can be heavily sedating, good for those who wake up in the middle of the night and cannot get back to sleep. This is a cooling and drying herb that can be aggravating to those who already lean that way constitutionally.

Topically, as a poultice, hops can bring relief to skin eruptions, spider bites, or wounds. The oil combines well in dreaming balms or can be used alone as a massage oil for its relaxing and antispasmodic properties. It can also be a pleasant oil in chest rubs meant to relieve coughing fits and relax the bronchials. Hops oil is a lovely relaxant and pain-relieving antispasmodic for muscular tension, pains, and twitching. It is often used for backaches, kinked necks, and menstrual pains.

Future harvest

No concerns here beyond the usual: never strip any one plant of all it offers the wildcrafter. The bines are weather-resilient and can be transplanted easily through spring cuttings.

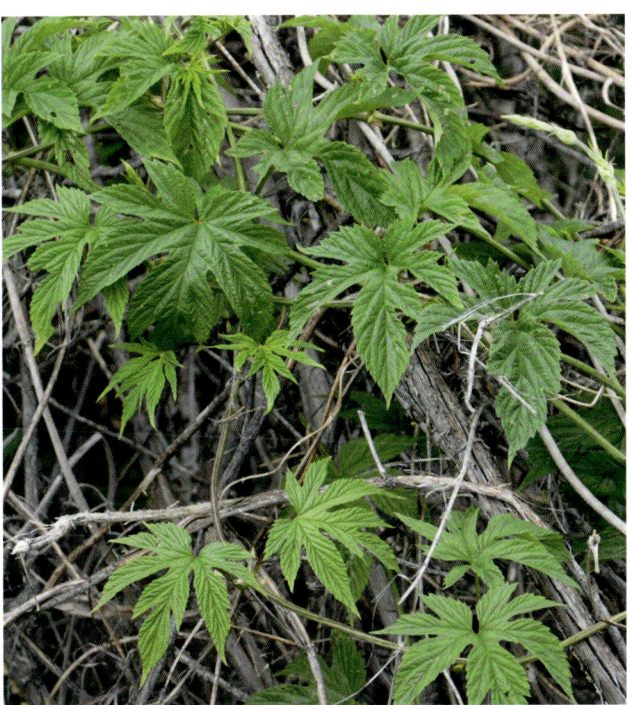

Several subspecies of hops can have more than three lobes around the leaf margins.

HERBAL PREPARATIONS

Tea
Hot infusion
2–3 tablespoons fresh or dried strobiles or
  leaves
1 cup water
Drink as needed.

Tincture
1 part fresh strobiles
2 parts menstruum (75% alcohol, 25%
  distilled water)
or
1 part dried strobiles
5 parts menstruum (60% alcohol, 40%
  distilled water)
Take 10–20 drops as needed.

Oil
Infuse with fresh or dried strobiles or leaves.

wild lettuce

Lactuca species

PARTS USED leaves, stems

The white latex is extremely bitter but useful at relieving pain.

How to identify

Wild lettuce leaves growing along the stem are lanceolate and arranged alternately, clasping the stalk closely. Leaf margins are toothed or prickly and may or may not be lobed. The underside of the midrib is noticeably barbed. The leaves start out in a basal rosette and could easily be confused with other similar-looking plants, like chicory, dandelion, or sow thistle, which all lack these small spines; however, all these plants have a milky white sap. The flowers of wild lettuce are small and yellow, with prominent green bracts. Wild lettuce can have a lot of branched flower stems coming off the main stalk. Seeds are small, brown, and attached to a fluffy white pappus.

Where, when, and how to wildcraft

Wild lettuce is a weedy foe to many in the mountain west, as it grows just about anywhere its seeds land. Find it in vacant lots and fields or lining sidewalks and parking lots. Gather the young leaves of the basal

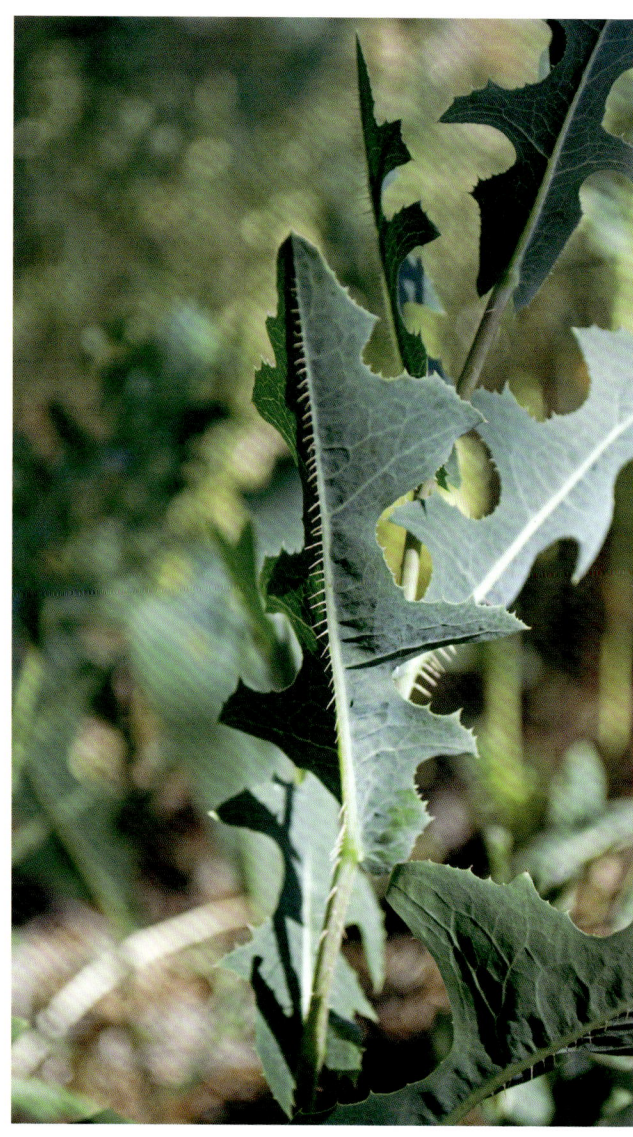

Leaves of wild lettuce have sharp tiny spines that line the back side of the midvein, as well as poky margins.

rosette in early spring and into summer, until the plant puts up a flowering stalk. You may also collect the young stalk and unopened flowerheads in summer.

Pick the choice-looking young leaves from the young rosette. Cut the stalk off at the base while it has fresh flowerbuds on it. The milky sap that exudes from the plant is the medicine we are after. It will coat your fingers and make your clippers sticky.

Medicinal uses

The bitter medicine of wild lettuce species helps to calm the nerves and soothe irritability in sick, restless children. It also acts as a mild sedative with an anodyne effect.

Tinctures can be made from the freshly cut plant parts leaking their milky latex. Fresh plant material is best, as the latex has the best medicine. The tincture can be included for fever formulations or for insomnia. It can also be used in formulas for pain relief of menstrual cramps, musculoskeletal issues like arthritis or injury, and wound care.

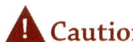 **Caution**

Wild lettuce is in the Asteraceae, and some people may have allergic reactions to this plant family.

Future harvest

Feel free to harvest vigorously—it's even fine to pull this easily spreading weed from the ground.

HERBAL PREPARATIONS

Tincture
1 part freshly cut leaves and stems
2 parts menstruum (90% alcohol, 10% distilled water)
Perform at least a triple maceration. Create your first tincture, letting the plant matter sit in the alcohol for a couple of days or so, and strain it. Add more freshly cut wild lettuce to the strained alcohol, let this sit for a few days, and strain again. Repeat this 3–5 times for a stronger tincture. You may prefer to sweeten with honey after your final strain. Take 5–10 drops as needed.

wild licorice

Glycyrrhiza lepidota
American licorice, sweet root

PARTS USED roots

*When combined with other herbs, wild licorice increases their vitality
and seems to seamlessly blend formulations, adding a slight sweet note to all.*

How to identify

The long leaves of wild licorice are compound and pinnate, always with an odd number of leaflets. The lanceolate leaflets grow opposite each other with a single leaflet at the tip. Leaf-stalks have a slight downward bend to them that deepens on hot days. A sticky, waxy coating can sometimes be felt on the entire plant. Wild licorice grows to about 2 feet tall and forms robust colonies, thanks to its creeping root system. It has small, pea-like flowers produced in a spike-like raceme, blooming in late spring and remaining through summer. Flowers are primarily white but can be yellow-green or purple tinged at times. Wild licorice is commonly confused with poisonous milk vetches (see caution), but the fruit of wild licorice is brown and burred. It is the only spiny-fruited member of the pea family (Fabaceae) in the mountain west.

Licorice can also be confused with *Xanthium* (cocklebur), which also has hook-bristled fruits, but cocklebur is a member of the sunflower family and a completely different medicine.

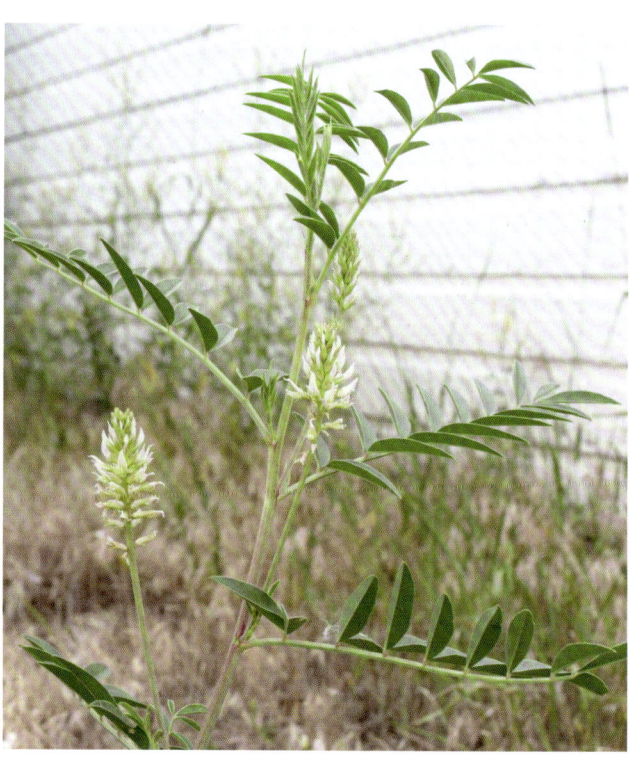

Find wild licorice sprawling in urban areas or inhabiting space in the wild hills.

Where, when, and how to wildcraft

Find wild licorice colonies skirting around cities, towns, and mountain drainages throughout our region, near mountain streams and irrigated fields and ditches. Gather roots in either spring or fall, when they hold the most flavor. The large taproots may be hard to dig up, as they can reach 3 feet in length; therefore, choose a location that has loose soil, such as a riverbank. In some places, roots are easily pulled up, complete with attached rhizomes.

Medicinal uses

The root of wild licorice is not as sweet as that of the cultivated species. It does however offer the same mucilaginous and anti-inflammatory properties. This makes it soothing for sore throats, coughs, or stomach irritations. The root can be chewed on fresh or dried and it will soothe or even heal up canker sores in the mouth. It can also work on ulcers in the stomach lining. Wild licorice has an affinity to help many conditions that are exacerbated by overdryness. This includes dry constipation, wheezing, or scratchy throats.

A cold infusion of the root can extract properties that are anti-inflammatory and support the immune system, which can be beneficial when a cold strikes and the bronchioles are inflamed.

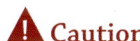 Caution

Wild licorice has a look similar to milk vetches (*Astragalus* species), which are poisonous. Be positive with your identification. Not for use in pregnancy, or by people with high blood pressure or kidney disease—wild licorice causes sodium retention.

Future harvest

This plant is stout and an aggressive grower; harvesting some roots should not hurt the stand. Don't harvest in areas where wild licorice is a bank stabilizer, helping to keep down erosion. Rhizomes transplant well and have been known to take over gardens.

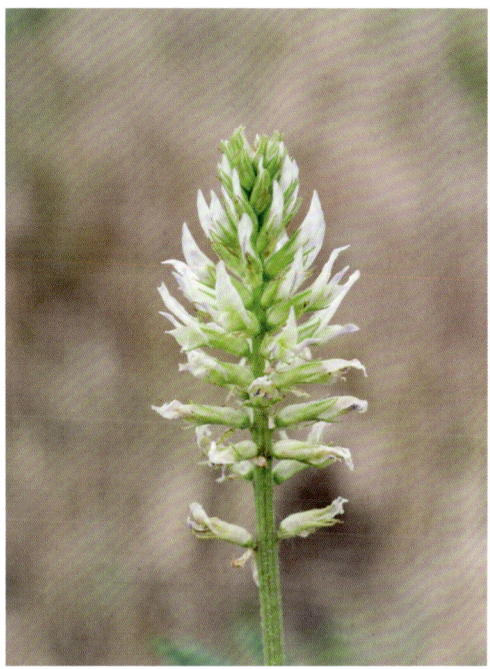

The flower of wild licorice will turn to a burred seedpod.

HERBAL PREPARATIONS

Tea
Hot or cold infusion
1–3 tablespoons fresh or dried chopped root
1 cup water
Decoction
1 ounce fresh or dried chopped root
1 quart water
Drink 1 cup 3 times a day.

Tincture
1 part fresh root
2 parts menstruum (75% alcohol, 25% distilled water)
or
1 part dried root
5 parts menstruum (60% alcohol, 40% distilled water)
Take 20–40 drops 3 times a day.

wild mint

Mentha species
poleo mint, field mint, cornmint
PARTS USED leaves, stems, flowers

Wild mints can usually be smelled before you realize you are walking on top of the plants, crushing them and releasing the aromatics.

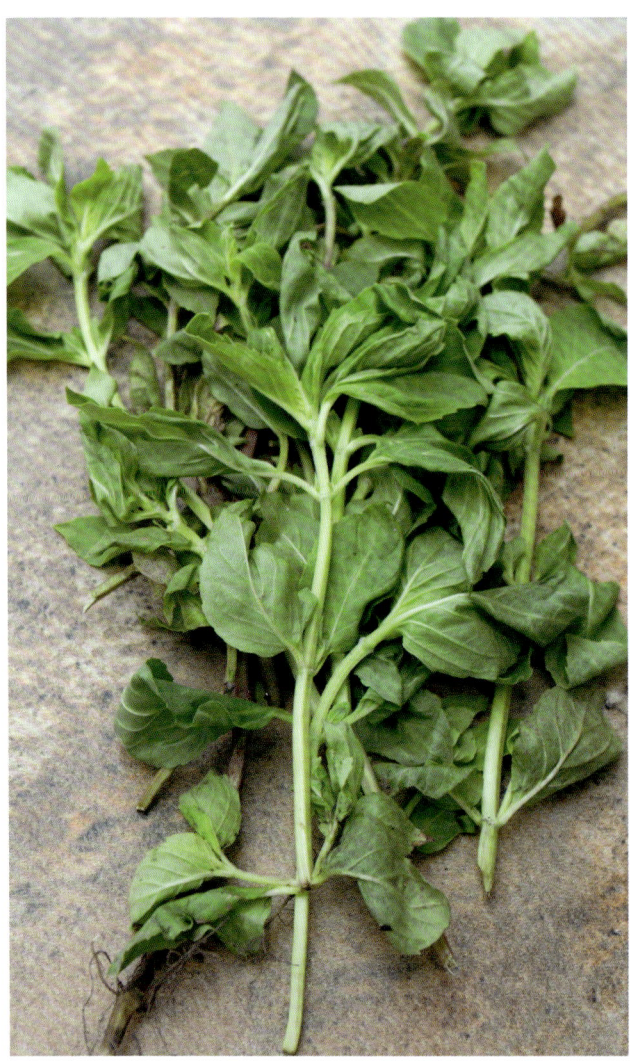

Freshly picked *Mentha arvensis* ready to be dried for tea.

How to identify

Mentha arvensis, our most common mint species, is almost always growing at the water's edge. For identification, pick a leaf—they are simple and grow in opposite pairs—crush it, and take a sniff. Mint will always smell like mint, and all mint stems are square. To be certain, roll the stem, feeling for the ridges of a square. The small flowers with long stamens grow around the stalk and look like light purple puffballs.

Where, when, and how to wildcraft

Along streams and riverbanks is a good place to start when looking for wild mint. You will find these plants from spring into fall anywhere with substantial moisture and a bit of shade. Young leaves are more tender; they get tougher and less potent as they age and begin to brown.

Walking along a riverbank or in a moist field, you can usually gather more than enough mint bundles for a season of medicinal use. I pinch off the top 4 inches of the plant, leaving plenty of leaves and flowers behind.

Medicinal uses

Wild mint tea can be a simple easy fix to an upset tummy or as a postdinner drink after overeating. It helps to dispel gas or calm gastrointestinal cramping. Blended into bitters formulas, wild mint can provide a cooling flavor that will help to stimulate the flow of bile.

The cooling combination of wild mint, yarrow, and elderflower is a useful tea for feverish children.

A double infusion of mint oil carries the tingliness of the mint, excellent in sore muscle rubs, lip balms, and massage oils.

Future harvest

Don't go tearing mint out of the soil; it acts as a stabilizer, protecting banks from erosion. Be gentle while harvesting this plant, and always leave enough for regrowth.

HERBAL PREPARATIONS

Tea
1 tablespoon fresh or dried leaves, stems, and flowers
1 cup water
Drink as needed.

Tincture
1 part fresh leaves, stems, and flowers
2 parts menstruum (75% alcohol, 25% alcohol)
or
1 part dried leaves, stems, and flowers
5 parts menstruum (60% alcohol, 40% distilled water)
Take 10–20 drops 3 times a day.

Oil
Infuse with fresh or dried leaves, stems, and flowers. After straining the first infusion, add more herbs and repeat the process until the oil is green and aromatic. A double infusion is usually enough.

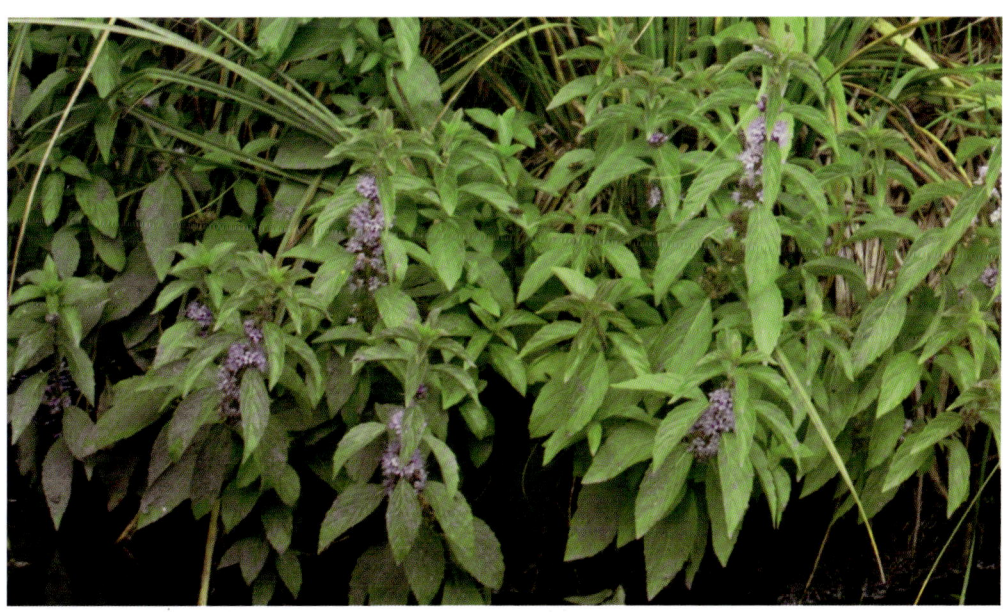

The delicate purple flowers of wild mint look just as lovely as the leaves smell.

Fragaria species

PARTS USED leaves, flowers, fruit

You'll hardly need the reminder, but do take the time to enjoy the berries while harvesting other parts of the strawberry plant. Better yet, find a way to incorporate the fruits into your medicine-making.

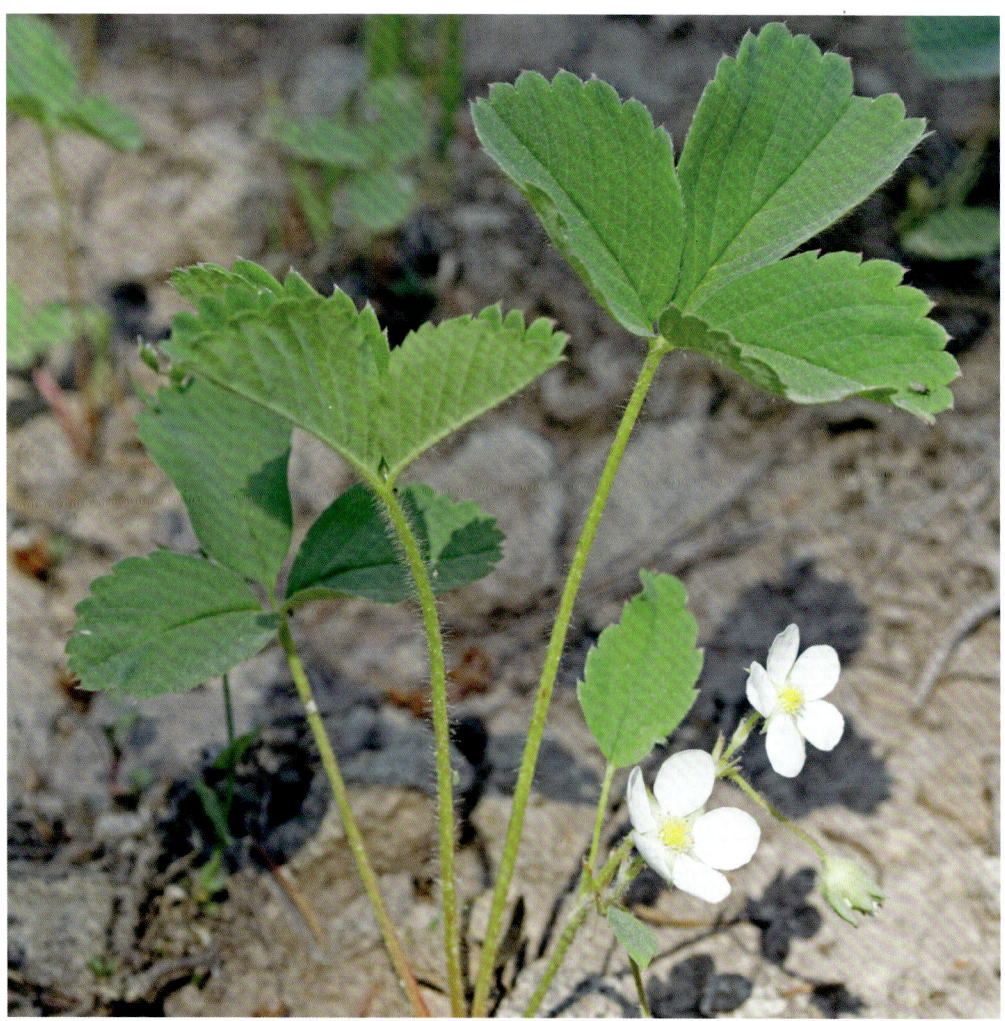

The trifoliate leaves of strawberry can be picked almost every season but winter, when they can be covered in snow.

How to identify

Wild strawberry grows horizontally, sprawling across the ground bearing white flowers and compound, three-part leaves. The leaflet edges are evenly jagged, giving them the distinctive strawberry look. Fine hairs may be present on the underside of the leaf and along the leafstalks. Five white petals make up the delicate flower that turns to fruit by midsummer. The stems of the fruits, flowers, and leaves are sometimes red, making them easy to spot. Another distinctive feature of strawberry is its reproductive use of stolons, creeping stems that root into the ground at regular intervals.

Where, when, and how to wildcraft

Strawberries dwell in meadows of varying elevations. They like moist but not wet, well-drained soil and are often surrounded by plants that won't completely crowd out sunlight. Find them near forest edges and riverbanks and along trails. Pick flowers in the spring and leaves through until fall. Berries can be gathered starting in early summer and continuing until late summer at higher elevations. They may grow bigger at lower elevations, and flavor can be dependent on habitat, but the tiny morsels at 11,000 feet are worth the scavenge.

Medicinal uses

Dry strawberry flowers and leaves for an astringing tea or sitz bath. This can be a tea used for young ones or those of any age experiencing diarrhea or stomach sensitivity. Chew up leaves for placement on gum injuries or mouth sores. The berries can be a flavorful accompaniment to tinctures, cordials, and elixirs. Dehydrated, the dried berries are a lovely addition to teas as well.

Future harvest

Harvest with care. Strawberries reproduce both by seed and by rooting from their stoloniferous spreading stems. Be sure to leave a good amount of fruit, both for the strawberries to reproduce and for the animals. To encourage next year's crop, be careful not to tread too heavily on the spreading stems.

HERBAL PREPARATIONS

Tea
Hot or cold infusion
2–3 tablespoons fresh or dried leaves, flowers, or fruit
1 cup water
Drink 1 cup 3 times a day.

Sitz bath infusion
3 ounces fresh or dried leaves and flowers
1 gallon water

Tincture
1 part fresh leaves, flowers, or fruit
3 parts menstruum (75% alcohol, 25% distilled water)
or
1 part dried leaves, flowers, or fruit
5 parts menstruum (60% alcohol, 40% distilled water)
Take 20–40 drops 3 times a day.

Oil
Infuse with fresh or dried leaves and flowers.

Salix species

PARTS USED bark, twigs, leaves

Salix *trees vary greatly, some species growing thin and small, others tall and hardy. Sample a few of your local species to find your favorites.*

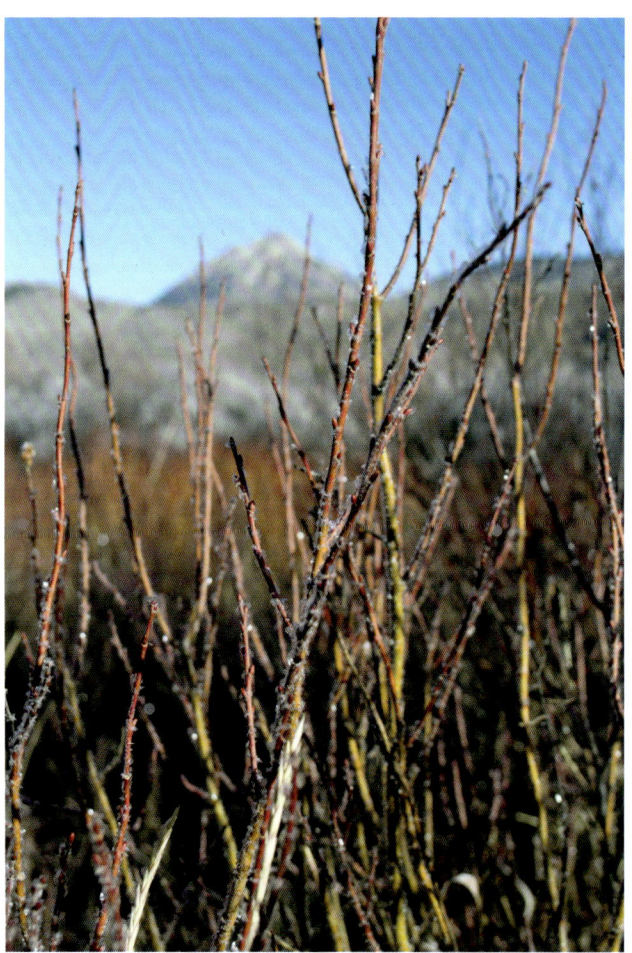

Frosted branches of willows in the fall. After they thaw a bit, trim the tips of the branches for tea or a soak to relieve pain or inflammation.

How to identify

There are so many *Salix* trees, and they can be found at any elevation. They range greatly in size. The genus includes one of the smallest "trees" or woody shrubs in the world—snow-bed willow varieties of *S. herbacea* that grow high in the alpines of eastern North America—and the countless shrubby willows you have to bushwhack through to get up or down a mountainside, and my favorite, the tall and glorious golden weeping willow *S. ×sepulcralis*. More than a few hundred *Salix* species grow throughout the world.

One major characteristic of willows is the narrow, lanceolate-ovate leaves, though some species, such as *Salix bebbiana*, are more rounded. The leaves usually have serrated margins, and all are pointed and grow alternately up thin bendy-brittle branches. The leafbuds that cling tightly to the branches in the wintertime are also a helpful indicator of species. Buds vary by species, but all have a single cap-like scale as a covering.

Willows are dioecious, meaning each plant has either all male flowers or all female flowers. The flowers consist of fluffy, upright, slightly dangling catkins.

Where, when, and how to wildcraft

Willow is one of the most common plants of the west and can be found in your neighborhood park, reviving riparian zones, and clustering on mountainsides. Harvest leaves and branches from willow trees when the sap is flowing in the spring and fall, but if the medicine is needed, you can also harvest on warm winter days or in the middle of summer. Bark can be peeled off branches or twigs and be chopped up to use fresh or for drying.

Medicinal uses

Willow is a long-standing pain reliever, revered for centuries for its powerful actions as an analgesic. Salicylic acid is perhaps the most useful constituent of willow; it acts as an anti-inflammatory and can be useful for inflammations all over the body, the gut, the bladder, or even for headaches.

The bark of willow, its twigs, or even leaves can be used in alcohol extractions, oils, sitz baths, decoctions, infusions, or vinegars. The tincture and tea of willow are drying, bitter, and astringent, which can help ease sore throats, fever and chills, or diarrhea.

The infused oil can be spread on the gums of a teething baby. Try combining it with equal parts pineapple weed for a calming pain relief. The oil can also be used as an eardrop, helping to dull the pain of a throbbing infection or virus. Mix it into warming oil with garlic, mullein flowers, and beebalm flowers or leaves.

The oil can be used for salves or massage oils that relieve sore or injured body parts.

Willow leaves can be used fresh for bug-bite poultices or chewed for relief of mouth pain.

⚠ Caution

If you are taking blood thinners, you should check first with your doctor before using willow, which has salicin in it. While willow does contain salicylic acid, it is not the same as aspirin and is therefore not an appropriate replacement.

Future harvest

Fresh willow branches can be picked from the grown tree and planted. They are incredibly vivacious and will happily root and grow where there is water or soil.

HERBAL PREPARATIONS

Tea
Decoction
1-3 ounces fresh or dried bark and twigs
1 quart water
Drink 1 cup 3 times a day. These proportions are also good for a sitz bath.

Tincture
1 part fresh bark and twigs
2 parts menstruum (75% alcohol, 25% distilled water)
or
1 part dried bark and twigs
5 parts menstruum (60% alcohol, 40% distilled water)
Take 20–40 drops 3 times a day.

Oil
Infuse with fresh or dried leaves, bark, or twigs.

willowherb

Epilobium species

PARTS USED leaves, flowers

Infused into oil, willowherb makes an antioxidant-rich face serum.

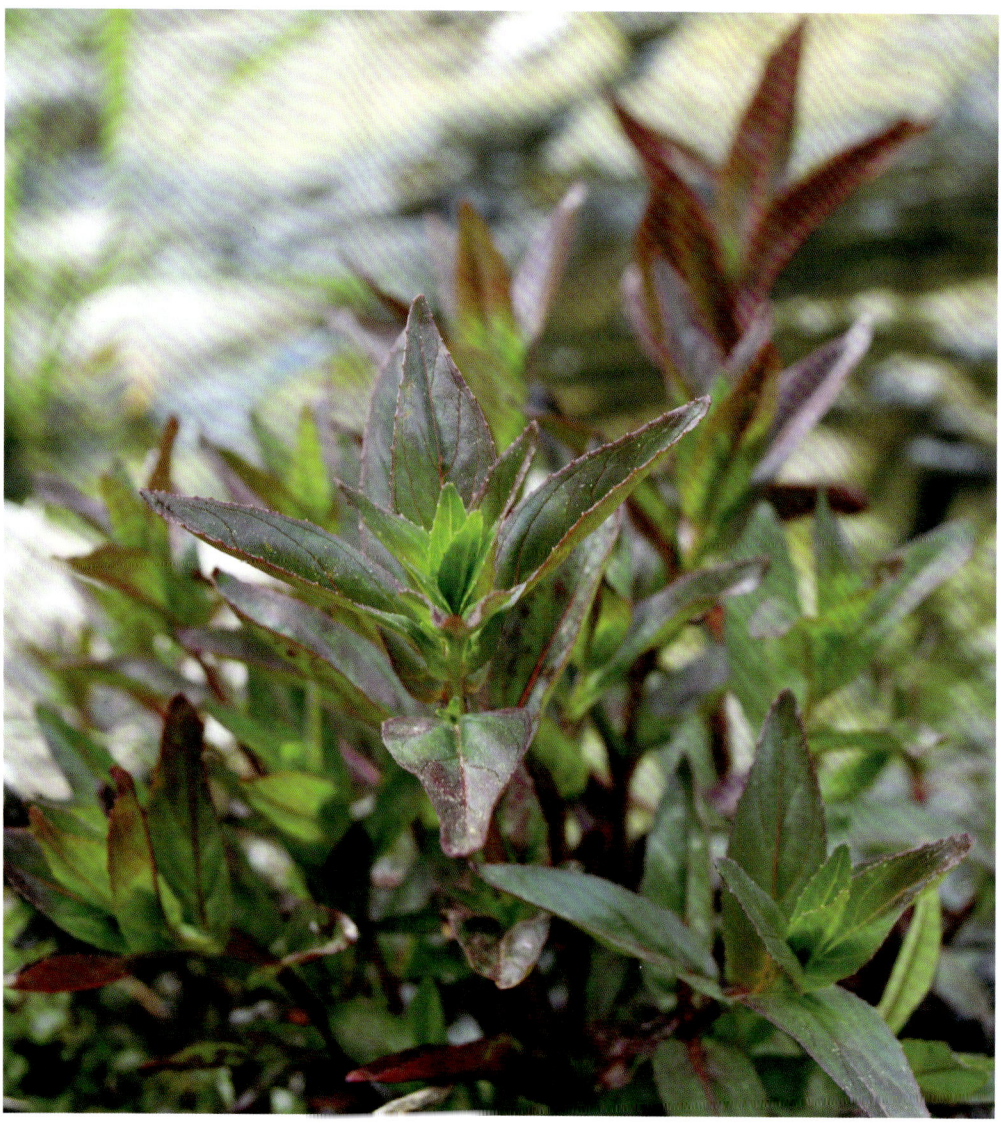

The young green and red leaves of willowherb growing along a creekside in late spring.

How to identify

Willowherb is closely related to our tall and radiant fireweed (*Chamerion* species). Its green leaves are tinged with red and grow oppositely along the slightly squared reddish-colored stem. Depending on the species, leaves are ovate to lanceolate in shape, and flowers are white, pink, or bluish purple in color and have four heart-shaped petals. The seedpods are elongated and filled with many tiny seeds that are attached to a plumed pappus, which helps them disperse by wind once the pods open.

Where, when, and how to wildcraft

Willowherb can be found in moist environments or near creeksides. Harvest in late spring when the leaves are a reddish green, or wait until the flowers have bloomed in the summer. Clip the top 6 inches of the plant, to get plenty of leaves and flowers in your harvest bundle. Take home to wilt or dry completely before making an infused oil. Fresh herb is best for tinctures.

Medicinal uses

Willowherb is very similar to fireweed in its medicinal actions. It has an affinity for helping lower inflammations of the pelvic region. As a tea or tincture, it can be beneficial for complaints of the gastrointestinal tract, from gut imbalances to acting as a mild laxative during a bout of constipation.

The freshly wilted plant makes an exquisite oil infusion for face serums. The plant is high in antioxidants and provides excellent nourishment for the skin. Blend with other herbs that treat the skin well, such as violet and elderflowers.

Future harvest

Clipping only the flowering tops or leaves from willowherb should not pose a threat to its survival and well-being in the wild.

HERBAL PREPARATIONS

Tea
Hot infusion
2 tablespoons fresh or dried leaves and
  flowers
1 cup water
Drink 1 cup 3 times a day.

Tincture
1 part freshly cut leaves and flowers
3 parts menstruum (75% alcohol, 25%
  distilled water)
or
1 part dried leaves and flowers
5 parts menstruum (60% alcohol, 40%
  distilled water)
Take 20–40 drops 3 times a day.

Oil
*Infuse with freshly wilted or dried leaves
and flowers.*

Artemisia absinthium
absinthe
PARTS USED leaves, flowers, stems

That's right. The infamous green drink called absinthe is made from this plant.

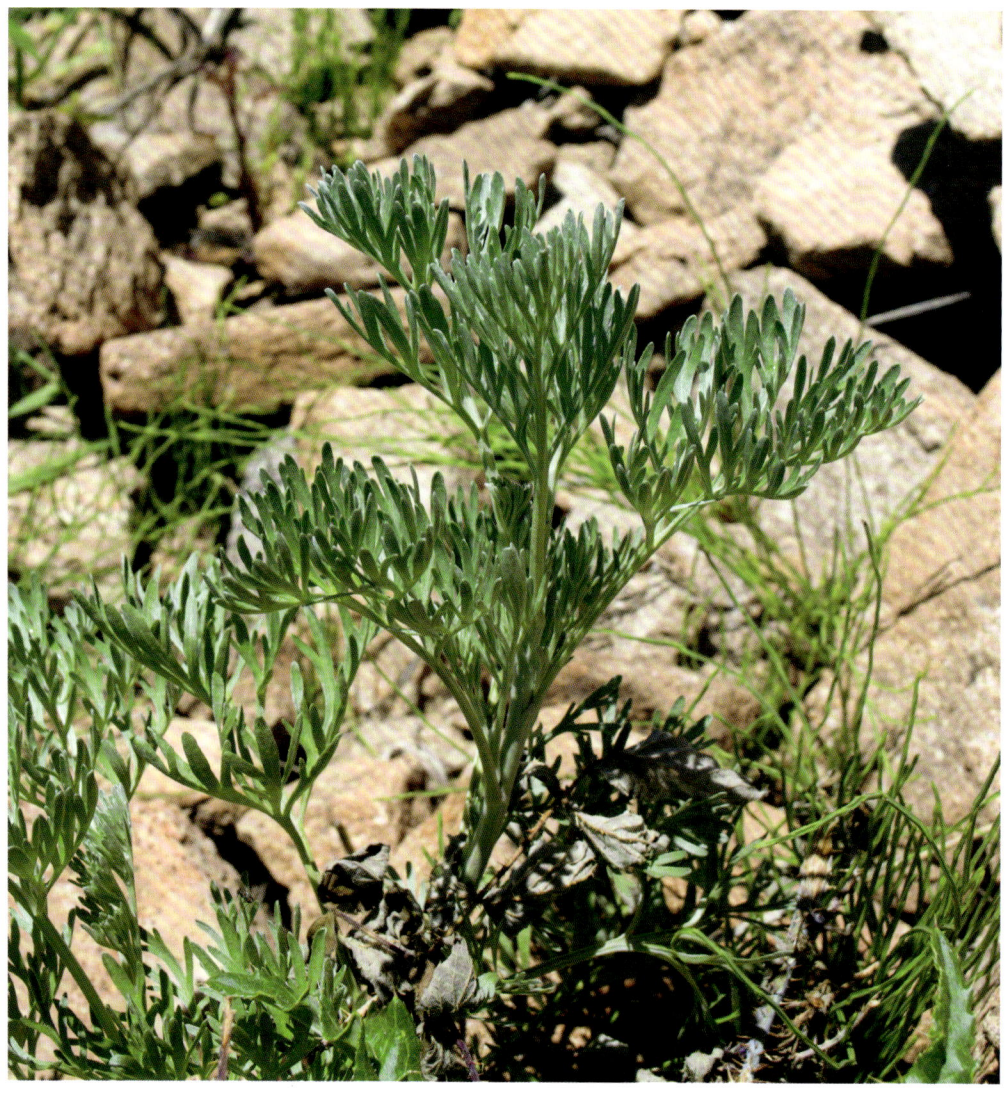

Take a leaf, crush it, and deeply inhale the aromatics of absinthe.

How to identify

Artemisia absinthium is a perennial that dies back each year. It has dark green leaves that have a teal to grayish silver color due to the fine hairs that cover the plant. Leaves are dissected several times and are divided into highly lobed leaflets, reaching a span of 2–5 inches. Flowers are small, yellow, inconspicuous, hanging buttons that grow in a spike-like inflorescence.

Where, when, and how to wildcraft

Discover wormwood growing as an invading artemisia, finding space on dry hillsides, in yards in mountain towns, and in poor, disturbed soils.

Tincture of the fresh leaves, stems, and flowers is strongest and harbors the most medicine. After the herb is dried, the most potent parts are the leaves and flowers. I crush these off the stem to use.

Medicinal uses

Wormwood tincture is something I don't travel without— it's the worst facing a stomach bug or parasite without it. It

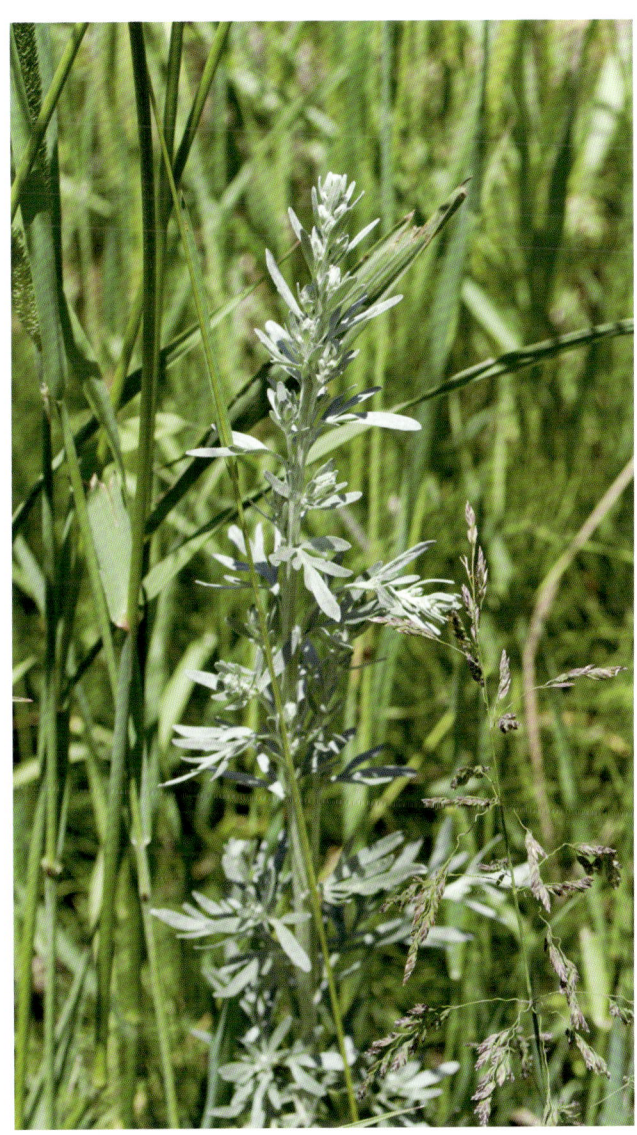

Wait for the stalks to grow tall to make it easier to gather bundles of wormwood.

has properties that will kill parasites or calm a rotten stomach. When the stomach viruses are going around and seem really contagious, this is also the bitter herb I reach for. It is extremely bitter and is needed only in doses as small as 3–10 drops. I like to put a few drops in my water bottle each day while visiting countries where the water is not reliable.

It combines well with black walnut, Oregon grape, and chaparral—topically as a soak, liniment, or oil for fungal or bacterial skin infections, and internally for intestinal dysbiosis and parasitic infection. This combination is especially helpful to combat athlete's foot, as this ailment is usually best addressed internally as well. Internally, take wormwood, black walnut, Oregon grape, and chaparral in combination with or without each other, depending on what you can harvest.

Tincture is the preferred format for consumption of wormwood. I would not like to take down a strong cup of tea, but a cold infusion is certainly much nicer than hot.

 ## Caution

Wormwood is not an herb to take for extended periods of time and should be taken in smaller doses, such as 3–20 drops 1–3 times a day for no longer than 6 weeks. This herb, especially when combined with other herbs such as black walnut, can be harsh on the gastrointestinal tract. Use in small doses unless consulting with an herbalist or other healthcare practitioner.

Future harvest

Watch where you harvest, as this plant can be targeted for spraying as a noxious weed.

HERBAL PREPARATIONS

Tea
Cold infusion
1 tablespoon fresh or dried leaves, stems, and flowers
1 cup water
Sip as needed.

Tincture
1 part fresh leaves, stems, and flowers
2 parts menstruum (75% alcohol, 25% distilled water)
or
1 part dried leaves and flowers
5 parts menstruum (60% alcohol, 40% distilled water)
Take 3–20 drops 1–3 times a day.

Oil
Infuse with fresh or dried leaves, stems, and flowers.

yarrow

Achillea millefolium

PARTS USED leaves, stems, flowers

A first-aid must, yarrow has a versatility that can help those wounded or sick while traveling in the woods.

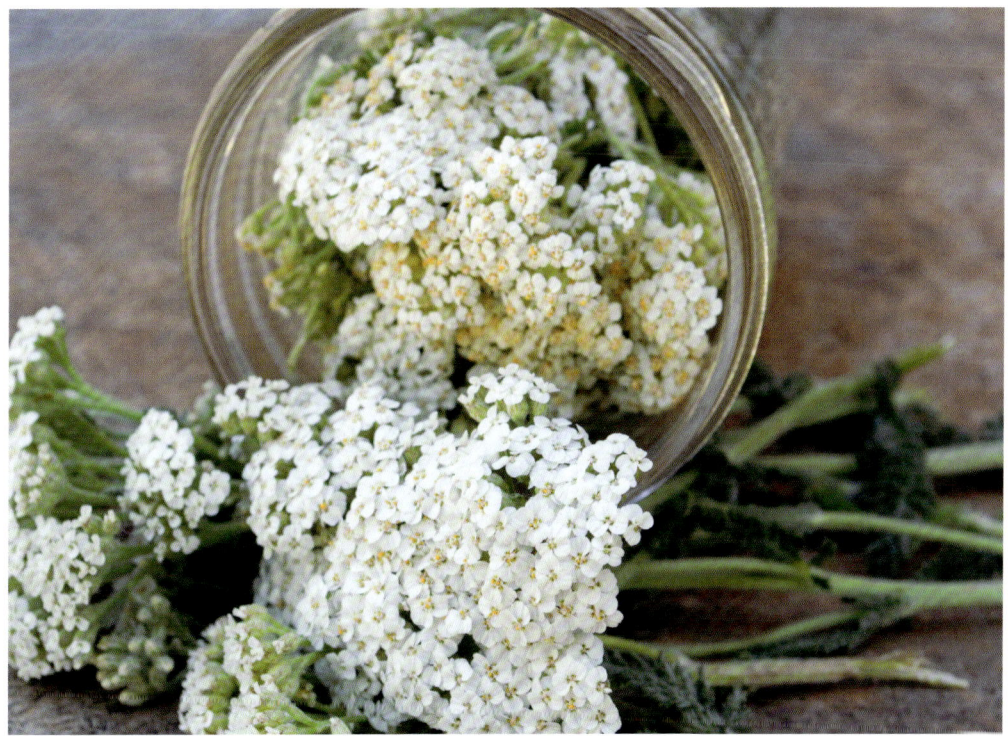
Gather flowering yarrow while fresh for tincture-making.

How to identify

Yarrow is a native perennial averaging heights of 1–3 feet. Plants can have one to several stems that arise from long, finely dissected basal leaves. Some stems may themselves be branched, and the leaves along the stem are small and especially feathery. Both basal and stem leaves are distinctly aromatic when crushed. Flowers form clusters that appear to be in an umbel; however, upon closer inspection you will find several separate flower clusters in heads which form a flat-topped corymb.

Where, when, and how to wildcraft

You can find yarrow almost anywhere in the mountain west. Gather leaves as you need them from spring through fall. Stems and flowers are best gathered while the flowers are at their most fragrant, in the heat of midsummer.

Gather leaves by plucking a few from each plant. If you have collected the whole stalk to use along with the flowers, first strip the stem of leaves, then finely chop it up, leaving the flowers still attached.

Medicinal uses

Yarrow is one of my top herbs, for almost everything. It has a gentle warmth that can help to soften and stimulate from the inside out. Dried yarrow is nice as a bath soak, respiratory steam, sitz bath, and tea. As infused oil it is warming to the skin and deeper. I often use it in massage oil—my

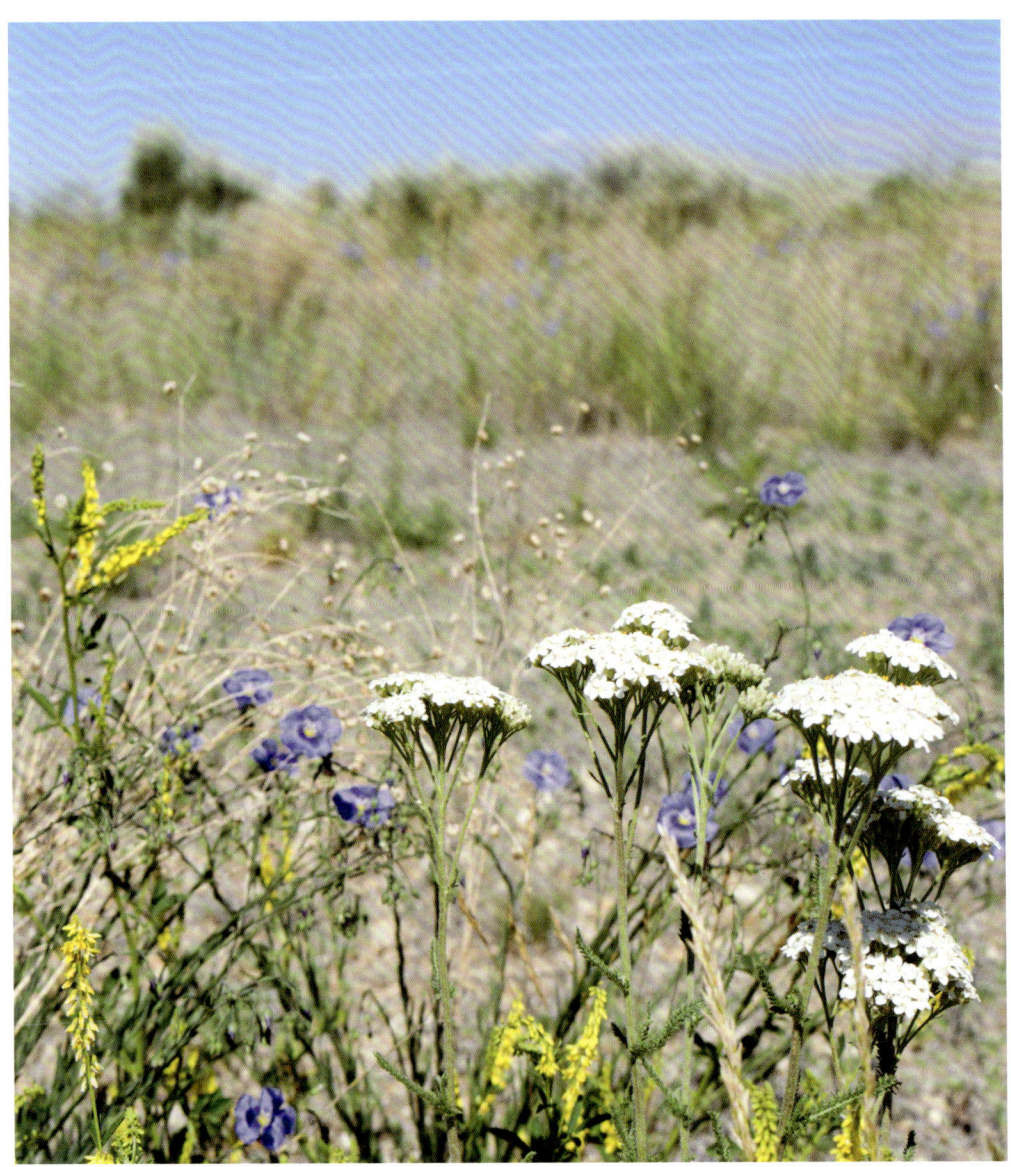

Aromatic hillsides of sagebrush, yarrow, and sweet clover offer a lofty whiff to passersby.

Wound Soak

Making a soak for external wounds can be like washing the extremities with tea. Soaks can be beneficial for dog bites, road rash, insect bites, or cuts and scrapes. The herbs used should be those that help to promote healing of the tissue while keeping it disinfected. Yarrow, plantain, and grindelia are a few of my favorites for this. Use the bark or twigs of aspen, cottonwood, or oak for their pain-relieving qualities.

Fill a pot with water, adding 1 ounce of herbs per quart of water. If using barks, decoct them first, throwing in leaves and flowers after removing the pot from the heat. Allow to steep for 15 minutes, while the water cools.

Soak a washcloth in the infusion if it is for a wound that cannot be submerged. For limbs that can be held in the water, do so for at least 10 minutes.

favorite blend is yarrow, arnica, and sweet clover, infused together in safflower oil. The smell is marvelous.

Stimulating circulation, yarrow helps with blood stagnation, blood blisters, old bruises that have hardened, or to decongest a stagnant and inflamed area. Oils, salves, and soaks are good for when there is bruising, hematomas, and trauma from an injury. Yarrow is useful in people with arthritis, gout, and rheumatism. It can be used on bug bites, stings, and itchy skin conditions.

The oil can be applied to children when they are feverish and chilled. It helps to warm them up while bringing stimulation to the sluggish sick body. The warmth acts as a diaphoretic, guiding the fever to a place that helps to better fight the infection, aiding in breaking it into a sweat. For feverish adults, yarrow makes a gentle, warming tea that will push the heat of the body out to the peripheries, so that the body can start to cool itself down.

Tincture or tea of yarrow can be beneficial for menses that are stagnant or need thinning out. A blend of yarrow, a demulcent herb (such as Siberian elm or mallow root), and rose can help stop the recurrent nosebleeds that come from too dry a climate or constitution.

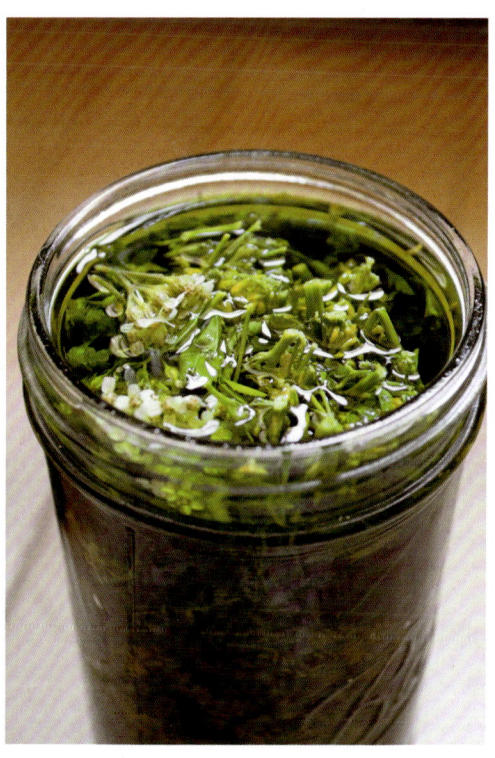

An alcohol-based tincture of yarrow after it has been left to macerate for weeks.

Chewing up the leaves for a spit poultice can help stop bleeding while in the backcountry. You can also mash the leaves between your fingers to activate the juices for coagulation without the saliva.

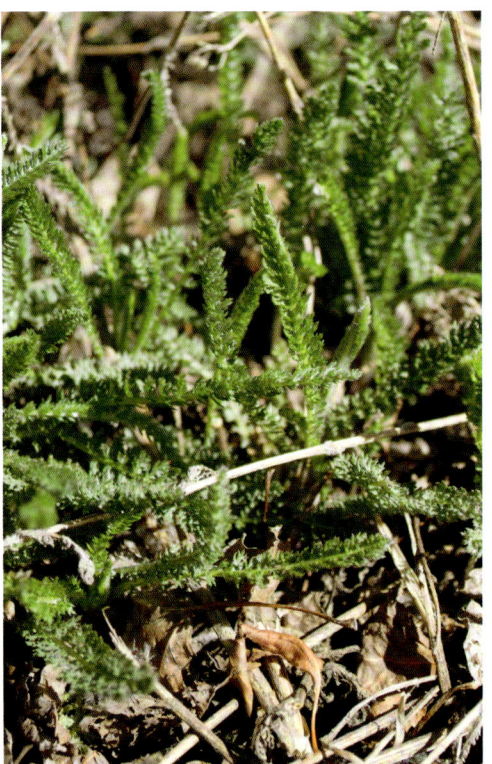

Many times you will be walking all over yarrow in the woods without even knowing it. These little feathery leaves can be picked for drying or to use fresh in a poultice.

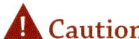 **Caution**

Yarrow is in the Asteraceae, and some people may have allergic reactions to this plant family. What's more, yarrow is often confused with water hemlock (*Cicuta* species) and poison hemlock (*Conium maculatum*) because its white-flowered corymb resembles an umbel. Be positive of your identification.

Future harvest

Yarrow is widespread throughout the mountain west. Always leave some flowerheads behind, and never strip a plant of all its leaves.

HERBAL PREPARATIONS

Tea
Hot infusion
2–3 tablespoons fresh or dried leaves, flowers, and stems
1 cup water
Drink 3 times a day.

Tincture
1 part fresh leaves, flowers, and stems
2 parts menstruum (75% alcohol, 25% distilled water)
or
1 part dried leaves, flowers, and stems
5 parts menstruum (60% alcohol, 40% distilled water)
Take 10–20 drops 3–5 times a day.

Oil
Infuse with fresh or dried leaves, flowers, and stems.

yerba mansa

Anemopsis californica
lizard tail
PARTS USED roots, leaves

*The warm and spicy root can help fight lung infections
while soothing the mucous membranes.*

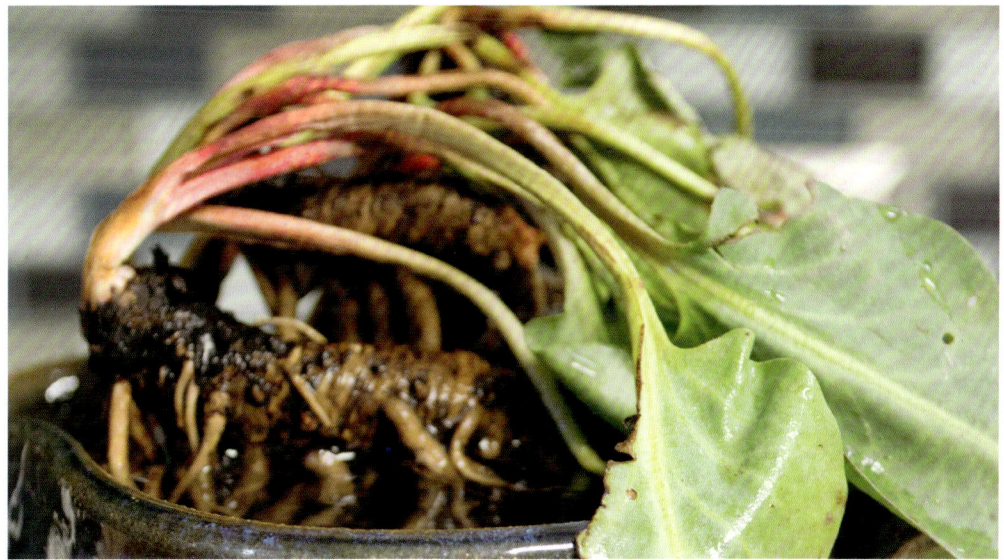

Yerba mansa is a water-loving plant that has been affected by humans changing the course of waterways, flooding out or drying up its habitat.

How to identify

Yerba mansa has one of the most gorgeously unique flowers with large white bracts posing as petals and a tall dense flowering spike that is made of many tiny white flowers. The leaves are basal and have a rounded arrow shape. They are green with thick, red-tinged petioles and are almost succulent or leathery feeling. Leaves turn a deep red in autumn.

Find yerba mansa growing as a perennial herb in stands and revitalizing certain riparian zones. The main rhizome has many thick fleshy rootlets. The interior of the root is orange.

Where, when, and how to wildcraft

The roots of yerba mansa can be harvested in the spring and fall, or in the middle of summer if that is when you can make it to the middle elevations of southern Nevada and southwestern Utah. It loves to inhabit continually wet, swampy areas. Leaves can be harvested throughout the spring until fall.

The roots propagate really well, and you

can also take fresh roots home to grow in a pot that stays damp. This way you can have your own harvest of yerba mansa either in a greenhouse or yard. I have a friend who grows this herb at 10,000 feet in a greenhouse, where it thrives!

When you harvest the roots, carefully dig around the base of a mature plant until you come upon the main root with runners that go deeper into the soil. Cut off the root between the mature plant and a sprout that is growing further along the root, taking a section as your medicine. Then, leaving at least a few inches of root attached to the sprout, replant it. This method allows you to harvest from one plant without taking too much life force, while simultaneously propagating another and helping increase the population.

Medicinal uses

Yerba mansa is a warming, drying, spicy, and aromatic root, providing circulation and stimulation. It has both anti-inflammatory and antimicrobial properties, which make it useful for both internal and topical infections.

Sinus and respiratory infections can be greatly relieved by yerba mansa, as it provides a warming circulatory flow that can help to expectorate coughs and move out congestion through toning and restoring mucous membranes.

The fresh root can be chewed on for a sore throat or lung infection when a viral infection is present. It will help to warm the body's temperature, acting as a diaphoretic. It can also be taken internally as a tincture or tea for a similar effect.

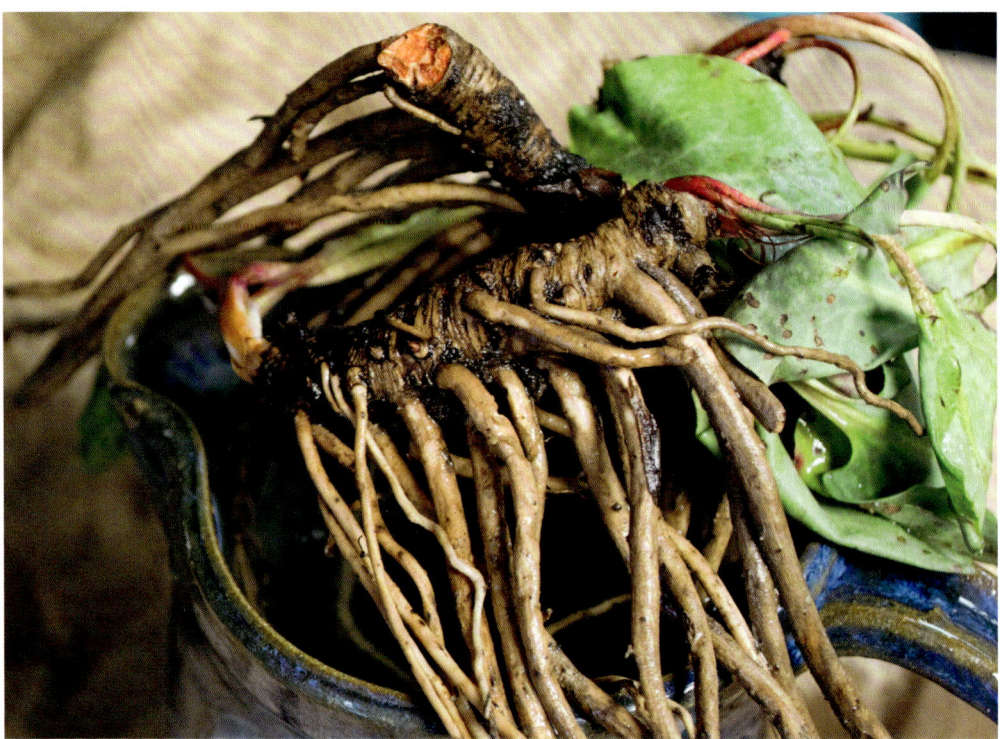

The inside of the yerba mansa root is orange, and it has long rootlets for reaching deep into the soils of the wetlands.

Chest Rub Oil

Chest rubs are a great way to help soothe the sick and tired. Herbs infused in oils penetrate the skin to help expectorate and settle coughs. They can also warm the body, support the flow of the lymphatic system, and soothe aches and pains. Some suggested herbs are cottonwood, conifer resin, yarrow, hops, alder, yerba mansa, and grindelia.

Apply oil as needed to the chest, back, and neck to help move a cold or respiratory infection out of the chest. You may also consider rubbing the oil on before or after a hot shower or steam bath. Dress in layers, preferably wool, to help the oil stay warm and absorb into the skin.

Yerba mansa smells amazing and is a lovely warming oil to apply to people who are sore and achy from a fever. It also blends well in a chest rub oil to help soothe and expectorate coughs; it can be applied to the front of the chest, back, and neck for this purpose. The infused oil can be used in salves for healing wounds. Oils can be made with the leaves and roots. Poultices can also be made of the leaves to place on sore or inflamed muscles.

Use yerba mansa in musculoskeletal issues where pain and inflammation are present. Combine it with antispasmodic herbs like hops, connective tissue healing herbs like *Maianthemum* species, or structural supporting herbs like mullein. Administer as an internal tincture or external liniment.

Future harvest

Yerba mansa's population can be greatly increased by human care and interaction. Take only a section of root and replant the remaining sprout.

HERBAL PREPARATIONS

Tea
Hot infusion
1 tablespoon fresh or dried chopped root or leaves
1 cup water
Decoction
1 ounce fresh or dried chopped root
1 quart water
Drink as needed.

Tincture
1 part fresh root and leaves
2 parts menstruum (80% alcohol, 20% distilled water)
or
1 part dried root
5 parts menstruum (70% alcohol, 30% distilled water)
Take 30–60 drops 3 times a day

Oil
Infuse with fresh or dried root and leaves.

yucca

Yucca species

PARTS USED roots, leaves

If you ever wanted a way to wash your hair in a river with the use of only a plant, then yucca root is your golden ticket.

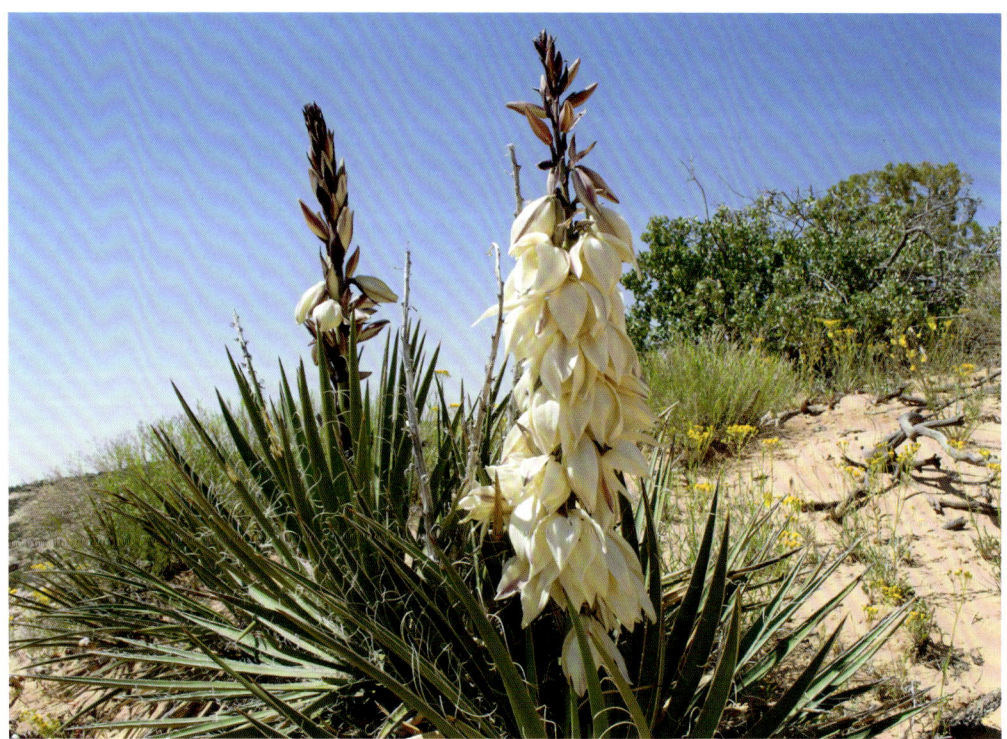

Flowers of yucca can be a nice nibble while out harvesting in sagebrush country, though keep it to only a few. After more than one or two, I have found them to be mildly irritating to the mucous membranes.

How to identify

Not many plants in the mountain west look anything like yucca. They are a distinct evergreen presence year-round—their tall brown flowerstalk and long green spine-tipped leaves can even protrude through the snow. Each plant usually has only one flowerstalk, and the rosette of leaves pokes out around its base. Leaves are stiff and sword-like, with fraying fibers along the edges. Flowers are bell-shaped and creamy white, with tints of purple or green. The oval seedpods are green or cream-colored.

Some of our common varieties of yucca are soapweed yucca (*Yucca glauca*), Spanish bayonet (*Y. harrimaniae*), and banana yucca

(*Y. baccata*). Narrow-leafed yucca (*Y. angustissima*) is also quite common on the Front Range of Colorado.

Where, when, and how to wildcraft

This plant can be found throughout the lower and middle elevations of the mountain west, usually below 8500 feet. It prefers the harsh climates of the desert, lack of water, and long, cold winters, growing among junipers, piñons, and ponderosas. The root can be harvested in the spring or fall. Be seriously careful, as the spiny leaves can puncture you and hurt like heck. Consider wearing eye-protection, such as sunglasses or snowboard goggles. Those poky leaves can be used to make twine or be spun into rope. This can be handy when bundling herbs.

Medicinal uses

Yucca is a moistening and cooling herb that can be used to relieve arthritis and inflammation in the musculoskeletal system. It has a mild analgesic effect, so it can be used in liniments for pain-relieving formulas. Internally, it is usually taken as a tincture.

The root of yucca has been used for its saponins to make soaps, detergents, or hair rinses. Those same saponins mean that yucca can be used as a moderate laxative as well as a mild emetic.

⚠ Caution

Too much tincture can result in a laxative effect. If this happens, decrease the amount. Do not confuse our native *Yucca* species with that of the edible yuca, or cassava root, found in some grocery stores. Definitely not the same plant!

Future harvest

Yucca grows prolifically in the west, but still, please, harvest with caution and care.

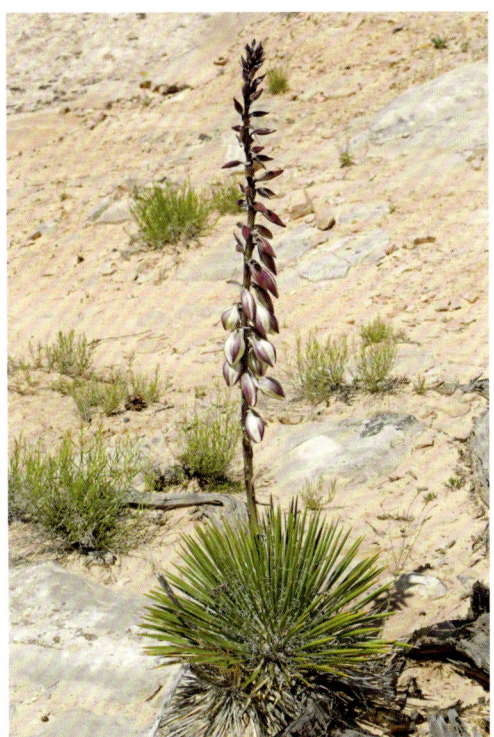

The sharp-pointed leaves of yucca can be stripped into thin, long pieces and spun together to make a strong cordage. This can be a nice rope for bundling herbs.

HERBAL PREPARATIONS

Hair Rinse
1–3 tablespoons fresh root
1 cup hot water
Combine in a jar and shake until suds appear.
Use as a shampooing rinse.

Tincture
1 part fresh root
2 parts menstruum (75% alcohol, 25% distilled water)
or
1 part dried root
5 parts menstruum (60% alcohol, 40% distilled water)
Take 10–20 drops 3 times a day.

METRIC CONVERSIONS

INCHES	CENTIMETERS		FEET	METERS
¼	0.6		1	0.3
⅜	1.0		2	0.6
½	1.3		3	0.9
¾	1.9		4	1.2
1	2.5		5	1.5
2	5.1		6	1.8
3	7.6		7	2.1
4	10.0		8	2.4
5	12.7		9	2.7
6	15.2		10	3
7	17.8			
8	20.3			
9	22.9			
10	25.4			

TO CONVERT LENGTH:	MULTIPLY BY
Yards to meters	0.90
Inches to centimeters	2.54
Inches to millimeters	25.40
Feet to centimeters	30.50

TEMPERATURES

Degrees Celsius = 5/9 × (degrees Fahrenheit − 32)

Degrees Fahrenheit = (9/5 × degrees Celsius) + 32

USEFUL RESOURCES

Wild medicine-making is a hands-on educational journey that requires the right resources. My guidance and inspiration have come from botanical teachers, field guides, plant keys, and herbalists across the country. Attending herbalism conferences and creating connections with other herbalists have been especially influential. My knowledge of herbal medicine has come from direct interaction with the plants that live near and far from my home in the central Colorado Rockies. Here is a list of references I have used in the past, resources I suggest you check out, and plant guides to help you in your identifications.

Medicinal plant references, resources, and guides for identification

Coffman, Sam. *The Herbal Medic*. San Antonio, TX: Herbal Medics, 2014.

Darrow, Katherine. *Wild About Wildflowers*. Glendale, AZ: WildKat Publishing Co., 2006.

Easley, Thomas, and Steven Horne. *Modern Herbal Medicine*. St. George, UT: The School of Modern Herbal Medicine, 2014.

———. *The Modern Herbal Dispensatory*. Berkeley, CA: North Atlantic Books, 2016.

Elpel, Thomas. *Botany in a Day: The Patterns Method of Plant Identification*. Pony, MT: HOPS Press, 1996.

Green, James. *The Herbal Medicine-Makers Handbook*. Berkeley, CA: The Crossing Press, 2000.

Hoffman, David. *Holistic Herbal*. Hammersmith, London: Thorsons, 2002.

Kane, Charles W. *Herbal Medicine of the American Southwest*. Lincoln Town Press, 2006.

———. *Herbal Medicine Trends and Traditions*. Lincoln Town Press, 2009.

Kershaw, Linda. *Edible and Medicinal Plants of the Rockies*. Auburn, WA: Lone Pine Publishing, 2000.

Kershner, Bruce. *National Wildlife Federation Field Guide to Trees of North America*. New York: Sterling Publishing, 2008.

Lesica, Peter. *Manual of Montana Vascular Plants*. Fort Worth, TX: Brit Press, 2012.

Martin, Corinne. *Herbal Remedies From the Wild*. Woodstock, VT: Countryman Press, 2000.

Moore, Michael. *Medicinal Plants of the Desert and Canyon West*. Sante Fe, NM: Museum of New Mexico Press, 1989.

———. *Medicinal Plants of the Mountain West*. Santa Fe, NM: Museum of New Mexico Press, 2003.

Schofield, Janice. *Discovering Wild Plants: Alaska, Western Canada, the Northwest*. Bothell, WA: Alaska Northwest Books, 1989.

Tierra, Michael. *The Way of Herbs*. New York, NY: Pocket Books, 1998.

Tilford, Gregory L. *Edible and Medicinal Plants of the West*. Missoula, MT: Mountain Press Publishing Company, 1997.

———. *From Earth to Herbalist*. Missoula, MT: Mountain Press Publishing Company, 1998.

Tilgner, Dr. Sharol Marie. *Herbal Medicine From the Heart of the Earth*. Pleasant Hill, OR: Wise Acres LLC, 2009.

Weber, William, and Ronald Wittmann. *Colorado Flora: Western Slope*. Boulder: University Press of Colorado, 2001.

Wiles, Briana. *Mountain States Foraging*. Portland, OR: Timber Press, 2016.

Williamson, Darcy. *Healing Plants of the Rocky Mountains*. McCall, ID: From the Forest, 2002.

Plant identification and location websites

bonap.org

plants.usda.gov

ACKNOWLEDGMENTS

To my family, who stuck with me through two books in three years, thank you for all your continual and unconditional support. Thank you to my mom, dad, brother, and sister, for the gift of life and for always putting up with my quirky passions. I am so grateful for my husband, Briant, who encourages me to chase my dreams. And to my son, Salix, and dog, Bella, who always bring more adventure to every wildcrafting trip—thank you for every ounce of patience.

To all my community tribal members, employees of Rooted Apothecary, and students—without my village helping to raise my child and grow a new store, this book would not have been possible. Special thanks to my photographer guru of a best friend, Kimbre Woods, for your help in every nook and cranny of my books.

I cannot begin to thank enough my number-one botanist, wild plant expert, teacher, and dear friend, Kat Mackinnon. Thank you for the countless hours we spent combing over this manuscript and making sure it was suitable for the world.

A muddled mess of teachers have inspired

and encouraged me to walk the path I follow. Without you all, I would have no idea how the plants speak, seek, and want their story to be told. Immense gratitude to jim mcdonald, Lisa Rose, Kiva Rose Bell-Hardin and Wolf Hardin, Lisa Ganora, Sean Donahue, Rebecca Altman, Holly Torgerson, Amanda Klenner-Labrow, Guido Mase, Paul Bergner, Tania Neubauer, Shelley Torgove, Sevensong, Howie Brounstein, Matthew Wood, Leslita Williams, Thomas Easley, Michael Cottingham, Peter May, and every teacher I am missing but took a class from. Each of you has taught me something that is present in this book through your findings and experiences as humans and herbalists.

Thank you to the team at Timber Press for all your hard work and dedication. And finally, thank you to all my friends and family who contributed to the photography in this book: Kimbre Woods, David Allen, Kiva Rose Bell-Hardin, Katy Able, Lisa Rose, Max Licher, John Slattery, and Briant Wiles.

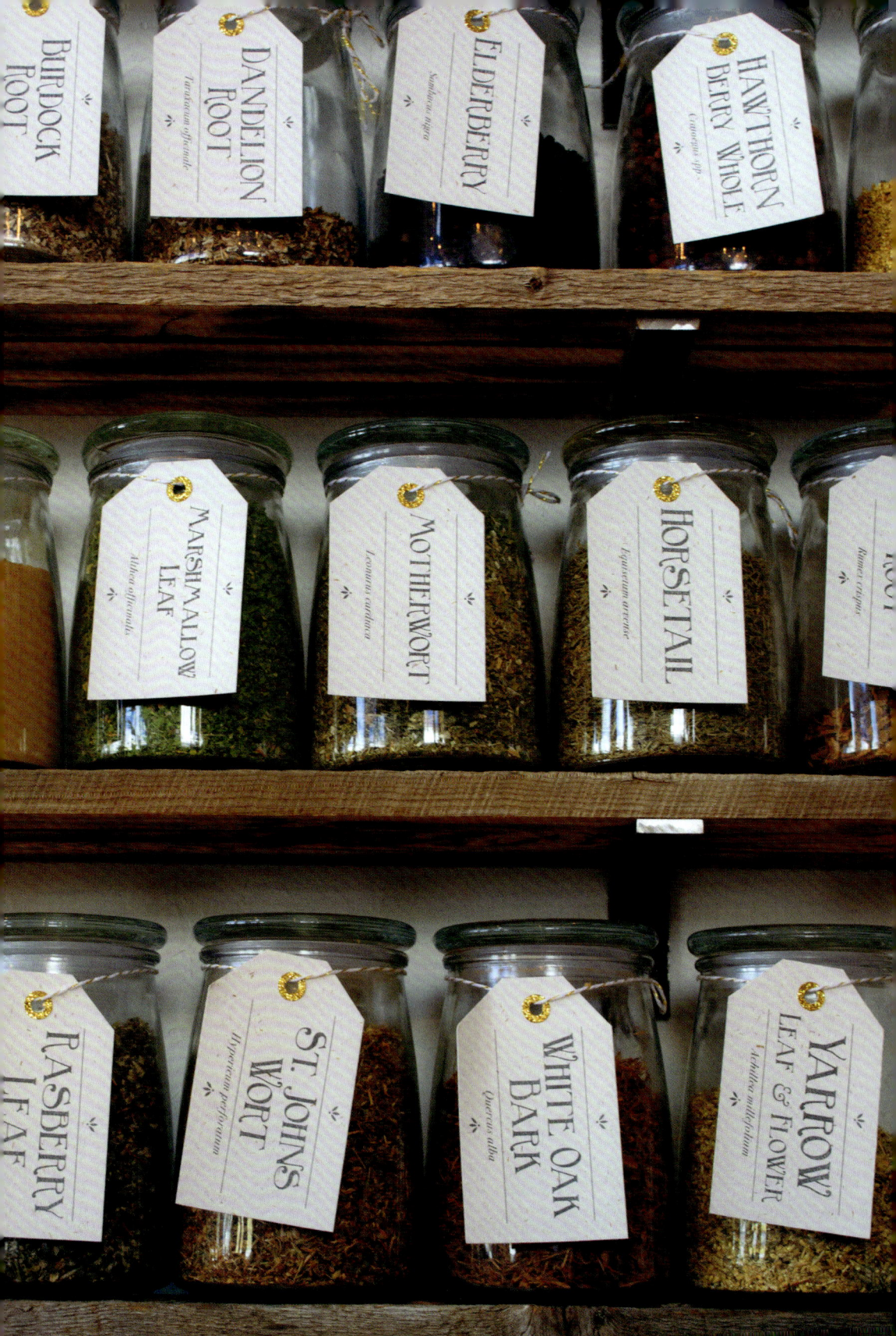

PHOTO CREDITS

Sarah Milhollin, pages 3, 5, 6, and 7.

Kimbre Woods, pages 8, 15 (bottom), 32, 60, 69 (top), 93, 109, 149 (right), 190, 218, 237 (top), and 244.

Lisa Rose, pages 14 (bottom) and 136.

David Allen, pages 15 (top), 67, and 243.

Max Licher, pages 16 (top), 84, 104, and 221 (left).

Katy Able, page 13.

John Slattery, pages 102, 193, 199, 209, and 210.

Kiva Rose Bell-Hardin, page 154.

Briant Wiles, pages 278 and 279.

All other photos were taken by the author.

INDEX

tobacco cessation, 152
tobacco root, 236
toenail fungus, 109, 151
tonics, 43, 148, 179, 228, 229, 248
tools and supplies for wildcrafting, 18
Toxicodendron species, 17
Toxicoscordion venenosum, 15
trembling aspen, 57
Trifolium pratense, 182
tumble mustard leaf shape, 20
twisted stalk, 20, 208
two-needle piñon, 167

U

ulcers. *See* mouth ulcers and sores; stomach ulcers
Ulmus pumila, 197
Ulmus rubra, 197
urinary tract, 71, 124, 135, 202, 234
Urtica dioica, 26, 217
usnea, 31, 33, 35, 37, 38, 232–233
Utah juniper, 127
uterus, 103, 137, 181, 216
uva-ursi, 31, 33, 35, 37, 234–235

V

Vaccinium species, 70
valerian, 31, 32, 35, 37, 236–238
Valeriana acutiloba, 236
Valeriana arizonica, 236
Valeriana dioica, 236
Valeriana edulis, 236
Valeriana occidentalis, 236
Valeriana sitchensis, 236
vanilla grass, 225
Veratrum species, 17
Verbascum thapsus, 140, 142
Verbena bracteata, 241, 242
Verbena hastata, 241
Verbena macdougalii, 241
Verbena stricta, 241
verdolagas, 177
veronica, 31, 33, 35, 239–240
Veronica americana, 240
vervain, 35, 37, 241–242
vinegar extractions, 25, 26
Viola adunca, 243
Viola canadensis, 243
Viola nuttallii, 243

Viola orbiculata, 243
violet, 31, 33, 35, 243–244
viruses, 100, 152, 181, 210, 270, 276
vitamins, 143–144, 163, 189, 212, 218, 220, 240
vomiting, 152, 242

W

warming herbs
  cough remedies, 169
  fever support, 62, 103, 163
  illnesses, 87–88, 98, 141, 148, 151, 163, 276–277
  infusions, 191–192
  injuries, 55–56, 272–273
  lung conditions, 210
water hemlock, 14, 48, 49–51, 160, 229, 249, 274
weeds, wildcrafting of, 18
western dock, 95
western mugwort, 102
wetlands harvest guide, 31, 33, 35, 37, 38
whitebark pine, 161
white fir, 104, 105
white sagebrush, 102
whorled leaf shape, 20, 83
whortleberry, 70
wild apple, 52
wild asparagus, 31, 33, 37, 245–246
wild bergamot, 62
wild caraway, 32, 34, 35, 37, 247–249
wild celery, 48
wild chamomile, 165
wild cherry, 31, 33, 35, 37, 38, 250–252
wildcrafting, 11–27
  making herbal preparations, 22–27
  permissions for, 13, 18
  respect for plants, 12–13
  seasonal harvest guides, 29–38
  tools and garb for, 18
wild geranium, 91
wild hops, 35, 253–255
wild lettuce, 31, 32, 35, 37, 256–257
wild licorice, 20, 31, 32, 37, 258–259

wild mint, 31, 33, 35, 260–261
wild raspberry, 179
wild sarsaparilla, 209
wild strawberry, 31, 33, 35, 37, 262–263
willow, 30, 31, 33, 37, 38, 264–265
willowherb, 31, 33, 35, 106, 240, 266–267
winnowing, 19
winter harvest guide, 37–38
witch hazel, 115
women
  hot flashes, 200
  menstruation, 50, 103, 137, 192, 237, 273
  nursing mothers, 42, 67, 77
  pelvic health, 181, 216
  pregnancy, 181, 218–219. *See also* Cautions *in plant profiles*
  reproductive tonics, 245–246
woodlands harvest guide, 31, 33, 35, 37, 38
woolly plantain, 171
wormwood, 33, 35, 37, 268–270
wound care
  astringent herbs, 45, 64–65, 146, 196
  poultices, 65, 110, 172, 198, 273–274
  salves and rubs, 233, 277
  wound soak, 273

X

Xanthium, 258

Y

yarrow, 31, 33, 35, 36, 37, 172, 271–274
yellow dock, 95–96
yerba la negrita, 110
yerba mansa, 31, 33, 35, 37, 172, 275–277
yucca, 15, 31, 33, 35, 37, 278–279
Yucca angustissima, 279
Yucca baccata, 279
Yucca glauca, 278
Yucca harrimaniae, 278

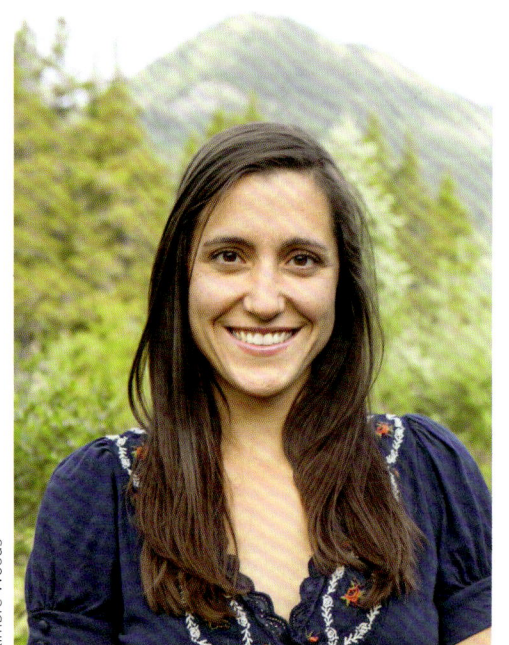

Kimbre Woods

Briana Wiles is a wild plant expert who loves expanding people's knowledge about the plants surrounding them. She teaches foraging and medicinal plant classes out of Rooted Apothecary, her shop in Crested Butte, Colorado, which offers her own line of body care products, remedies, and potions made with foraged botanicals. She resides in the central Rockies of Colorado with her husband, son, and Alaskan malamute. In her spare time, she enjoys rock climbing, snowboarding, hiking, white-water rafting, and figuring out how to wildcraft while doing the aforementioned. Visit her at rooted-apothecary.com.